Emerging Infectious Uveitis

Soon-Phaik Chee • Moncef Khairallah
Editors

Emerging Infectious Uveitis

Springer

Editors
Soon-Phaik Chee
Singapore National Eye Center
Singapore
Singapore

Moncef Khairallah
Department of Ophthalmology
Fattouma Bourguiba University Hospital
Faculty of Medicine
Monastir, Tunisia

ISBN 978-3-319-23415-1 ISBN 978-3-319-23416-8 (eBook)
DOI 10.1007/978-3-319-23416-8

Library of Congress Control Number: 2017934343

Printed on acid-free paper

This Springer imprint is published by Springer Nature
The registered company is Springer International Publishing AG
The registered company address is: Gewerbestrasse 11, 6330 Cham, Switzerland

Contents

1 Global Variations and Changes in Patterns of Infectious Uveitis

François Willermain, Yves Van Laethem, and Laure Caspers

1.1 Introduction

Before 1940, most uveitis cases were supposed to be due to infectious agents, mainly syphilis or tuberculosis [1]. Progress in the understanding of intraocular inflammation led to the discovery that uveitis can be of infectious and noninfectious origin and that many pathogens can cause infectious uveitis. Theoretically, Koch postulates must be fulfilled, in order to formerly demonstrate that a disease is due to an infectious agent. However, in infectious uveitis, most often, serological evidence, molecular or histological demonstration, and treatment response are usually the only available elements to suggest the infectious origin of the uveitis. Using these evidence a large number of infectious organisms have been demonstrated to cause infectious uveitis. Some have a global importance around the world, while others have more limited niches. Many of them have been considered as emerging pathogens.

F. Willermain (✉)
Department of Ophthalmology, CHU St-Pierre, Bruxelles, Belgium
e-mail: fwillerm@ulb.ac.be

Department of Ophthalmology, CHU Brugmann, Bruxelles, Belgium

Y. Van Laethem
Department of infectious diseases, CHU St-Pierre, Bruxelles, Belgium

L. Caspers
Department of Ophthalmology, CHU St-Pierre, Bruxelles, Belgium

According to Woolhouse, an emerging pathogen can be defined as an infectious agent whose incidence is increasing following its introduction into a new host population. A pathogen will be reemerging when its incidence increases in an existing host population [2]. However, in practice, both expressions are likely used by many authors regardless of those biological and epidemiological criteria. The term emerging disease will thus also be used in situation of increase awareness or discovery of pathogen in previously supposed non-infectious diseases [2]. As far as we know, most emerging infectious uveitis agents fall into the two last categories.

1.2 Emerging Disease

1.2.1 Origin of Human Infectious Disease

By definition, the question of emerging infectious disease addresses how a microbe becomes a pathogen in the human species. Emerging infectious disease thus resumes the origin of human infectious disease. Most of the emerging infections discovered during the last decades are zoonosis. Major modifications in human behavior have facilitated their jump from animals to humans. The global population has increased from 600 million humans around 1700 to 1.5 to 1.8 billion in 1900, 6 billion in 1998, and more than 7 billion in 2015. More than 50 % of those people reside in urban areas (from 40 % in

S.-P. Chee, M. Khairallah (eds.), *Emerging Infectious Uveitis*, DOI 10.1007/978-3-319-23416-8_1

Africa to 80 % in the Americas), in contrast with only 30 % in 1950. Environmental modifications were mandatory to build those cities, with deforestation or other forms of land use than in the past. Therefore, and also linked to widespread international trade of goods and animals, microbes have received a new and rapid access to an ever larger human population. In addition, the population is globally more mobile also; international travel rose above one billion people in 2012, further increasing pathogen dissemination around the globe.

In the past decades, most new pathogens were acute respiratory viruses. For instance, human metapneumovirus (first reported in 2001 in the Netherlands but demonstrated thereafter in specimens stored since the 1950s at least) is a paramyxovirus leading to very frequent and sometimes very severe respiratory tract infections in small children [3]. A new betacoronavirus is the agent of SARS (severe acute respiratory syndrome), discovered in 2003 after a physician infected a dozen patients in Hong Kong, with subsequent more than 8,000 cases in 29 countries and 774 deaths [4]. Another new coronavirus (MERS-CoV, Middle East respiratory syndrome coronavirus) has been demonstrated as the causative agent of a deadly respiratory tract infection in the Middle East since 2012, with more than 1,000 cases and 400 deaths [5]. But of all these emerging pathogens, the flu viruses, are the most widespread and deadly. Influenza A is a zoonose, with viruses mutating and mixing in swine and birds. If the Spanish flu (new H1N1 influenza A virus) killed more than 50 million people in 1917–1918, several pandemics (H2N2 in 1957, H3N2 in 1968, and new H1N1 in 2009) appeared in the more recent decades, with a lower but consequent mortality. In more restricted areas, non-pandemic strains of influenza A as H5N1 (Asia and Egypt) or H7N9 (China) are still potential deadly sword of Damocles [6].

1.2.2 The Birth of a Human Infectious Disease: Example of the AIDS Story

One of the most severe emerging infections of the last centuries is obviously AIDS (acquired immunodeficiency syndrome) linked to the HIV1 (and rarely HIV2) [7]. If it was first recognized in 1981 in the United States, its emergence in the human world is older and faraway from our Western World. Indeed, the oldest known case (a posteriori) is a man in the present Democratic Republic of Congo, in 1959. Analysis of the virus in his frozen serum as well as others suggests that HIV1 and HIV2 were separately acquired from monkeys in the 1930s, in the western part of Central Africa. In more than 40 SIV (simian immunodeficiency viruses) presently known, only HIV1 and HIV2 were able to infect humans and to establish persistent human to human transmission. Here again, urbanization and increasing local/regional trade, with all the sociologic modifications that it implicated, have largely contributed to the dissemination of the disease in sub-Saharan Africa. In a second time, international travel, sexual behaviors, and IV drug abuse have been keystone factors in the worldwide propagation of AIDS [8].

1.3 Re-emerging Disease

If emerging disease brings us to the origin of infectious disease, re-emerging disease deals with the evolution of infectious disease and the impact of the human society on it. Most of those reemerging infections are also zoonoses, often linked to a vector. Climatic changes (global warming) have allowed ticks to reach higher latitudes as well as altitudes, with transmission of Lyme disease or tick-borne encephalitis more in the north of Scandinavia or at higher altitude in Central Europe [9–11]. Similarly, mosquitos as *Aedes albopictus* are now found in the south of Europe (as France and Italy), with several local transmissions during the summer of dengue or chikungunya from imported cases. Chikungunya virus was discovered 60 years ago in Tanzania and since that time has spread to several parts of Africa and in all Indian Ocean/Western Pacific countries [12, 13]. Due to the introduction by an international traveler of an Asian strain in the Caribbean in 2014, Chikungunya is now an important public health problem not only in those islands but already also in Central and South America [14]. West Nile virus infection was unknown in the Americas until 1999. Due to migration from the Old World of birds wearing infected ticks, the infection was introduced in the northeast of the United States, and in a few years, it spread to all the States [15].

1.4 Variation in Patterns of Infectious Uveitis

1.4.1 Introduction

Few studies, and mainly from the occidental world, address the incidence and prevalence of uveitis [16]. It is therefore difficult to raise conclusions on global variations or evolution of this epidemiological aspect of intraocular inflammation. This contrasts with the important literature describing the causes of uveitis in different center and location in world which clearly shows important variations of the distribution of different etiologies around the globe. Those differences are mainly due to genetic and environmental factors and often grouped between the so-called developed and developing worlds. Accordingly, the distribution of both specific infectious and noninfectious causes varies greatly around the world.

In the context of infectious uveitis, some uveitis type is logically limited to endemic regions. Onchocerciasis, for example, has a limited distribution in Africa, South America, and Yemen [17]. Lyme disease is almost exclusively found in the Northern Hemisphere. Leptospirosis occurs most frequently in tropical and subtropical area. Brucellosis remains prevalent in the developing world, mostly in the Mediterranean Basin, the Arabic Gulf countries, India, and Central America. HTLV-1 infection is endemic in the Caribbean, Central and South America, South and Intertropical Africa, and Japan. Similarly other infectious agents such as dengue, West Nile virus, Rift Valley fever, or chikungunya virus, as well as rickettsia only infect patients in limited endemic regions. There are thus only reported as causes of uveitis in studies from those regions. In the series of Rathinam SR and Namperumalsamy from India, leptospirosis was the most frequent cause of infectious uveitis but remains very rare in the United States and Europe [18, 19]. However, due to evolution in our societies, such as globalization, those causes of infectious uveitis begin to emerge in non-endemic regions in patients having traveled in endemic regions (see Sect. 1.4.2.3) [20].

In contrast some *organisms* have spread worldwide, some with a relative stable incidence and others with period of increase and/or decrease incidence. For example, across the world, toxoplasmosis and herpesvirus remain major causes of posterior and anterior uveitis, respectively [21–26]. Tuberculosis and syphilis are discussed in the next paragraph as classic examples of worldwide cause of uveitis with period of burden and decrease. An important example of decreased incidence of a ubiquitous infectious uveitis is CMV retinitis which made a steep decline in incidence following the introduction of HAART [27].

1.4.2 Emerging Infectious Uveitis

1.4.2.1 Emerging Infectious Uveitis Secondary to Pathogen Incidence Increase

In Europe, it is believed that syphilis has emerged around 1495. Interestingly, it has been reported that in its early years, the disease was much more severe that nowadays, suggesting the selection of a milder strain of *Treponema pallidum* occurred. Since that time, syphilis has continued to spread around the world and became one of the major health problems, illustrated by the fact that, in the nineteenth century, an entire medical subspecialty, syphilology, was devoted to its study [28, 29]. The discovery of penicillin has been associated with a significant decrease of syphilis rate to the point that some authors have postulated that the disease might disappear. Unfortunately, this was not the case and the incidence of syphilis has been the subject of important variation with frequent outbreak [29, 30]. For example, in the United Kingdom, there has been a 1032 % increase in the incidence of syphilis between 1999 and 2008. This exponential increase has been attributed to unsafe sexual practices mainly among men who have sex with men (MSMs) [31]. The same trend was found in other countries. As a consequence, many reports have warned the uveitis community of what was called by Narsing Rao and colleague "the reemergence of an old adversary" [32, 33]. Meanwhile, a tremendous number of studies have been published improving our knowledge on the epidemiology and clinical presentation of ocular syphilis. Acute syphilitic posterior placoid chorioretinitis was in this context rediscovered with an exponential rate of publication from 1990, the year of its publication by Gass, to 2014 [34].

Tuberculosis is another old infectious disease which had a major impact on global human health. Overall, the worldwide burden of tuberculosis is still growing, as control of the disease in many regions of the world is offset by the increase incidence in another part, mainly sub-Saharan [35]. Tuberculosis remains one of the most important infectious causes of morbidity and mortality worldwide. In contrast with syphilitic uveitis, where the diagnosis can be easily made based on serological evidences, there is a great confusion regarding the diagnosis and treatment of ocular tuberculosis. Progress in systemic and ophthalmological investigation together with a more accurate description of clinical signs has permitted to better define guidelines for the diagnosis and treatment of intraocular tuberculosis [36, 37]. Nowadays, tuberculosis is a leading cause of uveitis in endemic countries, but tuberculosis uveitis can also be found in non-endemic countries with a probable recent increased frequency [24, 38–40]. This recent increment of tuberculosis uveitis in non-endemic countries is mainly attributed to the development of immigration and postulated by Llorenc and coworkers to be one of the challenges of globalization [39, 40]. There is thus an increased awareness of ocular tuberculosis among uveitis specialists all around the globe.

1.4.2.2 Emerging Infectious Uveitis Secondary to Pathogen Identification

One of the major recent breakthroughs in the uveitis field was the discovery that two entities, namely, Posner-Schlossman syndrome (PSS) and Fuchs heterochromic iridocyclitis (FHI), previously considered as idiopathic, were actually due to virus infection. Fuchs heterochromic iridocyclitis is characterized by a series of clinical signs (FHI making its classical presentation almost pathognomonic. The origin of FHI remains elusive until 2004 when Quentin CD and Reiber H elegantly demonstrated an elevated intraocular rubella antibody production in FHI, suggesting that FHI is a rubella-driven disease [41]. Four years later, de Visser et al. confirmed that rubella-positive patients presented a clinical syndrome similar to FHI [42]. As both a proof of concept and an illustration of the impact of human society on uveitis infectious epidemiology, Birnbaum et al. have demonstrated that FHI is less common in patients born since the introduction of the US rubella vaccination program [43]. At the same time, a study from the Singapore National Eye Centre, using PCR, found that CMV can also be detected in eyes with FHI [44]. More recently, Babu et al. have found in addition the presence of HSV and chikungunya virus in FHI eyes [45].

A possible role played by CMV infection in the development of PSS was suggested by early work of Bloch-Michel in the eighties [46]. Since that time, several works have confirmed this hypothesis [44, 47, 48]. In addition to PSS, it was found in those studies that CMV-positive anterior uveitis can also present the clinical characteristics of FHI or chronic granulomatous uveitis. Altogether, those data indicate that several previously thought idiopathic uveitis (PSS, FHI, and some chronic granulomatous anterior uveitis) have indeed a viral origin. This evidence has not only important implications for the epidemiology but, of course, also for the management of uveitis.

1.4.2.3 Emerging Infectious Uveitis Secondary to Increase Awareness and Better Disease Description

We have seen earlier that the success of humanity in terms of demographic expansion has create favorable conditions to increase the speed for the emergence and spreading of infectious diseases. In other terms, diseases might quickly jump between very distant part of the world and confront clinicians with diseases unusual in their region. Fortunately, the dissemination of information has also been progressively accelerated allowing a quick exchange of information between specialist from endemic regions and recently affected countries. In this context, a series of infectious uveitis, mainly rickettsioses, West Nile virus, dengue, or chikungunya, has been the subject of an increase awareness and careful descriptions from both endemic and non-endemic regions [20, 49, 50].

The recent outbreaks of Ebola and Zika virus have been similarly associated with uveitis cases and those pathogens should be now included in the list of emerging infectious uveitis agents [51, 52].

Conclusions

The epidemiology of infectious uveitis is a dynamic process and the consequence of the complex relationship between microbes and human. On one hand, some pathogens such as toxoplasmosis or herpesvirus remain major causes of uveitis, while others, such as tuberculosis, seem to progress despite our efforts to eradicate them. On the other hand, infectious uveitis previously limited to particular geographical niches can now be found almost all around the globe. This is clearly due to evolution of our lifestyle which has also important impact on the emergence of new infectious diseases which might become someday new uveitis causes. The decrease of CMV retinitis among AIDS patients following HAART highlights that, in addition to this negative aspect, our civilization also has a positive impact on infectious uveitis epidemiology and is able to reduce the incidence of some devastating infectious uveitis causes. Indeed, we should not forget that the development of our human society has also created better ways to diagnose, control, and eventually eradicate infectious diseases.

Core Messages

The cause of infectious uveitis varies greatly around the world. Some widespread microbes continue to threaten vision in almost every part of the globe. Some infectious uveitis previously limited to particular geographical niches can now be found almost all around the globe. This evolution is the consequence of changing in our lifestyle which has also important impact on the emergence of new infectious diseases as well as their diagnosis and management.

References

1. Samson CM, Foster CS (2002) Syphillis. In: Foster CS, Vitale AT (eds) Diagnosis and treatment of uveitis. WB Sauders Company, Philadelphia
2. Woolhouse MEJ (2002) Population biology of emerging and re-emerging pathogens? Trends Microbiol 10:S3–S7
3. Hamelin ME, Boivin G (2005) Human metapneumovirus: a ubiquitous and long standing respiratory pathogen. Pediatr Infect Dis J 24:S203–S207
4. World Health Organisation (2003) Consensus document on the epidemiology of SARS. http://www.who.int/csr/sars/en/WHOconsensus.pdf
5. ECDC. Severe Respiratory Disease associated with Middle East respiratory syndrome coronavirus (MERS-CoV) 14th update Feb 2015. http://www.ecdc.europa.eu/en/publications/_layouts/forms/Publication_DispForm.aspx?List=4f55ad51-4aed-4d32-b960-af70113dbb90&ID=1264
6. ECDC. Communicable disease threats report 15–21 February 2015 week 8. http://www.ecdc.europa.eu/en/publications/_layouts/forms/Publication_DispForm.aspx?List=4f55ad51-4aed-4d32-b960-af70113dbb90&ID=1263
7. Barré-Sinoussi F, Chermann JC, Rey F, Nugeyre MT, Chamaret S, Gruest J et al (1983) Isolation of a T-lymphotropic retrovirus from a patient at risk for acquired immune deficiency syndrome (AIDS). Science 220:868–871
8. De Cock KM, Jaffe HW, Curran JW (2011) Reflections on 30 years of AIDS. Emerg Infect Dis 17:1044–1048
9. WHO/ECDC. Joint factsheet on Lyme borreliosis. http://www.ecdc.europa.eu/en/healthtopics/vectors/world-health-day-2014/Documents/factsheet-lyme-borreliosis.pdf
10. WHO/ECDC factsheet on TBE. http://www.ecdc.europa.eu/en/healthtopics/vectors/world-health-day-2014/Documents/factsheet-tick-borne-encephalitis.pdf
11. Shuman EK (2011) Global climate change and infectious diseases. Int J Occup Environ Med 2:11–19
12. Chretien J-P, Linthicum K (2007) Chikungunya in Europe: what's next? Lancet 70:1805–1806

13. Burt FJ, Rolph MS, Rulli NE, Mahalingam S, Heise MT (2012) Chikungunya: a re-emerging virus. Lancet 379:662–671
14. Chikungunya outbreak in Caribbean region. http://www.ecdc.europa.eu/en/publications/_layouts/forms/Publication_DispForm.aspx?List=4f55ad51-4aed-4d32-b960-af70113dbb90&ID=1127
15. Jones KE, Patel NG, Levy MA, Storeygard A, Balk D, Gittleman JL et al (2008) Global trends in emerging infectious diseases. Nature 451:990–994
16. Daudin JB (2010) Epidémiologie. In: Brezin AP (ed) Les uvéites. Société Française d'Ophtalmologie: Elsevier Masson, Paris
17. Mackenzie CD, Homeida MM, Hopkins AD, Lawrence JC (2012) Elimination of onchocerciasis from Africa: possible? Trends Parasitol 28:16–22
18. Rathinam SR, Namperumalsamy P (2007) Global variation and pattern changes in epidemiology of uveitis. Indian J Ophthalmol 55:173–183
19. Shukla D, Rathinam SR, Cunningham ET (2010) Leptospiral uveitis in the developing world. Int Ophthalmol Clin 50:113–124
20. Khairallah M, Jelliti B, Jenzeri S (2009) Emergent infectious uveitis. Middle East Afr J Ophthalmol 16:225–238
21. Petersen E, Kijlstra A, Stanford M (2012) Epidemiology of ocular toxoplasmosis. Ocul Immunol Inflamm 20:68–75
22. Islam SM, Tabbara KF (2002) Causes of uveitis at the eye center in Saudi Arabia: a retrospective review. Ophthalmic Epidemiol 9:239–249
23. Khairallah M, Yahia SB, Ladjimi A, Messaoud R, Zaouali S, Attia S et al (2007) Pattern of uveitis in a referral centre in Tunisia, North Africa. Eye 21:33–39
24. Abdulaal M, Antonios R, Barikian A, Jaroudi M, Hamam RN (2014) Etiology and clinical features of ocular inflammatory diseases in a tertiary center in Lebanon. Ocul Immunol Inflamm 9:1–7
25. Jakob E, Reuland MS, Mackensen F, Harsch N, Fleckenstein M, Lorenz HM et al (2009) Uveitis subtypes in a German interdisciplinary uveitis center – analysis of 1916 patients. J Rheumatol 36:127–136
26. Sittivarakul W, Bhurayanontachai P, Ratanasukon M (2013) Pattern of uveitis in a university-based referral center in southern Thailand. Ocul Immunol Inflamm 21:53–60
27. Schwarcz L, Chen MJ, Vittinghoff E, Hsu L, Schwarcz S (2013) Declining incidence of AIDS-defining opportunistic illnesses: results from 16 years of population-based AIDS surveillance. AIDS 27:597–605
28. Knell RJ (2004) Syphilis in renaissance Europe: rapid evolution of an introduced sexually transmitted disease? Proc R Soc Lond 271:S174–S176
29. Shockman S, Buescher L, Stone SP (2014) Syphilis in the United States. Clin Dermatol 32:213–218
30. Mattei PL, Beachkofsky TM, Gilson RT, Wisco OJ (2012) Syphillis: a reemerging infection. Am Fam Physician 86:433–440
31. Mathew RG, Goh BT, Westcott MC (2014) British ocular syphilis study (BOSS): 2-year national surveillance study of intraocular inflammation secondary to syphilis. Invest Ophthalmol Vis Sci 55:5394–5400
32. Chao JR, Khurana RN, Fawzi AA, Reddy HS, Rao NA (2006) Syphilis: reemergence of an old adversary. Ophthalmology 113:2074–2079
33. Cunningham ET, Eandi CM, Pichi F (2014) Syphilitic uveitis. Ocul Immunol Inflamm 22:2–3
34. Gass JD, Braunstein RA, Chenoweth RG (1990) Acute syphilitic posterior placoid chorioretinitis. Ophthalmology 97:1288–1297
35. Maartens G, Wilkinson RJ (2007) Tuberculosis. Lancet 370:2030–2043
36. Gupta V, Gupta A, Rao NA (2007) Intraocular tuberculosis – an update. Surv Ophthalmol 52:561–587
37. Gupta A, Sharma A, Bansal R, Sharma K (2015) Classification of intraocular tuberculosis. Ocul Immunol Inflamm 23:7–13
38. Al Mezaine HS, Kangrave D, Abu El-Asrar AM (2010) Patterns of uveitis in patients admitted to a university hospital in Riyadh, Saudi Arabia. Ocul Immunol Inflamm 18:424–431
39. Jones NP (2013) The Manchester uveitis clinic: the first 3000 patients-epidemiology and casemix. Ocul Immunol Inflamm 23(2):118–126
40. Llorenç V, Mesquida M, Sainz de la Maza M, Keller J, Molins B, Espinosa G et al (2015) Epidemiology of uveitis in a Western urban multiethnic population. The challenge of globalization. Acta Ophthalmol 93(6):561–567
41. Quentin CD, Reiber H (2004) Fuchs heterochromic cyclitis: rubella virus antibodies and genome in aqueous humor. Am J Ophthalmol 138:46–54
42. de Visser L, Braakenburg A, Rothova A, de Boer JH (2008) Rubella virus-associated uveitis: clinical manifestations and visual prognosis. Am J Ophthalmol 146:292–297
43. Birnbaum AD, Tessler HH, Schultz KL, Farber MD, Gao W, Lin P et al (2007) Epidemiologic relationship between Fuchs heterochromic iridocyclitis and the United States rubella vaccination program. Am J Ophthalmol 144:424–428
44. Chee SP, Bacsal K, Jap A, Se-Thoe SY, Cheng CL, Tan BH (2008) Clinical features of cytomegalovirus anterior uveitis in immunocompetent patients. Am J Ophthalmol 145:834–840
45. Babu K, Adiga M, Govekar SR, Kumar BR, Murthy KR (2013) Associations of Fuchs heterochromic iridocyclitis in a South Indian patient population. J Ophthalmic Inflamm Infect 15:3–14
46. Bloch-Michel E, Dussaix E, Cerqueti P, Patarin D (1987) Possible role of cytomegalovirus infection in the etiology of the Posner-Schlossman syndrome. Int Ophthalmol 11:95–96
47. Sobolewska B, Deuter C, Doycheva D, Zierhut M (2014) Long-term oral therapy with valganciclovir in patients with Posner-Schlossman syndrome. Graefes Arch Clin Exp Ophthalmol 252:117–124

48. Accorinti M, Gilardi M, Pirraglia MP, Amorelli GM, Nardella C, Abicca I et al (2014) Cytomegalovirus anterior uveitis: long-term follow-up of immunocompetent patients. Graefes Arch Clin Exp Ophthalmol 252:1817–1824
49. Anninger WV, Lomeo MD, Dingle J, Epstein AD, Lubow M (2003) West Nile virus-associated optic neuritis and chorioretinitis. Am J Ophthalmol 136:1183–1185
50. Ng AW, Teoh SC (2015) Dengue eye disease. Surv Ophthalmol 60:106–114
51. Shantha JG, Yeh S, Nguyen QD (2016) Ebola virus disease and the eye. Curr Opin Ophthalmol. 27:538–544
52. Furtado JM, Espósito DL, Klein TM, Teixeira-Pinto T, da Fonseca BA (2016). Uveitis Associated with Zika Virus Infection. N Engl J Med. 375:394–6

2 The Role of Infectious Agents in the Pathogenesis of Autoimmune Diseases

Merih Oray and Ilknur Tugal-Tutkun

2.1 Introduction

Uveitis is classified as noninfectious when there is no known active systemic or intraocular infection, and the pathogenesis is presumed to be immune mediated [1–4]. Both autoimmune and autoinflammatory mechanisms are involved in the development of noninfectious uveitis [1–3, 5].

However, infectious triggers are increasingly recognized in the etiopathogenesis of immune-mediated inflammatory disorders in general and immune-mediated uveitis in particular [1, 2, 6–8].

A constant interplay between the innate and adaptive immune systems is required for maximum protection of the organism against invading pathogens while maintaining immunological tolerance to self as well as to the commensal microbiota that mostly have a symbiotic relationship with the host. Innate and adaptive arms of the immune system are thought to play a predominant role in the autoinflammatory and autoimmune mechanisms, respectively [6, 9, 10].

The innate immune system provides a fast and robust first-line defense against a wide range of pathogens that constitutively express pathogen-associated molecular patterns (PAMPs), including lipopolysaccharide (LPS), peptidoglycan, bacterial DNA/heat shock proteins (HSP), and viral DNA/RNA [1, 6]. Effector cells of the innate immune system include dendritic cells, monocytes/macrophages, natural killer (NK) cells, and neutrophils. Germline-encoded pattern recognition receptors (PRR) of the innate immune cells are capable of immediately recognizing PAMPs as well as danger-associated molecular patterns (DAMPs) expressed by damaged cells. Pattern recognition receptors such as Toll-like receptors (TLRs) and C-type lectins (CTLs) expressed on the plasma membranes or NOD-like receptors and RigI-helicases in the cytoplasm, once activated by their ligands, lead to the activation of intracellular signal transduction pathways and induction of proinflammatory cytokines such as IL-1, IL-6, IL-12, IL-18, tumor necrosis factor (TNF), and interferons (IFN) which in turn regulate the adaptive immune response [1, 6, 11]. While the innate immune response has been traditionally defined as a nonspecific rapid response without memory, recent studies have shown that recognition of various PAMPs by different PRRs enables identification of pathogens [11], and especially NK cells can deliver specific memory responses [12]. A long-term enhanced state of innate immunity through epigenetic reprogramming has been recently identified as a significant property of innate host defense mechanisms [12]. Hereditary autoinflammatory disorders are associated with

M. Oray, MD • I. Tugal-Tutkun, MD (✉)
Department of Ophthalmology,
Istanbul Faculty of Medicine,
Istanbul University, Istanbul, Turkey
e-mail: itutkun@istanbul.edu.tr

S.-P. Chee, M. Khairallah (eds.), *Emerging Infectious Uveitis*, DOI 10.1007/978-3-319-23416-8_2

mutations of genes coding for proteins involved in the regulation of innate immunity [9, 10, 13]. These rare disorders are characterized by seemingly unprovoked episodes of inflammation and absence of autoreactive T cell or B cell responses [9, 10, 13]. There are also an increasing number of complex inflammatory disorders where autoinflammatory mechanisms are mainly involved in the pathogenesis, but adaptive immunity also plays a significant role in the chronicity of inflammation and target organ damage [1, 9, 14, 15].

The adaptive immune system cells, T and B lymphocytes, can specifically recognize pathogens and build memory for protection against reinfection. Specific recognition of pathogenic microorganisms by T cell receptors (TCR) and B cell receptors (BCR) is mediated by a variable-diversity-joining (V-D-J) gene recombination process [1, 6]. This process enables generation of a vast repertoire of TCR and BCR that can recognize an unlimited number of foreign antigens but also carries the risk of self-antigen recognition. Self-damage is normally prevented by central and peripheral tolerance mechanisms. Loss of tolerance to self-antigens and development of autoantibodies and autoreactive antigen-specific T cells lead to autoimmune disorders [6].

Environmental factors, most importantly, bacteria, viruses, other pathogens, as well as vaccines, are thought to play a central role in the induction and perpetuation of autoinflammatory and autoimmune disorders in genetically susceptible individuals [6, 7, 16, 17]. Several putative mechanisms have been postulated to explain triggering of autoimmune disorders by infectious agents [7, 16]. Antigen-specific mechanisms include molecular mimicry and cross-reactivity between foreign and self-antigens; activation of autoreactive T cells by superantigens produced by bacteria, mycoplasmae, or virus-infected cells; and expression of modified self-epitopes secondary to infection-mediated inflammation. Bystander activation and epitope spreading may also lead to a nonspecific immune response toward different self-antigens [7, 16]. It is difficult to incriminate a given infectious agent in an immune-mediated disease because the triggering infection may have taken place years before the clinical expression of the disease, latent infection or seroprevalence may be high in the healthy population, and laboratory identification of triggering infection may be limited. Furthermore, several different pathogens can trigger a single autoimmune disease, and a given pathogen can trigger various immune-mediated diseases. Complex interactions between immunogenetic factors and various infectious agents have not been completely understood yet.

Based on experimental models of autoimmune uveitis (EAU), the inciting event in human uveitis is most likely the activation of innate immunity outside the eye [2–4]. The activation of effector T cell subsets depends on the conditions under which exposure to a retinal or cross-reactive antigen occurs. In the classic EAU, immunization with interphotoreceptor retinoid-binding protein (IRBP) emulsified in complete Freund's adjuvant (CFA), which contains heat-killed tuberculosis bacteria, derives differentiation of effector T cells toward Th17 phenotype, and a monocytic inflammatory response develops in the eye [2–4, 18]. In the more recent EAU model, injection of IRBP pulsed in dendritic cells matured in vitro with bacterial LPS derives a Th1 effector phenotype response, and the nature of inflammatory infiltrate in the eye is granulocytic, producing a fundus picture different from that seen in classic EAU [2, 3, 18]. Thus, quality and quantity of innate receptor stimulation by exogenous stimuli (infectious agents) seem to determine the immunological response profile as well as pathological and clinical features of intraocular inflammation. These findings in EAU may help explain the role of inciting stimuli on the heterogeneity of human uveitis.

2.2 Behçet Disease

Behçet disease (BD) is a multisystem inflammatory disorder characterized by oral and genital ulcerations, skin lesions, and uveitis, as well as involvement of joints, blood vessels, central nervous system, and gastrointestinal system [19]. Patients with BD have seemingly unprovoked recurrent inflammatory episodes in all organ systems involved

[20]. Ocular involvement is characterized by a recurrent nongranulomatous panuveitis and occlusive retinal vasculitis and tends to be more severe and sight-threatening than most of the other forms of noninfectious uveitis [21, 22].

Pathogenetic mechanisms underlying BD include complex interactions between genetic factors, environmental factors, and immunological aberrations [20, 23–25]. Genome-wide association studies (GWAS) have confirmed that the known association with HLA-B51 is the strongest genetic factor for the development of BD. Recent GWAS have also identified novel susceptibility genes within the HLA class I region and variants in IL-10, IL23R-IL12RB2, STAT4, CCR1, and ERAP-1 [26–30]. BD-associated noncoding CCR1 allele is implicated in impaired microbial clearance [26, 31]. Epistasis was found between HLA-B51 and ERAP-1 variants which is an enzyme that trims peptides for proper loading onto the HLA class I molecule [26]. Additional associations with rare variants were discovered, including TLR4, MEFV, and NOD2 genes, which are associated with an increased responsiveness to bacterial products [30, 31]. These findings implicate defects in sensing and processing of pathogen and danger signals as well as in genes encoding pivotal proteins involved in Th1 and Th17 regulation [30]. A more recent genetic imputation study implicated the role of peptide-MHC-I binding and involvement of NK and cytotoxic T cell activation by MHC in the pathogenesis of BD [32].

Environmental factors, mainly infectious agents, have long been considered in the pathogenesis of BD. Infections are suspected in the initial triggering of the disease as well as in relapses of its manifestations [33]. However, there is no single microorganism that can be blamed as the specific etiologic agent. Oral microbial flora, especially *Streptococcus* species, colonizing in the oral cavity, may be the trigger of oral ulcers, the most common initial manifestation of the disease [23–25, 33, 34]. *Streptococcus sanguis*, *S. salivarius*, *S. mitis*, and *S. mutans* are associated with frequent oral infections [23]. Clinical observations of poor oral hygiene, dental caries, periodontitis in BD patients, and initiation or relapses of the disease following dental procedures or tonsillitis suggest the role of oral microbiota and *Streptococcus* [23, 24]. Behçet patients have high serum antibody titers and increased T cell reactivity and skin hypersensitivity to *Streptococcus* antigens. Furthermore, a favorable disease course is observed following improvement of oral hygiene and long-term control of dental and periodontal problems as well as following prophylactic penicillin treatment [23, 33]. Other bacteria that have been implicated as potential triggers include mycobacteria, *Borrelia burgdorferi*, *Escherichia coli*, *Staphylococcus aureus*, *Mycoplasma fermentans,* and *Helicobacter pylori* [25].

A triggering role of viruses has also been postulated, and especially the role of herpes simplex virus (HSV) has been the main focus of research [35]. An HSV-induced BD mouse model has been developed, based on the induction of several inflammatory lesions resembling manifestations of BD after inoculation of scratched earlobes with HSV 1 [35]. Other viruses that have been implied in the pathogenesis of BD include herpes virus 6 and 7, varicella-zoster virus (VZV), cytomegalovirus (CMV), parvovirus, Epstein-Barr virus (EBV), and hepatitis A, B, and C virus (HCV) [23, 25, 35]. Tripartite motif-containing (TRIM) proteins have key roles in antiviral immunity either by restriction of viral replication cycle or by regulating pathways mediated by pattern recognition of viral RNA/DNA and the inflammasome [36]. TRIM proteins induce production of type I interferons and proinflammatory cytokines such as IL-1β and thus may be involved in the pathogenesis of autoimmune and autoinflammatory responses [36]. TRIM proteins that have been specifically implicated in the pathogenesis of BD include TRIM39 and TRIM19 which functions in innate defense mechanisms against HSV [35].

It is thought that an aberrant immune response may be generated to different microorganisms recognized by pattern receptors in genetically susceptible individuals. Heat shock proteins are highly conserved molecules inducible by any form of cellular stress and act as intracellular scavenger and adjuvant [37]. Human HSP60, included in the DAMPs, has a high sequence homology with the mycobacterial HSP65 and also cross-reacts with streptococcal HSPs [23, 33]. Innate immune cells as well as γδT cells are stimulated by HSPs, through TLR2 and TLR4 expression. Differential TLR stimulation by microbial agents and their products and subsequent cytokine production by innate immune cells may lead to the skewed T cell responses observed in BD [34, 37, 38]. Alternatively, cross-reactivity of human HSPs with bacterial or viral HSP may derive the selection of autoreactive T cells resulting in perpetuation and chronicity of inflammation [37]. In summary, an impaired microbial clearance and exuberant innate and adaptive immune responses to microbial products may have a major contribution to the pathogenesis of BD.

2.3 Sarcoidosis

Sarcoidosis is a multisystem chronic inflammatory disorder characterized by formation of noncaseating granulomas. Although the lungs and thoracic lymph nodes are most commonly affected, other lymph nodes, skin, salivary glands, liver, spleen, kidneys, heart, joints, nervous system, orbit, and eyes may also be involved [39]. Patients may also present with bilateral granulomatous intraocular inflammation in the absence of extraocular manifestations [40]. Characteristic features of ocular sarcoidosis include mutton-fat granulomatous keratic precipitates, iris and trabecular meshwork nodules, snowball vitreous opacities, chorioretinal lesions, nodular and/or segmental periphlebitis, retinal arterial macroaneurysms, and optic disc or choroidal nodules [40].

The etiology of sarcoidosis is not known. Genetic susceptibility, noninfectious environmental agents, and infectious triggers have been considered in the pathogenesis. In genetically susceptible individuals, a dysregulated immune response to one or more antigens may lead to a granulomatous inflammation characterized by infiltration of monocytes, macrophages, and activated T lymphocytes [41]. Genetic studies have shown class I HLA-B7 and HLA-B8 associations as well as associations with class II HLA-DRB1 and HLA-DQB1 that have been confirmed by recent GWAS. Immunologically relevant non-HLA genes have also been identified, including CARD15 (NOD2), butyrophilin-like protein 2 (BTNL2), and annexin A11 (ANXA11) [39, 41, 42]. CARD15 (NOD2) is an intracellular PRR, and polymorphisms of this gene are associated especially with early-onset sarcoidosis or Blau syndrome. BTNL2 is a member of the immunoglobulin superfamily and functions as a negative costimulatory molecule downregulating T cell activation. BTNL2 G16071A polymorphism found in sarcoidosis patients leads to loss of function of BTNL2 and thus could result in amplified T cell activation [41, 42]. ANXA11 is presumed to be a regulator of cell division and apoptosis; and interactions between ANXA11 and class II HLA genotypes have been identified in sarcoidosis [43].

Several noninfective environmental and occupational risk factors have been implicated, such as exposure to rural irritants, insecticides, inorganic particles, nanoparticles, metals, moldy environments, and fire [41, 44, 45]. However, no single cause of sarcoidosis was identified in ACCESS (a case-control etiologic study of sarcoidosis), although positive associations were found with agricultural employment, insecticides at work, moldy environments with possible exposures to microbial bioaerosols, and occupational exposure to insecticides [46]. Inappropriate processing of ubiquitous foreign agents may be the cause of chronic granulomatous inflammation in sarcoidosis patients.

Among infectious triggers, *Mycobacterium tuberculosis* has been suggested as the major causative agent [42, 44, 47]. Sarcoid specimens do not classically contain live *M. tuberculosis* organisms. Cell wall-deficient mycobacterial remnants have been shown in some specimens, and PCR studies have shown presence of mycobacterium DNA in sarcoidosis tissues [44, 47]. In a meta-analysis of studies reporting PCR identification of mycobacteria in sarcoid samples, the overall rate of positivity was 26 % and suggested a 9- to 19-fold increased odds compared to non-sarcoidosis controls [48]. The presence of *Mycobacterium tuberculosis* catalase–peroxidase (mKatG) and *katG* DNA in sarcoidosis tissues and almost half of sarcoidosis patients having serum antibodies to mKatG are further evidence to a mycobacterial etiology in at least a subset of sarcoidosis patients [44, 49]. mKatG is a virulence factor that allows prolonged survival of mycobacteria inside macrophages, and dysfunctional mKatG is associated with isoniazid resistance [49]. It has been hypothesized that mKatG may only be a component of mycobacterial antigens that form a nidus in sarcoid granulomas [49]. The potential of nontuberculous mycobacteria to cause sarcoidosis has been suggested as well [42, 47]. *Propionibacterium acnes*, *Borrelia burgdorferi*, herpes viruses, and EBV have also been implicated as potential causes of sarcoidosis, mostly based on an increased seroprevalence of these agents in the patient populations [44]. However, nonspecific polyclonal hypergammaglobulinemia is a feature of sarcoidosis and may account for increased antibody titers. Notably, Yasuhara et al. [50] have identified *P. acnes* and *P. granulosum* DNA by PCR analysis of vitreous specimens in six patients with sarcoid uveitis.

In summary, it is currently thought that multiple different antigens may be capable of inducing an aberrant immune response leading to manifestations of sarcoidosis in genetically susceptible individuals.

2.4 Vogt-Koyanagi-Harada Disease

Vogt-Koyanagi-Harada (VKH) disease is a systemic autoimmune disorder that affects tissues containing melanin such as the eye, inner ear, meninges, and skin. The disease is characterized by chronic bilateral panuveitis associated with exudative retinal detachment along with a varying constellation of auditory, neurological, and cutaneous manifestations [51, 52].

While the exact etiology of VKH disease is unknown, it is thought to be a T cell-mediated immune process that is directed at the melanocytes [53–55]. Vogt-Koyanagi-Harada disease has a prodromal phase characterized by vague systemic symptoms suggestive of viral infection; therefore, infectious agents are thought to be the inciting factors for this autoimmune disease. Molecular mimicry and cross-reaction are the mechanisms used to explain the association of autoimmunity and viral infection [53]. The presence of EBV genome in cerebrospinal fluid and vitreous of patients with VKH has been shown [56]. A cross-reactive T cell response between tyrosinase peptides, which are postulated as target antigens on melanocytes and CMV antigen in patients with VKH disease, has also been described [57, 58]. It is assumed that there may be a molecular mimicry between some viruses and melanocytes; however, a clear association between a specific viral agent and the disease has not been established yet.

2.5 HLA-B27-Associated Anterior Uveitis

HLA-B27-associated anterior uveitis is a distinct clinical entity which has frequent associations with a group of systemic diseases called seronegative spondyloarthropathies (SSpAs). Seronegative spondyloarthropathies are a group of chronic inflammatory disorders characterized by an absence of serum rheumatoid factor and a strong association with the HLA-B27 antigen. Ankylosing spondylitis, reactive arthritis, psoriatic arthritis, arthritis and inflammatory bowel disease, and juvenile-onset spondyloarthropathy as a form of juvenile chronic arthritis are included in the spectrum of SSpAs. Uveitis is the most common extra-articular manifestation of seronegative arthritis [59].

HLA-B27-associated anterior uveitis is characterized by unilateral, alternating, recurrent, nongranulomatous acute anterior uveitis with significant protein and cellular extravasation into the aqueous humor that may be associated with fibrin and hypopyon formation [60–64].

In this group of uveitis patients, HLA-B27 positivity allows naming the entity; however, the precise molecular and pathogenic mechanisms linking HLA-B27 and uveitis are not completely understood. The expression of HLA antigens was found to be upregulated in the iris of patients with anterior uveitis, and this induction of HLA-antigen expression on iris cells may play a role in the pathogenesis of HLA-B27-associated anterior uveitis [65].

The underlying pathogenic mechanism is believed to be an interaction between genetic and environmental factors. Triggering role of bacterial infections in the pathogenesis of anterior uveitis and other HLA-B27-associated disease is suggested. In the well-characterized transgenic B27 model of SSpAs, the presence of normal microbial gut flora is required to induce disease. The finding that animals raised in germ-free conditions do not develop disease in this model also confirms the role of infections [66]. Endotoxin-induced uveitis in animal models is based on the induction of uveitis by bacterial products [67]. There is also evidence that links gastrointestinal tract infective and inflammatory abnormalities to extraintestinal manifestations of SSpAs such as uveitis and arthritis in humans [66].

Chang et al. [68] demonstrated the presence of toll-like receptor 4 and its associated lipopolysaccharide receptor complex in the human uvea. This study gives molecular insights into the potential mechanisms in which Gram-negative bacterial triggers may be involved in the development of anterior uveitis. Bacteria that have been implicated as potential triggers include *Chlamydia trachomatis* [69], *Helicobacter pylori* [70], and the Gram-negative enterobacteria including *Klebsiella* [71–74], *Salmonella* [75–77], *Yersinia* [78–82], and *Campylobacter jejuni* [60, 78, 83]. However, there are also some studies which have failed to show an association between these microorganisms and the etiology of anterior uveitis [84–87].

The fact that several infective etiologies appear to play a role in the pathogenesis of SSpAs has led to several hypotheses regarding etiopathogenesis. According to molecular mimicry hypothesis, there is an antigenic similarity between HLA-B27 and certain bacterial microorganisms, which may result in development of pathogen- or autoreactive T cells and consequently formation of an autoimmune chronic disease [88, 89]. Another postulated hypothesis suggests that HLA-B27 molecule may function as a receptor. Exogenous peptide derived from bacteria or endogenous protein produced as a result of an infection might be presented to cytotoxic T cells by the HLA-B27 molecule, activating the immune response [90].

In summary, HLA-B27-associated anterior uveitis is a common form of inflammatory eye disease, and recent advances in clinical and experimental research have shown the triggering role of bacteria in the etiopathogenesis of this disease. However, still many questions remain unanswered, and the cause of HLA-B27-associated anterior uveitis remains unclear.

2.6 Fuchs Uveitis Syndrome

Fuchs uveitis syndrome (FUS) is a low-grade, chronic, intraocular inflammatory disease of unknown origin. The disease has well-defined characteristics such as diffuse, scattered, and small- and medium-sized keratic precipitates with mild anterior chamber flare and minimal cells along with iris atrophy which may lead to acquired heterochromia in the absence of posterior synechiae and macular edema. Unlike other uveitis entities, FUS does not respond to corticosteroid therapy. Cataract formation and glaucoma are the main complications that may develop during the course of the disease [91–94].

The etiopathogenic mechanism of FUS remains elusive. Many theories regarding the etiology have been proposed, including genetic, sympathetic, infectious, neurogenic, and immunologic-inflammatory, but none of them was able to explain the whole pathogenesis [95, 96]. After recent improvements in diagnostic laboratory techniques for identification of infectious agents, the infectious theory has become of major interest to the researchers. A number of infectious causes have been proposed, including toxoplasma, rubella, CMV, and HSV [97, 98]. There are also some sporadic cases showing FUS following ocular *Toxocara canis* [99, 100], chikungunya [101, 102], and ophthalmomyiasis [103] infections.

Initially Fuchs [104] and Kimura et al. [105] described the association of peripheral retinochoroidal scars with FUS, which raised the possibility of ocular toxoplasmosis as an etiologic factor. Toledo de Abreu et al. [106] have reported the first study in the literature in which an association between ocular toxoplasmosis and FUS has been based on the clinical findings by showing presence of retinochoroidal scars in 56.5 % of FUS patients. In the vast majority of studies, an assumed association between FUS and ocular toxoplasmosis was implicated based on presence of retinochoroidal scars at variable frequencies [104–108]. Nevertheless, a few sporadic cases of FUS in congenital ocular toxoplasmosis [109] and at the time of an active toxoplasmic retinochoroiditis in the same eye [106, 110, 111] or in contralateral eye [112] have also been reported.

Ocular toxoplasmosis in all these different presentations may be responsible for triggering the onset of FUS via a complex pathway by inducing autoimmunity directed against retinal or choroidal antigens. However, at what level the connection exists is a matter for debate. Different theories have been postulated. The most recent immunological theory suggests that FUS may develop over a period of time after congenital or acquired ocular toxoplasmosis and it may be a secondary immune reaction with a past antigenic stimulation to a previous infection rather than reactivation of ocular toxoplasmosis [107]. On the other hand, in FUS cases with active ocular toxoplasmosis, immunologic antigens may be released into general circulation due to retinal destruction by proliferating organism, which may also result in sensitization, thereby causing inflammation in the same eye or in contralateral eye [107].

In more recent studies, viral etiologies including rubella and CMV have also been postulated in the pathogenesis of FUS. The presence of rubella virus genome and demonstration of intraocular production of antibodies against the rubella virus point out toward the possibility of rubella virus as a possible etiological agent [113, 114]. In 2004, Quentin and Reiber [113] were the first to find an evidence of intraocular synthesis of rubella antibodies in the aqueous humor of all of 52 patients with FUS and rubella genome in 18 % of the tested aqueous humor samples. Groot-Mijnes et al. [114] also confirmed the presence of rubella infection by showing a positive Goldmann-Witmer index for rubella virus in 93 % of FUS patients. Similarly a number of other groups also conducted independent studies confirming these findings [115–117]. Another indirect evidence supporting this hypothesis is that the incidence of FUS has been shown to decline significantly among the vaccinated population in a tertiary center after the initiation of measles-mumps-rubella vaccination program in the United States [118]. Still the relationship between the rubella virus and FUS is not clear. It is hypothesized that the intraocular immune response against the rubella virus as a result of delayed manifestations of a congenital or acquired rubella infection may be the inciting factor for the development of FUS [115].

Chee et al. [119, 120] were the first to postulate CMV as another possible etiological agent in the pathogenesis of FUS by showing presence of CMV DNA in aqueous humor of eyes with presumed FUS. It is possible that different infectious agents may be the triggering cause of FUS in different geographic regions.

In summary, none of these pathogens has been fully linked to FUS. Fuchs uveitis syndrome may be a secondary phenomenon or a final common pathway following an initiating event caused by various triggers.

2.7 Serpiginous Choroiditis and Serpiginoid Choroiditis

Serpiginous choroiditis is a chronic, progressive, recurrent, and usually bilateral intraocular inflammatory disease of unknown origin. It is characterized by a geographic pattern of choroiditis, which typically extends from the peripapillary area and affects the overlying retinal pigment epithelium and the outer retina [121, 122].

Serpiginoid choroiditis, also described as serpiginous-like choroiditis, multifocal serpiginous choroiditis, multifocal serpiginoid choroiditis, or ampiginous choroiditis, may present as multifocal progressive or diffuse choroiditis resembling serpiginous choroiditis [123–128]. However, unlike serpiginous choroiditis, ocular involvement in serpiginoid choroiditis is usually unilateral, with multifocal irregular serpiginoid lesions involving the posterior pole, mid-periphery, and periphery sparing the juxtapapillary area. There is typically a prominent inflammatory cellular reaction in the vitreous and/or anterior chamber in this form [121].

Serpiginous choroiditis is primarily considered as an immune-mediated disease. An increased frequency of HLA-B7 and retinal S antigen association has been reported [129, 130]. Infectious triggers have also been postulated in the etiopathogenesis. Despite an association with syphilis has been shown [131, 132], the most often considered triggering bacterial infection is *Mycobacterium tuberculosis* [133–135]. However, antituberculosis chemotherapy has been shown to fail to halt the progression of the disease [136]. Furthermore, in contrast to serpiginoid choroiditis, patients with serpiginous choroiditis are usually from areas where tuberculosis is not endemic and patients mostly reveal negative results for tuberculin skin test, interferon gamma release assay, and chest x-ray [121].

In serpiginous choroiditis patients, a possible association with herpes viruses has also been postulated [137–139]. In PCR studies, VZV, HSV, CMV, and EBV genome has been shown to be positive in the aqueous humor of patients with serpiginous choroiditis; however, it is not clear whether antiviral treatment can halt choroiditis progression or recurrence [137, 138]. Interestingly, *Candida* species were also postulated as another possible etiological agent in a case series, which has not been confirmed by any other studies [140]. Still, evidence suggests that serpiginous choroiditis is primarily an idiopathic or autoimmune disease which can be treated with a combined regimen of oral corticosteroids along with immunomodulatory agents and not with anti-infectious agents [121].

Mycobacterium tuberculosis DNA was shown to be positive in the aqueous and vitreous humor of patients with serpiginoid choroiditis, and unlike serpiginous choroiditis, the disease shows good response to systemic antituberculosis chemotherapy [123, 124, 141]. Interestingly, in a recent PCR study, EBV DNA was also shown to be positive in the aqueous humor of patients with serpiginoid choroiditis [138].

Although various infections may be the inciting factors, serpiginous choroiditis and serpiginoid choroiditis are two different entities with different clinical morphology and management. The precise etiopathogenesis of each of these disorders remains unknown.

2.8 Birdshot Chorioretinopathy

Birdshot chorioretinopathy is an uncommon form of idiopathic bilateral posterior uveitis characterized by multiple, distinctive, hypopigmented choroidal lesions which are typically seen in middle-aged women of Caucasian origin [142, 143].

The disease has a strong genetic association with the HLA-A29 antigen, which suggests that genes for major histocompatibility antigens may play a role in the pathogenesis of the disease. Still, the immune mechanism involved in the pathogenesis remains unclear [144]. It is presumed that an infectious agent may initiate an immune response either by itself or through molecular mimicry in a genetically predisposed person by facilitating the presentation of autoantigen to T cells by the HLA-A29 molecule [142, 145]. *Borrelia burgdorferi* and *Coxiella burnetii* are the two organisms postulated as potential etiologic agents; however, there is still no study showing the direct role of infectious agents in the pathogenesis [146–148].

2.9 White Dot Syndromes

Inflammatory chorioretinopathies, referred to as “white dot syndromes,” are a group of disorders of unknown etiology characterized by multiple discrete whitish-yellow inflammatory lesions located at the various levels of the retina, outer retina, retinal pigment epithelium, choriocapillaris, and choroid [149, 150]. Acute posterior multifocal placoid pigment epitheliopathy (APMPPE), multiple evanescent white dot syndrome (MEWDS), multifocal choroiditis with panuveitis (MFC), and punctate inner choroiditis (PIC) are the disease entities included in the spectrum of white dot syndromes [151]. Common presenting symptoms include photopsias, blurred vision, floaters, nyctalopia, and visual field loss (blind spot enlargement), and some of these syndromes are also associated with an antecedent prodromal illness characterized by flu-like symptoms. Most of these entities are more commonly seen in myopic young women [149].

While the etiology of the white dot syndromes is not completely understood, various mechanisms have been postulated including infectious and noninfectious causes. Jampol et al. [152] suggested that a variety of relatively common susceptibility genes which probably also correspond to the ones that have been identified for systemic autoimmune diseases are present in patients with white dot syndromes. These loci are thought to be not disease specific and environmental triggers such as infections, immunizations, stress, and other factors (age, other genetic factors, sex) interact to predispose these individuals to particular ocular disorders. Since these patients have underlying shared susceptibility genes, they may also develop more than one of these disease entities and are also predisposed to recurrences [152]. An infectious cause, viral in particular, as an environmental trigger has been suggested based upon suspected or documented infections for some of these disorders.

The underlying pathology of APMPPE is presumed to be an abnormal immune response to an inciting agent. An association with HLA subtypes B7 and DR2 has also been shown [153]. The occurrence of APMPPE following influenza, varicella, or hepatitis B vaccination supports the hypothesis that the ocular disease may be caused by a delayed type hypersensitivity reaction due to activation of sensitized T lymphocytes by vaccination [154–157]. APMPPE has also been described in association with various infectious conditions including mumps, group A streptococcal infection, tuberculosis, and Lyme disease [158–161]. Furthermore, in some cases of recurrent disease, a hypersensitivity reaction to antimicrobial agents has been postulated as an etiologic factor. On the other hand, some noninfectious conditions may also present with clinical features of APMMPE including sarcoidosis, Wegener's granulomatosis, polyarteritis nodosa, and ulcerative colitis [162–165].

MEWDS is preceded by a viral-like illness in about one third of cases, and an association with HLA-B51 has been reported [166, 167]. Since a significant number of patients have a preceding flu-like illness and increased serum levels of IgM and IgG have been found during the acute phase of MEWDS, it is again hypothesized that the underlying inflammatory immune reaction to either a virus or a vaccine occurs in genetically susceptible persons [168–171]. Gass [172] suggested that infectious agents, viruses in particular, may gain entrance into the receptor cells at the edge of the optic disc and the ora serrata and finally trigger a subsequent autoimmune disease.

Like the other entities included in the spectrum of white dot syndromes, the etiology of MFC also remains uncertain; however, it has been hypothesized that an exogenous pathogen may sensitize the antigens in the retinal photoreceptors, retinal pigment epithelium, or choroid [173]. Some investigators have suggested a viral etiology such as HSV, VZV, and EBV; however, there is no conclusive evidence [174–176]. It is also unclear whether MFC and PIC represent two distinct disorders or should be included in the same clinical spectrum [177].

In summary, although various infections are thought to be the triggering factors in susceptible persons, the precise etiopathogenesis of the disease entities included in the spectrum of white dot syndromes remains unknown.

Core Messages

- Environmental factors, especially infectious triggers, including bacteria, viruses, and vaccines are thought to play an important role in the induction and perpetuation of some immune-mediated uveitis entities in genetically susceptible individuals.
- Oral microbiota, especially *Streptococcus* species, have been postulated as the

predominant infectious triggers in Behçet disease.

- In sarcoidosis, *Mycobacterium tuberculosis* has been suggested as the major triggering agent.
- In Vogt-Koyanagi-Harada disease, a viral infection, especially Epstein-Barr virus, may be the inciting factor.
- Gram-negative bacterial triggers may be involved in the development of HLA-B27-associated anterior uveitis.
- Rubella virus has been identified as the main cause of Fuchs uveitis syndrome.
- The major association of serpiginoid choroiditis has been found to be latent *Mycobacterium tuberculosis* infection.
- Viral infections and vaccinations have been postulated as possible triggers of white dot syndromes.

References

1. Willermain F, Rosenbaum JT, Bodaghi B et al (2012) Interplay between innate and adaptive immunity in the development of non-infectious uveitis. Prog Retin Eye Res 31:182–194
2. Caspi RR (2010) A look at autoimmunity and inflammation in the eye. J Clin Invest 120:3073–3083
3. Caspi RR (2014) Understanding autoimmunity in the eye: from animal models to novel therapies. Discov Med 17:155–162
4. Forrester JV, Klaska IP, Yu T, Kuffova L (2013) Uveitis in mouse and man. Int Rev Immunol 32:76–96
5. Tarabishy AB, Hise AG, Traboulsi EI (2012) Ocular manifestations of the autoinflammatory syndromes. Ophthalmic Genet 33:179–186
6. Doria A, Zen M, Bettio S et al (2012) Autoinflammation and autoimmunity: bridging the divide. Autoimmun Rev 12:22–30
7. J-F B (2005) Infections and autoimmune diseases. J Autoimmun 25:74–80
8. Tlaskalova-Hogenova H, Tuckova L, Stepankova R et al (2005) Involvement of innate immunity in the development of inflammatory and autoimmune diseases. Ann N Y Acad Sci 1051:787–798
9. Jesus AA, Goldbach-Mansky R (2014) IL-1 blockade in autoinflammatory syndromes. Annu Rev Med 65:223–244
10. Savic S, Dickie LJ, Wittmann M, McDermott MF (2012) Autoinflammatory syndromes and cellular responses to stress: pathophysiology, diagnosis and new treatment perspectives. Best Pract Res Clin Rheumatol 26:505–533
11. Abdelsadik A, Trad A (2011) Toll-like receptors on the fork roads between innate and adaptive immunity. Hum Immunol 72:1188–1193
12. Netea MG (2013) Training innate immunity: the changing concept of immunological memory in innate host defense. Eur J Clin Invest 43:881–884
13. Rubartelli A (2014) Autoinflammatory diseases. Immunol Lett 161:226–230
14. Lachman HJ, Quartier P, So A, Hawkins PN (2011) The emerging role of IL-1 in autoinflammatory diseases. Arthritis Rheum 63:314–324
15. Dinarello CA, van der Meer WM (2013) Treating inflammation by blocking interleukin-1 in humans. Semin Immunol 25:469–484
16. Samarkos M, Vaiopoulos G (2005) The role of infections in the pathogenesis of autoimmune diseases. Curr Drug Targets Inflamm Allergy 4:99–103
17. Chervonsky AV (2010) Influence of microbial environment on autoimmunity. Nat Immunol 11:28–35
18. Caspi RR (2011) Understanding autoimmune uveitis through animal models. The Friedenwald lecture. Invest Ophthalmol Vis Sci 52:1872–1879
19. Mat MC, Sevim A, Fresko İ, Tüzün Y (2014) Behçet's disease as a systemic disease. Clin Dermatol 32:435–442
20. Gül A (2005) Behçet's disease as an autoinflammatory disorder. Curr Drug Targets Inflamm Allergy 4:81–83
21. Tugal-Tutkun I, Onal S, Altan-Yaycioglu R, Altunbas HH, Urgancioglu M (2004) Uveitis in Behçet disease: an analysis of 880 patients. Am J Ophthalmol 138:373–380
22. Tugal-Tutkun I (2009) Behçet's uveitis. Middle East Afr J Ophthalmol 16:219–224
23. Kapsimali VD, Kanakis MA, Vaiopoulos GA, Kaklamanis PG (2010) Etiopathogenesis of Behçet's disease with emphasis on the role of immunological aberrations. Clin Rheumatol 29:1211–1216
24. Emmi G, Silvestri E, Squatrito D et al (2014) Behçet's syndrome pathophysiology and potential therapeutic targets. Intern Emerg Med 9:257–265
25. Galeone M, Colucci R, D'Erme AM, Moretti S, Lotti T (2012) Potential infectious etiology of Behçet's disease. Pathol Res Int 2012:595380
26. Kirino Y, Bertsias G, Ishigatsubo Y et al (2013) Genome-wide association analysis identifies new susceptibility loci for Behçet's disease and epistasis between HLA-B*51 and ERAP1. Nat Genet 45:202–207
27. Remmers EF, Cosan F, Kirino Y et al (2010) Genome-wide association study identifies variants in the MHC class I, IL10 and IL23R-IL12RB2 regions associated with Behçet's disease. Nat Genet 42:698–702

28. Mizuki N, Meguro A, Ota M, Ohno S, Shiota T, Kawagoe T (2010) Genome-wide association studies identify IL23R-IL12RB2 and IL10 as Behçet's disease susceptibility loci. Nat Genet 42:703–706
29. Hou S, Yang Z, Du L et al (2012) Identification of a susceptibility locus in STAT4 for Behçet's disease in Han Chinese in a genome-wide association study. Arthritis Rheum 64:4104–4113
30. Gül A (2014) Genetics of Behçet's disease: lessons learned from genomewide association studies. Curr Opin Rheumatol 26:56–63
31. Kirino Y, Zhou Q, Ishigatsubo Y et al (2013) Targeted resequencing implicates the familial Mediterranean fever gene MEFV and the toll-like receptor 4 gene TLR4 in Behçet disease. Proc Natl Acad Sci U S A 110:8134–8139
32. Ombrello MJ, Kirino Y, de Bakker PI, Gül A, Kastner DL, Remmers EF (2014) Behçet disease-associated MHC class I residues implicate antigen binding and regulation of cell-mediated cytotoxicity. Proc Natl Acad Sci U S A 111:8867–8872
33. Mazzoccoli G, Matarangolo A, Rubino R, Inglese M, De Cata A 2014 Behçet syndrome: from pathogenesis to novel therapies. Clin Exp Med [Epub ahead of print]
34. Hamzaoui K, Hamzaoui A (2012) Immunological responses in patients with Behçet's disease: advances in understanding. Expert Rev Ophthalmol 7:261–270
35. Kim DY, Cho S, Choi MJ, Sohn S, Lee ES, Bang D (2013) Immunopathogenic role of herpes simplex virus in Behçets's disease. Genet Res Int 2013:638273
36. Jefferies C, Wynne C, Higgs R (2011) Antiviral TRIMs: friend or foe in autoimmune and autoinflammatory disease? Nat Rev Immunol 25(11):617–625
37. Direskeneli H (2013) Innate and adaptive responses to heat shock proteins in Behçet's disease. Genet Res Int 2013:249157
38. Shimizu J, Kaneko F, Suzuki N (2013) Skewed helper T-cell responses to IL-12 family cytokines produced by antigen-presenting cells and the genetic background in Behcet's disease. Genet Res Int 2013:363859
39. Kawagoe T, Mizuki N (2011) Sarcoidosis. Curr Opin Ophthalmol 22:502–507
40. Herbort CP, Rao NA, Mochizuki M, Members of Scientific Committee of First International Workshop on Ocular Sarcoidosis (2009) International criteria for the diagnosis of ocular sarcoidosis: results of the first International Workshop on Ocular Sarcoidosis (IWOS). Ocul Immunol Inflamm 17:160–169
41. Iannuzzi MC, Rybicki BA, Teirstein AS (2007) Sarcoidosis. N Engl J Med 357:2153–2165
42. Mortaz E, Masjedi MR, Tabarsi P, Pourabdollah M, Adcock IM (2014) Immunopathology of sarcoidosis. Iran J Allergy Asthma Immunol 13:300–306
43. Levin AM, Iannuzzi MC, Montgomery CG et al (2013) Association of *ANXA11* genetic variation with sarcoidosis in African Americans and European Americans. Genes Immun 14:13–18
44. Saidha S, Sotirchos ES, Eckstein C (2012) Etiology of sarcoidosis: does infection play a role? Yale J Biol Med 85:133–141
45. Newman KL, Newman LS (2012) Occupational causes of sarcoidosis. Curr Opin Allergy Clin Immunol 12:145–150
46. Newman LS, Rose CS, Bresnitz EA, ACCESS Research Group et al (2004) A case control etiologic study of sarcoidosis: environmental and occupational risk factors. Am J Respir Crit Care Med 170:1324–1330
47. Brownell I, Ramírez-Valle F, Sanchez M, Prystowsky S (2011) Evidence for mycobacteria in sarcoidosis. Am J Respir Cell Mol Biol 45:899–905
48. Gupta D, Agarwal R, Aggarwal AN, Jindal SK (2007) Molecular evidence for the role of mycobacteria in sarcoidosis: a meta-analysis. Eur Respir J 30:508–516
49. Moller DR (2007) Potential etiologic agents in sarcoidosis. Proc Am Thorac Soc 4:465–468
50. Yasuhara T, Tada R, Nakano Y et al (2005) The presence of Propionibacterium spp. In the vitreous fluid of uveitis patients with sarcoidosis. Acta Ophthalmol Scand 83:364–369
51. Moorthy RS, Inomata H, Rao NA (1995) Vogt-Koyanagi-Harada syndrome. Surv Ophthalmol 39:265–292
52. Greco A, Fusconi M, Gallo A et al (2013) Vogt-Koyanagi-Harada syndrome. Autoimmun Rev 12:1033–1038
53. Yamaki K, Gocho K, Hayakawa K, Kondo I, Sakuragi S (2000) Tyrosinase family proteins are antigens specific to Vogt–Koyanagi–Harada disease. J Immunol 165:7323–7329
54. Matsuda H, Sugiura S (1971) Ultrastructural changes of the melanocyte in Vogt-Koyanagi-Harada syndrome and sympathetic ophthalmia. Jpn J Ophthalmol 15:69–80
55. Damico FM, Bezerra FT, Silva GC, Gasparin F, Yamamoto JH (2009) New insights into Vogt–Koyanagi–Harada disease. Arq Bras Oftalmol 72:413–420
56. Minoda H, Sakai J, Sugiura M, Imai S, Osato T, Usui M (1999) High inducibility of Epstein-Barr vírus replication in B lymphocytes in Vogt-Koyanagi-Harada disease. Nippon Ganka Gakkai Zasshi 103:289–96, Japanese
57. Sugita S, Takase H, Imai Y, Mochizuki M (2002) Immunopathogenic mechanisms of a melanocyte-specific autoimmune disease: a cross-reaction between tyrosinase peptides and cytomegalovirus antigen. Invest Ophthalmol Vis Sci 43:E-abstract 1529
58. Sugita S, Takase H, Kawaguchi T et al (2007) Cross-reaction between tyrosinase peptides and

cytomegalovirus antigen by T cells from patients with Vogt-Koyanagi-Harada disease. Int Ophthalmol 27:87–95
59. Ali A, Samson MC (2007) Seronegative spondyloarthropathies and the eye. Curr Opin Ophthalmol 18:476–480
60. Wakefield D, Montanaro A, Mc Cluskey P (1991) Acute anterior uveitis and HLA-B27. Surv Ophthalmol 36:223–232
61. Chang JH, McCluskey PJ, Wakefield D (2005) Acute anterior uveitis and HLA-B27. Surv Ophthalmol 50:364–388
62. Tuncer S, Adam YS, Urgancioglu M, Tugal-Tutkun I (2005) Clinical features and outcomes of HLA-B27-positive and HLA-B27-negative acute anterior uveitis in a Turkish patient population. Ocul Immunol Inflamm 13:367–373
63. Rothova A, van Veenedaal WG, Linssen A et al (1987) Clinical features of acute anterior uveitis. Am J Ophthalmol 103:137–145
64. Feltkamp TEW, Ringrose JH (1998) Acute anterior uveitis and spondyloarthropathies. Curr Opin Rheumatol 10:314–318
65. Abi-Hanna D, McCluskey P, Wakefield D (1989) HLA antigens in the iris and aqueous humor gamma interferon levels in anterior uveitis. Invest Ophthalmol Vis Sci 30:990–994
66. Wakefield D, Chang JH, Amjadi S et al (2011) What is new HLA-B27 acute anterior uveitis? Ocul Immunol Inflamm 19:139–144
67. Rosenbaum JT, Rosenzweig HL, Smith JR, Martin TM, Planck SR (2008) Uveitis secondary to bacterial products. Ophthalmic Res 40:165–168
68. Chang JH, McCluskey P, Wakefield D (2004) Expression of toll-like receptor 4 and its associated lipopolysaccharide receptor complex by resident antigen-presenting cells in the human uvea. Invest Ophthalmol Vis Sci 45:1871–1878
69. Wakefield D, Robinson P, Easter J et al (1985) Decreased chemiluminescent associated phagocytic response of peripheral blood mononuclear cells to Chlamydia trachomatis in patients with HLA-B27+ anterior uveitis. Br J Rheumatol 24:332–339
70. Otasevic L, Zlatanovic G, Stanojevic-Paovic A et al (2007) Helicobacter pylori: an underestimated factor in acute anterior uveitis and spondyloarthropathies? Ophthalmologica 221:6–13
71. Ebringer R, Cawdell D, Ebringer A (1979) Klebsiella pneumoniae and acute anterior uveitis in ankylosing spondylitis. Br Med J 1:383
72. Ebringer A, Baines M, Ptaszynska T (1985) Spondyloarthritis, uveitis, HLA-B27 and Klebsiella. Immunol Rev 86:101–115
73. White L, McCoy R, Tait B et al (1984) A search for Gram-negative enteric microorganisms in acute anterior uveitis: association of Klebsiella with recent onset of disease, HLA-B27 and B7CREG. Br J Ophthalmol 68:750–755
74. Blankenberg-Sprenkels SH, Fielder M, Feltkamp TE, Tiwana H, Wilson C, Ebringer A (1998) Antibodies to Klebsiella pneumoniae in Dutch patients with ankylosing spondylitis and acute anterior uveitis and to Proteus mirabilis in rheumatoid arthritis. J Rheumatol 25:742–747
75. Saari KM, Vilppula A, Lassus A et al (1980) Ocular inflammation in Reiter's disease after Salmonella enteritis. Am J Ophthalmol 90:63–68
76. McCluskey PJ, Wakefield D (1988) Anterior uveitis following Salmonella immunization in a patient with HLA-B27. Arthritis Rheum 31:1454
77. Aihara Y, Shimizu C, Fujiwara Y, Yakoto S (1996) Acute anterior uveitis in a child with HLAB60 after Salmonella enteritidis associated with the transient appearance of auto-antibody. Acta Paediatr Jpn 38:286–287
78. Saari KM, Laitinen O, Leirisalo M, Saari R (1980) Ocular inflammation associated with Yersinia infection. Am J Ophthalmol 89:84–95
79. Mattila L, Granfors K, Toivanen A (1982) Acute anterior uveitis after Yersinia infection. Br J Ophthalmol 66:209–212
80. Larkin DF, Cafferkey MT, Eustace P (1988) Yersinia-induced uveitis in Ireland. Br J Ophthalmol 72:938–941
81. Wakefield D, Stahlberg TH, Toivanen A, Granfors K, Tennant C (1990) Serologic evidence of Yersinia infection in patients with anterior uveitis. Arch Ophthalmol 108:219–221
82. Careless DJ, Chui B, Rabinovitch T, Wade Y, Inman RD (1997) Immunogenetic and microbial factors in acute anterior uveitis. J Rheumatol 24:102–108
83. Rosenbaum JT (1996) HLA B27-associated diseases. In: Pepose JS, Holland GN, Wilhelmus KR (eds) Ocular infection and immunity. Mosby-Yearbook, St Louis, pp 475–484
84. Onal S, Kazokoglu H, Demiralp EE, Yavuz S (2006) Prevalence and levels of serum antibodies to gram negative microorganisms in Turkish patients with HLA-B27 positive acute anterior uveitis and controls. Ocul Immunol Inflamm 14:293–299
85. Sprenkels SH, Uksila J, Vainionpaa R, Toivanen P, Feltkamp TE (1996) IgA antibodies in HLA-B27 associated acute anterior uveitis and ankylosing spondylitis. Clin Rheumatol Suppl 1:52–56
86. Sprenkels SH, Van Kregten E, Feltkamp TE (1996) IgA antibodies against Klebsiella and other Gram-negative bacteria in ankylosing spondylitis and acute anterior uveitis. Clin Rheumatol 15(Suppl 1):48–51
87. Huhtinen M, Laasila K, Granfors K et al (2002) Infectious background of patients with a history of acute anterior uveitis. Ann Rheum Dis 61:1012–1016
88. Lahesmas R, Skurnik M, Vaars M et al (1991) Molecular mimicry between HLA-B27 and Yersinia, Salmonella, Shigella and Klebsiella within the same region of HLA alpha-I helix. Clin Exp Immunol 86:399–404
89. Granfors K, Märker-Hermann E, de Keyser F et al (2002) The cutting edge of spondylarthropathy research in the millennium. Arthritis Rheum 46:606–613

90. Urvater JA, Hickman H, Dzuris JL et al (2001) Gorillas with spondyloarthropathies express an MHC class I molecule with only limited sequence similarity to HLA-B27 that binds peptides with arginine at P2. J Immunol 166:3334–3344
91. Bonfioli AA, Curi AL, Orefice F (2005) Fuchs' heterochromic cyclitis. Semin Ophthalmol 20(3):143–146
92. Jones NP (1991) Fuchs' heterochromic uveitis: a reappraisal of the clinical spectrum. Eye 5:649–661
93. Jones NP (1991) Glaucoma in Fuchs' heterochromic uveitis: aetiology, management and outcome. Eye 5:662–667
94. Tugal-Tutkun I, Guney-Tefekli E, Kamacı-Duman F, Corum I (2009) A cross-sectional and longitudinal study of Fuchs uveitis syndrome in Turkish patients. Am J Ophthalmol 148:510–515
95. Van Gelder RN (2008) Idiopathic no more: clues to the pathogenesis of Fuchs heterochromic iridocyclitis and glaucomatocyclitic crisis. Am J Ophthalmol 145:769–771
96. La Hey E, de Jong PT, Kijlstra A (1994) Fuchs' heterochromic cyclitis: review of the literature on the pathogenic mechanisms. Br J Ophthalmol 78:307–312
97. Babu K, Adiga M, Govekar SR, Kumar BVR, Murthy KR (2013) Associations of Fuchs heterochromic iridocyclitis in a south Indian patient population. J Ophthalmic Inflamm Infect 3:14
98. Barequet IS, Li Q, Wang Y, O'Brein TP, Hooks JJ, Stark WJ (2000) Herpes simplex virus DNA identification from aqueous fluid in Fuchs heterochromic iridocyclitis. Am J Ophthalmol 129:672–673
99. Hashida N, Ohguro N, Maruyama H (2011) Fuchs' heterochromic iridocyclitis associated with ocular toxocariasis. Jpn J Ophthalmol 55(1):76–78
100. Teyssot N, Cassoux N, Lehoang P, Bodaghi B (2005) Fuchs heterochromic cyclitis and ocular toxocariasis. Am J Ophthalmol 139:915–916
101. Mahendradas P, Shetty R, Malathi J, Madhavan HN (2010) Chikungunya virus iridocyclitis in Fuchs' heterochromic iridocyclitis. Indian J Ophthalmol 58:545–547
102. Babu K, Murthy GJ (2012) Chikungunya virus iridocyclitis in Fuchs' heterochromic iridocyclitis. Indian J Ophthalmol 60:73–74
103. Spirn MJ, Hubbard GB, Bergstrom C et al (2006) Ophthalmomyiasis associated Fuchs heterochromic iridocyclitis. Retina 26:973–974
104. Fuchs E (1906) Über komplicationen der heterochromie. Z Augenheilkd 15:191–212
105. Kimura SJ, Hogan MJ, Tygeson P (1955) Fuchs' syndrome of heterochromic cyclitis. Arch Ophthalmol 54:179–186
106. Toledo de Abreu M, Belfort R Jr, Hirata PS (1982) Fuchs' heterochromic cyclitis and ocular toxoplasmosis. Am J Ophthalmol 93:739–744
107. Jad A, Celine T, Bahram B, Phuc L, Nathalie C (2013) Fuchs' heterochromic cyclitis: a post-infectious manifestation of ocular toxoplasmosis? Int Ophthalmol 33:189–194
108. Arffa RC, Schlaegel TF (1984) Chorioretinal scars in Fuchs' heterochromic iridocyclitis. Arch Ophthalmol 102:1153–1155
109. La Hey E, Rothova A (1991) Fuchs's heterochromic cyclitis in congenital ocular toxoplasmosis. Br J Ophthalmol 75:372–373
110. Saraux H, Laroche L, Le Hoang P (1985) Secondary Fuch's heterochromic cyclitis: a new approach to an old disease. Ophthalmologica 190:193–198
111. Schwab JR (1991) The epidemiologic association of Fuchs' heterochromic iridocyclitis and ocular toxoplasmosis. Am J Ophthalmol 111:356–362
112. La Hey E, Baarsma GS (1993) Contrlateral active ocular toxoplasmosis in Fuchs' heterochromic cyclitis. Br J Ophthalmol 77:455–456
113. Quentin CD, Reiber H (2004) Fuchs heterochromic cyclitis: rubella virus antibodies and genome in aqueous humor. Am J Ophthalmol 138:46–54
114. de Groot-Mijnes JD, de Visser L, Rothova A, Schuller M, van Loon AM, Weersink AJ (2006) Rubella virus is associated with Fuchs heterochromic iridocyclitis. Am J Ophthalmol 141:212–214
115. Liu Y, Takusagawa HL, Chen TC, Pasquale LR (2011) Fuchs heterochromic iridocyclitis and the rubella virus. Int Ophthalmol Clin 51:1–12
116. Ruokonen PC, Metzner S, Ucer A et al (2010) Intraocular antibody synthesis against rubella virus and other microorganisms in Fuchs' heterochromic cyclitis. Graefes Arch Clin Exp Ophthalmol 248:565–571
117. Suzuki J, Goto H, Komase K et al (2010) Rubella virus as a possible etiological agent of Fuchs heterochromic iridocyclitis. Graefes Arch Clin Exp Ophthalmol 248:1487–1491
118. Birnbaum AD, Tessler HH, Schultz KL et al (2007) Epidemiologic relationship between Fuchs heterochromic iridocyclitis and the United States rubella vaccination program. Am J Ophthalmol 144:424–428
119. Chee SP, Jap A (2008) Presumed Fuchs heterochromic iridocyclitis and Posner-Schlossman syndrome: comparison of cytomegalovirus-positive and negative eyes. Am J Ophthalmol 146:883–889
120. Chee SP, Bacsal K, Jap A, Se-Thoe SY, Cheng CL, Tan BH (2008) Clinical features of cytomegalovirus anterior uveitis in immunocompetent patients. Am J Ophthalmol 145:834–840
121. Nazari H, Rao NA (2013) Serpiginous choroiditis and infectious multifocal serpiginoid choroiditis. Surv Ophthalmol 58:203–232
122. Lim WK, Buggage RR, Nussenblatt RB (2005) Serpiginous choroiditis. Surv Ophthalmol 50:231–244
123. Gupta V, Gupta A, Arora S, Bambery P, Dogra MR, Agarwal A (2003) Presumed tubercular serpiginous-like choroiditis: clinical presentations and management. Ophthalmology 110:1744–1749

124. Bansal R, Gupta A, Gupta V, Dogra MR, Sharma A, Bambery P (2012) Tubercular serpiginous-like choroiditis presenting as multifocal serpiginoid chorodiditis. Ophthalmology 119:2334–2342
125. Gupta A, Sharma A, Bansal R, Sharma K (2015) Classification of intraocular tuberculosis. Ocul Immunol Inflamm 23:7–15
126. Cunningham ET, Gupta A, Zierhut M (2014) The creeping choroiditides – serpiginous and multifocal serpiginoid choroiditis. Ocul Immunol Inflamm 22:345–348
127. De Luigi G, Mantovani A, Papadia M, Herbort CP (2012) Tuberculosis-related choriocapillaritis (multifocal-serpiginous choroiditis): follow-up and precise monitoring of therapy by indocyanine green angiography. Int Ophthalmol 32:55–60
128. Bhuibhar SS, Biswas J (2012) Nested PCR-positive tubercular ampiginous choroiditis: a case report. Ocul Immunol Inflamm 20:303–305
129. Broekhuyse RM, van Herck M, Pinckers AJ et al (1988) Immune responsiveness to retinal S-antigen and opsin in serpiginous choroiditis and other retinal diseases. Doc Ophthalmol 69:83–93
130. Erkkila H, Laatikainen L, Jokinen E (1982) Immunological studies on serpiginous choroiditis. Graefes Arch Clin Exp Ophthalmol 219:131–134
131. Gass JD, Braunstein RA, Chenoweth RG (1990) Acute syphilitic posterior placoid chorioretinitis. Ophthalmology 97:1288–1297
132. Hooper PL, Kaplan HJ (1991) Triple agent immunosuppression in serpiginous choroiditis. Ophthalmology 98:944–951
133. Witmer R (1952) Fine spezielle form rezidivierendir choroiditis. Ophthalmologica 123:353–354
134. Schlaegel TF (1969) Metastatic nonsuppurative uveitis. In: TF S (ed) Essentials of uveitis. Little Brown, Boston, p 77
135. Maumenee AE (1970) Clinical entities in "uveitis". An approach to the study of intraocular inflammation. Am J Ophthalmol 69:1–27
136. Karagiannis DA, Sampat FV, Dowler J (2007) Serpiginous choroidopathy with bilateral foveal sparing and good visual acuity after 18 years of disease. Retina 27:989–990
137. Priya K, Madhavan HN, Reiser BJ et al (2002) Association of herpesviruses in the aqueous humor of patients with serpiginous choroiditis: a polymerase chain reaction-based study. Ocul Immunol Inflamm 10:247–261
138. Janani MK, Malathi J, Biswas J, Sridharan S, Madhavan HN (2014) Genotyping detection of ebstein barr virus from clinically suspected viral retinitis patients in a tertiary eye care center, India. Ocul Immunol Inflamm :1–8 [Ebub ahead of print]
139. Rodman J, Pizzimenti J (2011) Serpiginous choroiditis in a herpes-positive patient. Optom Vis Sci 88:776–780
140. Pisa D, Ramos M, García P et al (2008) Fungal infection in patients with serpiginous choroiditis or acute zonal occult outer retinopathy. J Clin Microbiol 41:130–135
141. Mackensen F, Becker MD, Wiehler U, Max R, Dalpke A, Zimmermann S (2008) QuantiFERON TB-Gold-A new test strengthening long-suspected tuberculous involvement in serpiginous-like choroditis. Am J Ophthalmol 146:761–766
142. Shah KH, Levinson RD, Yu F et al (2005) Birdshot chorioretinopathy. Surv Ophthalmol 50(6):519–541
143. Shao EH, Manezo V, Taylor SRJ (2014) Birdshot chorioretinopathy. Curr Opin Ophthalmol 25:488–489
144. Levinson RD, Brezin A, Rothova A et al (2006) Research criteria for the diagnosis of birdshot chorioretinopathy: results of an international consensus conference. Am J Ophthalmol 141:185–187
145. Gasch AT, Smith JA, Whitcup SM (1999) Birdshot retinochoroidopathy. Br J Ophthalmol 83:241–249
146. Kuhne F, Morlat P, Riss I et al (1992) Is A29, B12 vasculitis caused by the Q fever agent? (*Coxiella Burnetti*). J Fr Ophhalmol 15:313–321
147. Kuiper H, de Jongh BM, Nauta AP et al (1991) Lyme borreliosis in Dutch forestry workers. J Infect 23:279–286
148. Suttorp-Schulten MS, Luyendijk L, van Dam AP et al (1993) Birdshot chorioretinopathy and Lyme borreliosis. Am J Ophthalmol 115:149–153
149. Quillen DA, Davis JB, Gottlieb JL (2004) The white dot syndromes. Am J Ophthalmol 137:538–550
150. Abu-Yaghi NE, Hartono SP, Hodge DO, Pulido JS, Bakri SJ (2011) White dot syndromes: a 20-year study of incidence, clinical features, and outcomes. Ocul Immunol Inflamm 19:426–430
151. Gass JDM (1997) Stereoscopic atlas of macular diseases: diagnosis and treatment, 4th edn. Mosby, St. Louis
152. Jampol LM, Becker K (2002) White spot syndromes of the retina: a hypothesis based on the common genetic hypothesis of autoimmune/inflammatory disease. Am J Ophthalmol 135:376–379
153. Wolf MD, Folk JC, Panknen CA, Goeken NE (1990) HLA-B7 and HLA-DR2 antigens and acute posterior multifocal placoid pigment epitheliopathy. Arch Ophthalmol 108:698–700
154. Park D, Schatz H, McDonald HR, Johnson RN (1995) Acute multifocal posterior placoid pigment epitheliopathy: a theory of pathogenesis. Retina 15:351–352
155. Fine HF, Kim E, Flynn TE, Gomes NL, Chang S (2010) Acute posterior multifocal placoid pigment epitheliopathy following varicella vaccination. Br J Ophthalmol 94:282–283
156. Mendrinos E, Baglivo E (2010) Acute posterior multifocal placoid pigment epitheliopathy following influenza vaccination. Eye 24:180–181
157. Bourges JL, Pisella PJ, Laurens C, Limon S (1998) Multifocal placoid epitheliopathy and anti-hepatitis B vaccination. J Fr Ophtalmol 21:696–700
158. Anderson K, Patel KR, Webb L, Dutton GN (1996) Acute posterior multifocal placoid pigment epitheli-

opathy associated with pulmonary tuberculosis. Br J Ophthalmol 80:186
159. Lowder CY, Foster RE, Gordon SM, Gutman FA (1996) Acute posterior multifocal placoid pigment epitheliopathy after acute group A streptococcal infection. Am J Ophthalmol 122:115–117
160. Borruat FX, Piguet B, Herbort CP (1998) Acute posterior multifocal placoid pigment epitheliopathy following mumps. Ocul Immunol Inflamm 6:189–193
161. Wolf MD, Folk JC, Nelson JA, Peeples ME (1992) Acute, posterior, multifocal, placoid, pigment epitheliopathy and Lyme disease. Arch Ophthalmol 110:750
162. Chiquet C, Lumbroso L, Denis P, Papo T, Durieu I, Lehoang P (1999) Acute posterior multifocal placoid pigment epitheliopathy associated with Wegener's granulomatosis. Retina 19:309–313
163. Crecchio D, Parodi MB, Saviano S, Ravalico G (2001) Acute posterior multifocal placoid pigment epitheliopathy and ulcerative colitis: a possible association. Acta Ophthalmol Scand 79:319–321
164. Hsu CT, Harlan JB, Goldberg MF, Dunn JP (2003) Acute posterior multifocal placoid pigment epitheliopathy associated with a systemic necrotizing vasculitis. Retina 23:64–68
165. Dick DJ, Neuman PK, Richardson J, Wilkinson R, Morley AR (1988) Acute posterior multifocal placoid pigment epitheliopathy and sarcoidosis. Br J Ophthalmol 72:74–77
166. Dell'Omo R, Pavesio C (2012) Multiple evanescent white dot syndrome (MEWDS). Int Ophthalmol Clin 52:221–228
167. Borruat FX, Herbort CP, Spertini F et al (1998) HLA typing in patients with multiple evanescent white dot syndrome (MEWDS). Ocul Immunol Inflamm 6:39–41
168. Goyal S, Nazarian SM, Thayi DR, Hammond F, Petrovic V (2013) Multiple evanescent white dot syndrome following recent influenza vaccination. Can J Ophthalmol 48:e115–e116
169. Fine L, Fine A, Cunningham ET Jr (2001) Multiple evanescent white dot syndrome following hepatitis A vaccination. Arch Ophthalmol 119:1856–1858
170. Baglivo E, Safran AB, Borruat FX (1996) Multiple evanescent white dot syndrome after hepatitis B vaccine. Am J Ophthalmol 122:431–432
171. Chung YM, Yeh TS, Liu JH (1987) Increased serum IgM and IgG in the multiple evanescent white-dot syndrome. Am J Ophthalmol 104:187–188
172. Gass JD (2003) Are acute zonal occult outer retinopathy and the white spot syndromes (AZOOR complex) specific autoimmune diseases? Am J Ophthalmol 135:380–381
173. Folk JC, Gehrs KM (2001) Multifocal choroiditis with panuveitis, diffuse subretinal fibrosis, and punctate choroidopathy. In: Retina, vol 2, 3rd edn. Andrew P. Schachat, St. Louis, pp 1709–1720
174. Grutzmacher RD, Henderson D, McDonald PJ et al (1983) Herpes simplex chorioretinitis in a healthy adult. Am J Ophthalmol 96:788–796
175. Frau E, Dussaix E, Offret H et al (1990) The possible role of herpes viruses in multifocal choroiditis and panuveitis. Int Ophthalmol 14:365–369
176. Tiedeman JS (1987) Ebstein-Barr virus antibodies in multifocal choroiditis and panuveitis. Am J Ophthalmol 103:659–663
177. Essex RW, Wong J, Jampol LM et al (2013) Idiopathic multifocal choroiditis: a comment on present and past nomenclature. Retina 33:1–4

Part I

Emerging Bacterial Infections

3 Rickettsioses

Sana Khochtali, Sonia Attia, and Moncef Khairallah

3.1 Introduction

Rickettsioses are worldwide distributed zoonoses due to obligate intracellular small Gram-negative bacteria. They are transmitted to humans by the bite of contaminated arthropods, including ticks, lice, mites, and fleas. Systemic involvement is typically characterized by a triad of high fever, headache, and general malaise and a maculopapular skin eruption in a patient living in or traveling back from a region endemic for rickettsiosis [1, 2]. Ocular involvement is common, but frequently asymptomatic and self-limited. Diagnosis of rickettsial disease is usually based on clinical features and is confirmed by positive serologic testing [3]. Doxycycline is the drug of choice for the treatment, but prevention is the mainstay of rickettsial infection control.

3.2 Epidemiology

Rickettsial agents have been classified into spotted fever and typhus groups [1, 2]. The spotted fever group mainly includes Mediterranean spotted fever (MSF), Rocky Mountain spotted fever (RMSF), and numerous other species. MSF, which is caused by *Rickettsia* (*R.*) *conorii*, is prevalent in Mediterranean countries and Central Asia, including India. Rocky Mountain spotted fever, which is caused by *R. rickettsii*, is endemic in parts of North, Central, and South America. The typhus syndromes include epidemic and endemic typhus that are due to infection with *R. prowazekii* and *R. typhi*, respectively. Epidemic typhus is usually encountered in areas of crowded population with poor hygiene conditions, as seen during wars and natural disasters. Murine typhus is found worldwide in warm-climate countries [1, 2]. A more recent classification has categorized more than 20 species within the genus *Rickettsia* into four groups, including the ancestral group, the typhus group, the spotted fever group, and a transitional group [4, 5].

3.3 Pathophysiology

Specific surface cells antigens play an important role in rickettsial adhesion to host cells and in their invasion. Rickettsiae, in vivo, preferentially infect microvascular endothelial cells in humans as well as in animal models. As a consequence, a host-immune response is triggered, leading to disseminated inflammation, impairment of endothelial barrier function, and altered vascular permeability. Infected endothelium will be induced to express prothrombotic, proadhesive, and

S. Khochtali • S. Attia • M. Khairallah, MD (✉)
Department of Ophthalmology,
Fattouma Bourguiba University Hospital, Faculty of Medicine, University of Monastir, Monastir, Tunisia
e-mail: moncef.khairallah@rns.tn

S.-P. Chee, M. Khairallah (eds.), *Emerging Infectious Uveitis*, DOI 10.1007/978-3-319-23416-8_3

proinflammatory genes, resulting in systemic vasculitis [1, 5]. Since the pathophysiologic basis for rickettsial disease is vasculitic, most common ocular lesions involve the retinal and optic disc vasculature [3, 6].

3.4 Clinical Features

3.4.1 Systemic Disease

Rickettsial disease usually occurs in late spring or summer, when the arthropod vectors, particularly ticks, are most active. A history of outdoor activities, occupational exposure, or tick attachment is frequent [1, 2]. After an incubation period of 5–7 days, the onset of the disease is abrupt, and typical cases present with high fever, headache, general malaise, and skin rash. The skin rash is usually generalized, maculopapular in type, often involving the palms and soles, but sparing the face (Fig. 3.1a). A local skin lesion, termed "tache noire" (black spot), may develop at the site of arthropod bite, mainly in patients with MSF (Fig. 3.1b). Most patients will recover within 10 days without any sequelae. However, severe life-threatening complications including major neurological manifestations and multiorgan involvement occur in 5 % to 6 % of patients, and the mortality rate is 2 % to 3 % [7–9]. Epidemic typhus is associated with more severe systemic disease and higher mortality rates than MSF [5].

3.4.2 Ocular Disease

Ocular involvement is common in patients with rickettsiosis, but because it is usually asymptomatic and self-limited, it may be easily overlooked [3, 10]. Affected patients, however, may present with ocular complaints, including vision blurring, scotomata, floaters, or redness. Retinitis, retinal vasculitis, and optic nerve involvement are the most common ocular findings, but an array of other ocular manifestations also may occur.

3.4.2.1 Adnexal and Anterior Segment Manifestations

Conjunctiva may be a portal of entry for *R. rickettsii*, as well as *R. conorii* infection, by a spurt of ticks blood. This may result in unilateral conjunctivitis that can accompany a Parinaud's oculoglandular syndrome (Fig. 3.2) [11, 12]. Bilateral conjunctivitis also has been described in patients with MSF, as well as RMSF [13]. Subconjunctival hemorrhages, conjunctival petechiae, keratitis, nongranulomatous anterior uveitis, and iris nodule have also been reported in association with rickettsial disease [11, 14, 15].

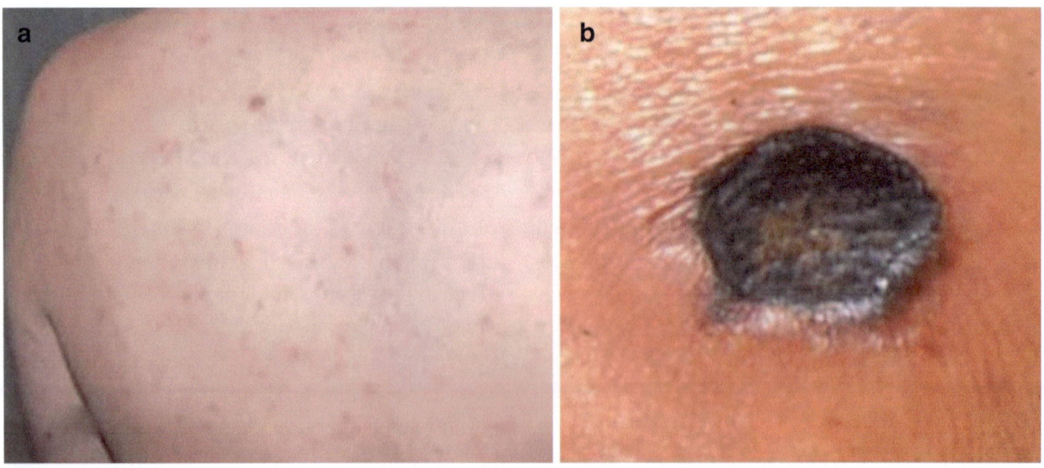

Fig. 3.1 (**a**) Maculopapular skin rash in a patient with Mediterranean spotted fever. (**b**) Dark spot, also called "tache noire," in a patient with Mediterranean spotted fever

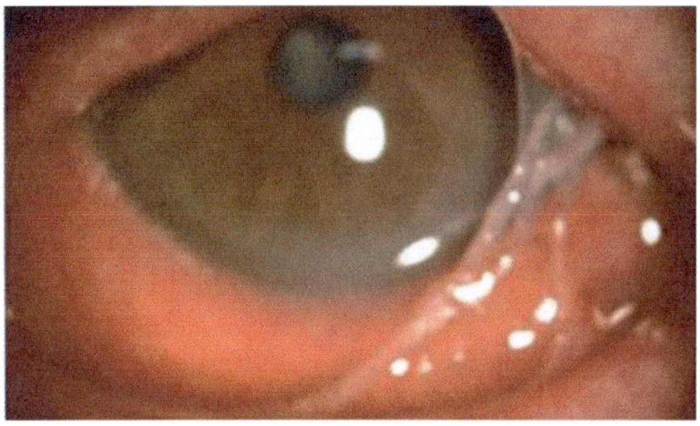

Fig. 3.2 Parinaud's oculoglandular syndrome in a patient with Mediterranean spotted fever. Slit-lamp photograph of the left eye shows unilateral conjunctivitis with purulent discharge. There was an associated ipsilateral swollen preauricular lymph node

3.4.2.2 Retinochoroidal Involvement

Retinochoroidal involvement is common, affecting, for instance, more than 80 % of patients with acute MSF [3]. However, it is often asymptomatic. Posterior segment manifestations typically include retinitis, retinal vascular changes, and optic disc involvement, with mild or no vitritis.

Retinitis

Retinitis, primarily involving the inner retinal layers, is the most common clinical finding, occurring in approximately one third of patients with acute MSF [3, 16–20]. It presents as white retinal lesions, variable in size and number, involving the posterior pole or the peripheral retina, typically adjacent to retinal vessels (Figs. 3.3a and 3.4a). Small lesions in the posterior fundus may strikingly resemble cotton-wool spots. Fluorescein angiography shows early hypofluorescence and late staining of large retinal lesions and isofluorescence or moderate hypofluorescence of small retinal lesions [3]. Optical coherence tomography (OCT) exhibits increased internal reflectivity of retinal lesions, with posterior shadowing. It also usually shows macular edema and serous retinal detachment in association with large white retinal lesions (Fig. 3.4b and c) [6].

There are reports of multiple small white retinal lesions in other rickettsioses including RMSF, Queensland tick typhus, and murine typhus [21–26]. Multiple retinal lesions similar to those seen in multiple white dot syndrome have also been reported [14, 27].

The pathogenesis of rickettsial retinal involvement remains speculative. Retinitis could develop as a consequence of multiplication of rickettsial microorganisms within retina. Alternatively, immune response to bacteremia might induce immune complexes and inflammatory cells to form white infiltrates through deposition in retinal vessels [3].

Rickettsial retinitis has a self-limited evolution in most patients with progressive resolution of white retinal lesions, within several weeks. There is usually no visible residual chorioretinal scarring [3].

Retinal Vascular Involvement

The marked tropism of rickettsial organisms for retinal vasculature is evidenced by the frequent occurrence of retinal vascular involvement. This may include focal or diffuse retinal vascular sheathing; arterial plaques similar to toxoplasmic Kyrieleis arteritis; superficial, deep, or white-centered retinal hemorrhages; and retinal vascular leakage on fluorescein angiography, mostly in the vicinity of white retinal lesions (Fig. 3.3). Vascular occlusive events may occur, usually in the form of asymptomatic or symptomatic branch retinal arteriolar occlusion that is usually intimately related to a white retinal inflammatory lesion. Central retinal artery occlusion and retinal vein occlusions have been less commonly reported [3, 10, 28–32].

Other Retinochoroidal Changes

Hypofluorescent choroidal lesions on fluorescein or indocyanine green angiography and endogenous endophthalmitis have been reported [3, 33, 34].

3.4.2.3 Neuro-ophthalmic Manifestations

Optic nerve involvement is common, reflecting the tropism of rickettsial organisms for optic disc vasculature besides retinal vasculature. It may include optic disc edema, optic disc hyperfluorescence, optic neuritis, neuroretinitis, and ischemic optic neuropathy. Third and sixth cranial nerve

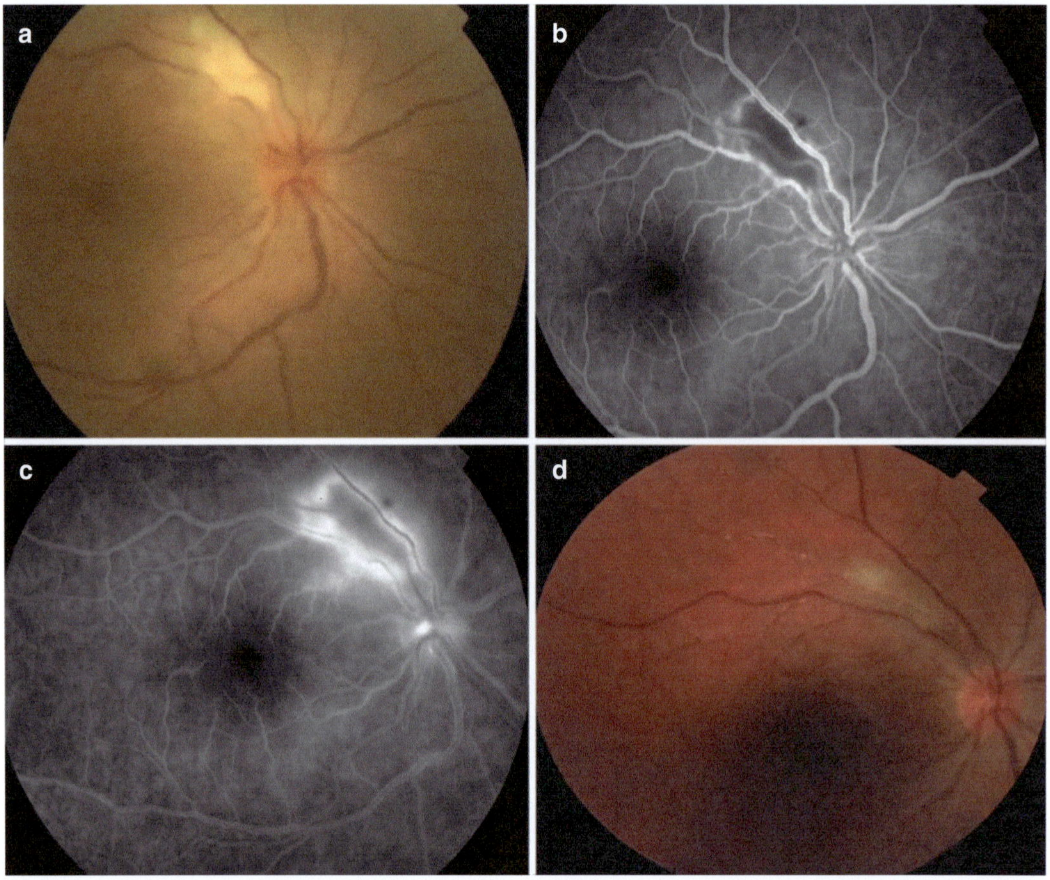

Fig. 3.3 A 43-year-old woman with a history of recent febrile illness complained of blurred vision in the right eye. Visual acuity was 20/20. (**a**) Fundus photograph of the right eye shows a juxtavascular white retinal lesion superotemporally, close to the optic disc. Note the presence of associated retinal vascular sheathing and optic disc hyperemia. Fluorescein angiography shows early hypofluorescence (**b**) and late staining (**c**) of the white retinal lesion, retinal vascular leakage, and mild optic disc hyperfluorescence. Serology was positive for *R. conorii*. The patient received doxycycline (100 mg twice a day) for 10 days. (**d**) Fundus photograph of the same eye, taken 2 months after initial presentation shows an almost complete resolution of the white retinal lesion without obvious chorioretinal scarring. Note the residual periarterial sheathing

palsies have also been reported in this setting [3, 10, 16–18, 33, 35–39].

3.5 Diagnosis

Diagnosis of rickettsial infection is usually suspected on the basis of clinical features (ocular and systemic) and epidemiological data. Serology is the most widely used method to confirm the diagnosis. Serum may be tested by immunofluorescence (IF) for rickettsial antigens, which is the gold standard for laboratory diagnosis. IF is considered positive when there is either initial high antibody titer or a fourfold rise of the titer in the convalescent serum. Case confirmation with IF might take 2–3 weeks. Other serological tests include Weil-Felix test, latex agglutination, indirect hemagglutination, immunoperoxidase assay, and ELISA. Cell culture systems and molecular methods for isolating rickettsial agents from human samples including quantitative PCR (qPCR) are less available techniques and performed only in selected cases [1, 17, 40].

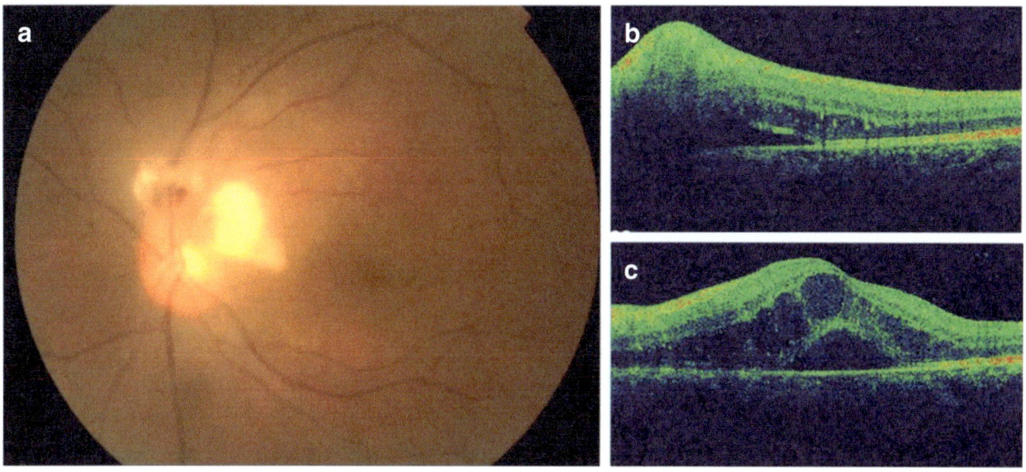

Fig. 3.4 A 37-year-old woman with Mediterranean spotted fever presented with vision loss in the left eye. Visual acuity was 20/200. (**a**) Fundus photograph of the left eye shows juxtapapillary white retinal lesions temporally and superiorly with associated small retinal hemorrhage. (**b, c**) OCT shows increased internal reflectivity with posterior shadowing corresponding to the temporal retinal lesion and associated cystoid macular edema and serous retinal detachment

In a patient suspected as having rickettsial systemic disease, a systematic fundus examination, revealing frequently abnormal, fairly typical findings, can help to establish the diagnosis while serologic testing is pending [3].

3.6 Differential Diagnosis

The differential diagnosis of rickettsiosis includes numerous systemic infectious and noninfectious diseases manifesting with acute febrile illness, such as typhoid fever, measles, rubella, enteroviral infection, meningococcemia, disseminated gonococcal infection, secondary syphilis, leptospirosis, cat scratch disease, infectious mononucleosis, arbovirus infection, Kawasaki disease, Behçet's disease and other systemic vasculitic disorders, idiopathic thrombocytopenic purpura, and drug reaction.

Specific epidemiological data, history, systemic symptoms and signs, and ocular findings can help differentiate rickettsial ocular disease from other infectious or noninfectious causes of retinitis, retinal vasculitis, or optic neuropathy. The differential diagnosis includes toxoplasmosis, cat scratch disease, syphilis, herpetic disease, chikungunya, Behçet's disease, and sarcoidosis. Small retinal infiltrates in the posterior fundus should be differentiated from cotton-wool spots that may be associated with a wide variety of ocular or systemic conditions [16–18].

3.7 Management

Early empirical antibiotic treatment should be given for any suspected rickettsiosis. Doxycycline (100 mg every 12 hours for 7–10 days) is the drug of choice for the treatment of rickettsial disease. Antibiotic treatment for systemic disease may be terminated 48 hours after the patient is afebrile. Other tetracyclines, chloramphenicol, and fluoroquinolones are also effective. Macrolides, including clarithromycin, azithromycin, and particularly josamycin can be used as alternative therapy in children and pregnant women [1, 41].

Additional therapeutic agents may be required for ocular disease: topical antibiotics for conjunctivitis or keratitis; topical corticosteroids and mydriatics for anterior uveitis; systemic corticosteroids for severe ophthalmic involvement, including extensive retinitis threatening the macula or optic disc, serous retinal detachment, macular edema, retinal vascular occlusion, severe vitritis, and optic neuropathy; and anticoagulant agents for retinal vascular occlusions. The role of antibiotic therapy, as well as that of oral steroids, on the course of posterior segment involvement, remain unknown. The effect of anticoagulants on the course of retinal occlusive complications is also unclear [3, 16–18].

Prevention is the mainstay of rickettsial disease control. It consists of personal protection against tick bites in endemic areas (repellents, protective clothing, and avoidance of dogs, detection and removal of an attached tick) and improvement of sanitary conditions including the control of rat reservoirs and of flea or lice vectors.

3.8 Prognosis

Although prognosis of systemic infection is usually good, rickettsioses may be severe and potentially lethal and therefore should be treated accordingly [1].

Ophthalmic manifestations of rickettsioses have a self-limited course in most patients, disappearing between the third and tenth week after the first examination. Posterior segment involvement associated with rickettsial disease has a good overall visual outcome. Causes of persistent visual impairment include residual central retinal pigment epithelial changes, retinal artery or vein occlusion, optic atrophy, and choroidal neovascularization [6].

Conclusion

The best diagnostic tool of rickettsial infection relies on a high index of suspicion in the presence of the triad of high fever, headache and general malaise, and skin rash in a patient living in or traveling back from a region endemic for rickettsiosis. Asymptomatic or symptomatic ocular involvement is common in patients with rickettsial disease. Retinitis presenting as small or large white retinal lesions in association with mild vitritis, retinal vasculitis, and optic nerve involvement are the most common and typical ocular findings.

A systematic fundus examination should be part of the routine evaluation of any patient who presents with fever and/or skin rash living in or returning from a specific endemic area. Fairly typical posterior segment findings can help to establish an early diagnosis of rickettsiosis, while serologic testing is pending.

Core Messages

- Systemic rickettsial disease: acute high fever, headache and general malaise, maculopapular skin rash
- Ocular symptoms: usually absent or mild, visual loss
- Ocular findings: focal or multifocal inner retinitis, retinal vasculitis, optic neuropathy, mild vitritis, nongranulomatous anterior uveitis, conjunctivitis, Parinaud's oculoglandular syndrome, others
- Laboratory diagnosis: serology (immunofluorescence), with initial high antibody titer or a fourfold rise of the titer in the convalescent serum, qPCR, cell culture
- Management: doxycycline, other antibiotics: macrolides, fluoroquinolones
- Prognosis: systemic disease: usually good, but potentially lethal
- Prognosis: ocular disease: usually self-limiting, rarely persistent visual loss
- Prevention: personal protection against tick bites, improvement of sanitary conditions

References

1. Parola P, Raoult D (1998) Rickettsioses éruptives. EMC (Elsevier Paris) Maladies infectieuses, 8-037-I-20, 24p
2. Mc Dade JE (1998) Rickettsial diseases. In: Hausler WJ, Sussman M (eds) Topley and Wilson's microbiology and microbial infections, vol 3, 9th edn. Arnold, London, pp 995–1011

3. Khairallah M, Ladjimi A, Chakroun M, Messaoud R, Ben Yahia S, Zaouali S, Ben Romdhane F, Bouzouaia N (2004) Posterior segment manifestations of Rickettsia conorii infection. Ophthalmology 111(3):529–534
4. Gillespie JJ, Beier MS, Rahman MS, Ammerman NC, Shallom JM, Purkayastha A, Sobral BS, Azad AF (2007) Plasmids and rickettsial evolution: insight from Rickettsia felis. PLoS One 2(3):e266
5. Sahni SK, Narra HP, Sahni A, Walker DK (2013) Recent molecular insights into rickettsial pathogenesis and immunity. Future Microbiol 8(10):1265–1288
6. Kahloun R, Gargouri S, Abroug N, Sellami D, Ben Yahia S, Feki J, Khairallah M (2014) Visual loss associated with rickettsial disease. Ocul Immunol Inflamm 22(5):373–378
7. Amaro M, Bacellar F, Franca A (2003) Report of eight cases of fatal and severe Mediterranean spotted fever in Portugal. Ann N Y Acad Sci 990:331–343
8. Renvoisé A, Raoult D (2009) L'actualité des rickettsioses. Med Mal Infect 39:71–81
9. Jemni L, Hamouda H, Chakroun M et al (1994) Mediterranean spotted fever in central Tunisia. J Travel Med 1:106–108
10. Alio J, Ruiz-Beltran R, Herrero-Herrero JI, Hernandez E (1987) Retinal manifestations of Mediterranean spotted fever. Ophthalmologica 195:31–37
11. Bazin R (2002) Rickettsial diseases. In: Foster F, Vitale A (eds) Diagnosis and treatment of uveitis. WB Saunders Company, Philadelphia, pp 297–304
12. Pinna A, Sotgiu M, Carta F, Zanetti S, Fadda G (1997) Oculoglandular syndrome in Mediterranean spotted fever acquired through the eye. Br J Ophthalmol 81:172
13. Helmick CG, Bernard KW, D'Angelo LJ (1984) Rocky Mountain spotted fever: clinical, laboratory, and epidemiological features of 262 cases. J Infect Dis 150:480–488
14. Alio J, Ruiz-Beltran R, Herrera I, Artola A, Ruiz-Moreno JM (1992) Rickettsial keratitis in a case of Mediterranean spotted fever. Eur J Ophthalmol 2:41–43
15. Cherubini TD, Spaeth GL (1969) Anterior nongranulomatous uveitis associated with Rocky Mountain spotted fever. First report of a case. Arch Ophthalmol 81:363–365
16. Khairallah M, Jelliti B, Jenzeri S (2009) Emergent infectious uveitis. Middle East Afr J Ophthalmol 16:225–238
17. Khairallah M, Chee SP, Rathinam SR, Attia S, Nadella V (2010) Novel infectious agents causing uveitis. Int Ophthalmol 30:465–483
18. Khairallah M, Ben Yahia S, Attia S (2010) Arthropod vector-borne uveitis in the developing world. Int Ophthalmol Clin 50:125–144
19. Khairallah M, Ben Yahia S, Toumi A, Jelliti B, Loussaief C, Romdhane FB, Messaoud R, Chakroun M (2009) Ocular manifestations associated with murine typhus. Br J Ophthalmol 93:938–942
20. Khairallah M, Ben Yahia S, Jelliti B, Ben Romdhane F, Loussaief C, Attia S, Toumi A, Messaoud R, Chakroun M (2009) Diagnostic value of ocular examination in Mediterranean spotted fever. Clin Microbiol Infect 15(Suppl 2):273–274
21. Raab EL, Leopold IH, Hodes HL (1969) Retinopathy in Rocky Mountain spotted fever. Am J Ophthalmol 68:42–46
22. Presley GD (1969) Fundus changes in Rocky Mountain spotted fever. Am J Ophthalmol 67:263–267
23. Smith TW, Burton TC (1977) The retinal manifestations of Rocky Mountain spotted fever. Am J Ophthalmol 84:259–262
24. Duffey RJ, Hammer ME (1987) The ocular manifestations of Rocky Mountain spotted fever. Ann Ophthalmol 19:301–306
25. Lukas JR, Egger S, Parschalk B, Stur M (1998) Bilateral small retinal infiltrates during rickettsial infection. Br J Ophthalmol 82:1215–1218
26. Hudson HL, Thach AB, Lopez PF (1997) Retinal manifestations of acute murine typhus. Int Ophthalmol 21:121–126
27. Esgin H, Akata F (2001) Bilateral multiple retinal hyperfluorescent dots in a presumed Rickettsia conorii infection. Retina 21:535–537
28. Lu TM, Kuo BI, Chung YM, Liu CY (1997) Murine typhus presenting with multiple white dots in the retina. Scand J Infect Dis 296:632–633
29. Paufique L, Bonnet M (1964) Thromboses vasculaires rétiniennes et rickettsioses. Bull Soc Ophtalmol Fr 64:410–415
30. Verdot S, Estavoyer JM, Prost F, Montard M (1986) Atteinte oculaire en phase aiguë de fièvre boutonneuse méditerranéenne. Bull Soc Ophtalmol Fr 86:429–431
31. Adan A, Lopez-Soto A, Moser C, Coca A (1998) Use of steroids and heparin to treat retinal arterial occlusion in Mediterranean spotted fever. J Infect Dis 158:1139–1140
32. Nagaki Y, Hayasaka S, Kadoi C, Matsumoto M, Sakagami T (2001) Branch retinal vein occlusion in the right eye and retinal hemorrhage in the left eye in a patient with classic Tsutsugamushi disease. Jpn J Ophthalmol 45:108–110
33. Vaphiades MS (2003) Rocky Mountain spotted fever as a cause of macular star figure. J Neuroophthalmol 23:276–278
34. Mendivil A, Cuartero V (1998) Endogenous endophthalmitis caused by Rickettsia conorii. Acta Ophthalmol Scand 76:121–122
35. Bronner A, Payeur G (1973) Hemorrhagic papillitis and rickettsiosis. Bull Soc Ophtalmol Fr 73:355–358
36. Castanet J, Costet C (1988) Neuropathie optique au cours d'une fièvre boutonneuse méditerranéenne. Presse Med 17:439–440
37. Granel B, Serratrice J, Rey J, Conrath J, Disdier P, Weiller PJ (2001) Impaired visual acuity in Mediterranean boutonneuse fever. Presse Med 30:859
38. Khairallah M, Zaouali S, Ben Yahia S, Ladjimi A, Messaoud R, Jenzeri S, Attia S (2005) Anterior isch-

emic optic neuropathy associated with Rickettsia conorii infection. J Neuroophthalmol 25:212–214
39. Rajadhyaksha A, Phatak S, Nolkha N, Pathan Y, Sonawale A (2013) Rickettsial fever presenting with isolated third nerve palsy. J Assoc Physicians India 61(2):144–145
40. Angelakis E, Richet H, Rolain JM, La Scola B, Raoult D (2012) Comparison of real time quantitative PCR and culture for the diagnosis of emerging Rickettsioses. PLoS Negl Trop Dis 6(3):e1540
41. Parola P, Paddock CD, Socolovschi C, Labruna MB, Mediannikov O, Kernif T, Abdad MY, Stenos J, Bitam I, Fournier PE, Raoult D (2013) Update on tick-borne rickettsioses around the world: a geographic approach. Clin Microbiol Rev 26(4):657–702

4 Syphilitic Uveitis

Sara J. Haug and Emmett T. Cunningham Jr.

4.1 Introduction

Syphilis is caused by infection by the spirochete *Treponema pallidum* and is, in the vast majority of cases, sexually transmitted. Although uncommon, syphilis and syphilitic uveitis continue to be an important cause of patient morbidity. Not only can vision and visual function be severely reduced by ocular involvement in syphilis, but severe and sustained non-ocular complications can also accompany infection. This latter point is particularly important given the high proportion of patients with syphilitic uveitis for whom ocular inflammation is the presenting sign of infection.

S.J. Haug, MD, PhD (✉)
West Coast Retina Medical Group,
San Francisco, CA, USA

Department of Ophthalmology, California Pacific Medical Center, San Francisco, CA, USA
e-mail: wcr@westcoastretina.com

E.T. Cunningham Jr., MD, PhD, MPH
West Coast Retina Medical Group,
San Francisco, CA, USA

Department of Ophthalmology, California Pacific Medical Center, San Francisco, CA, USA

Department of Ophthalmology, Stanford University School of Medicine, Stanford, CA, USA

The Francis I. Proctor Foundation,
UCSF School of Medicine,
San Francisco, CA, USA

4.2 Epidemiology

Recognized for over 150 years as an important cause of both iritis and chorioretinitis, the prevalence of confirmed cases of syphilitic uveitis has decreased dramatically over this time – first as a result of improved serologic testing and later with the introduction of effective antibiotic therapy [1]. This decline was particularly dramatic in the developed world in the latter half of the twentieth century such that by 2000 the annual rate of primary and secondary syphilis in the United States reached its lowest recorded level of 2.1 cases per 100,000 population [2–4]. Since 2000, however, the rate of primary and secondary syphilis in the United States has more than doubled to 5.3 cases per 100,000 population in 2013 [5]. Estimates in the United Kingdom indicate the incidence of syphilis between 1999 and 2008 have increased 1032 % [4]. This dramatic increase has occurred largely in men, who accounted for 91.1 % of reported early syphilis cases in 2013. The greatest percentage increases were among men having sex with men (MSM), most probably linked to the practice of unprotected sex in the era of effective antiretroviral therapy [4–7].

The British Ocular Syphilis Study utilized a national reporting system (the British Ocular Surveillance Unit) to collect new cases of syphilitic uveitis from 2009 to 2011. They found the annual incidence of ocular syphilis to be 0.3 cases per 1,000,000 persons and that syphilitic uveitis affected 0.6 % of all those affected with

S.-P. Chee, M. Khairallah (eds.), *Emerging Infectious Uveitis*, DOI 10.1007/978-3-319-23416-8_4

infectious syphilis every year [4]. This prevalence of ocular syphilis was lower than expected and may have been due to increased awareness of the resurgence of syphilis and, consequently, more prompt treatment. Another study out of Nantes, France, studied 36 patients hospitalized for syphilis from 2000 to 2010. All but one of the patients were MSM and 50 % were HIV positive. Of the 36 patients with severe syphilitic infection requiring hospitalization, 11 (30.6 %) had syphilitic uveitis [8].

4.3 Pathophysiology

Humans are the only known reservoir for syphilis. The spirochete typically enters the body through intact mucosa, whereafter invasion of local and distant tissues ensues. The bacteria do not produce an intrinsic toxin; rather, tissue damage results predominantly from the ensuing adaptive immune response in the host. *T. pallidum* initially elicits a prominent B-cell response, with T-cell-mediated immunity playing a key role in elimination from infected hosts [9]. Dissemination occurs despite the humoral and cellular response of the host, and, without treatment, the bacteria can persist in the body for decades [9, 10].

4.4 Clinical Features

4.4.1 Systemic Manifestations

The systemic manifestations of syphilis have been divided into three clinical stages. Primary syphilis is the first stage of syphilitic infection and occurs about 3 weeks after exposure. It is characterized by an ulcerative chancre at the contact point and is associated with regional lymphadenopathy. Although there is systemic dissemination shortly after inoculation through the lymphatics and blood stream, flu-like systemic symptoms are rarely associated with primary syphilis. The chancre is usually painless and heals spontaneously within a few weeks and, therefore, is often unnoticed.

Untreated, the infection progresses to secondary syphilis 2–12 weeks after initial inoculation. Systemic manifestations such as arthralgias, headache, low-grade fever, and a maculopapular rash can occur and last for a few weeks or linger over many months. After secondary syphilitic infection, the disease moves to a latent stage that can continue for years.

The tertiary phase of syphilis refers to the occurrence of sequelae of infection months or years after the untreated resolution of the signs of secondary syphilis, complications that can affect 15–30 % of those infected [11] and can include focal inflammatory lesions known as gummas, vasa vasorum of the aorta, tabes dorsalis, and general paresis. Although involvement of the central nervous system (CNS) can result in severe manifestations in tertiary syphilis, CNS infection, or neurosyphilis, may be demonstrated at any stage. Ocular involvement, which can also occur either during secondary or latent syphilitic infection, elevates the suspicion of nervous system involvement and is usually treated as such.

Congenital syphilis may manifest at any time throughout life. Symptoms occurring at the age of 2 years or younger are considered early onset of congenital syphilis; symptoms after age 2 are termed late onset of congenital syphilis.

4.4.2 Ocular Manifestations

While direct conjunctival inoculation resulting in primary ocular syphilis is possible [12], ocular syphilis occurs most often during the secondary and latent stages of infection.

4.4.2.1 External Examination

The conjunctiva may be involved in several ways in syphilis. In primary syphilis, an ulcerative conjunctival lesion with a rounded edge and surrounding conjunctival injection may be seen, very similar to chancres seen at a genital inoculation site. There tends to be little or no discharge associated with a primary conjunctival lesion. A nonspecific conjunctivitis usually consisting of a primary papillary reaction can present in secondary syphilis and is usually mild and often overlooked. In tertiary syphilis, there can be a granulomatous conjunctivitis with secondary necrosis and gumma formation [11].

Scleritis and episcleritis can be seen in conjunction with other ocular findings of syphilitic uveitis however are uncommon in isolation [13, 14]. Anterior nodular scleritis is the most common form of direct scleral involvement and tends not to progress to necrosis. Syphilitic scleritis should show rapid improvement to appropriate antimicrobial treatment [13].

4.4.2.2 Anterior Segment

Corneal manifestations of congenital and acquired syphilis are probably the most recognized ocular findings in syphilis. Nonulcerative stromal keratitis is most commonly a manifestation of late congenital syphilis, appearing between 5 and 15 years of age [15, 16]. However, as the rates of congenital syphilis decrease and the rate of acquired syphilis increases, more cases of adult stromal keratitis are being reported [15–17]. Nonulcerative stromal keratitis presents in adults with syphilis as marginal, central, or multifocal stromal inflammation with neovascularization, usually immediately anterior to Descemet's membrane. The keratitis responds to corticosteroid therapy, but occasionally can recur [16]. With inactive interstitial keratitis, ghost vessels may be seen and can be associated with stromal scarring.

Iritis and iridocyclitis is a nonspecific finding in syphilitic uveitis and may be granulomatous (Fig. 4.1) or nongranulomatous. Hypopyon may be present, but is uncommon. Dilated iris capillaries (iris roseola) are thought to be highly suggestive of syphilitic infection (Fig. 4.2). The classic pupillary finding in syphilis is the Argyll Robertson pupil, usually seen in latent syphilis and diagnostic for neurosyphilis. The pupils are unequal in size, irregular, and miotic, and while the pupil will accommodate, it will not react to light. The pathologic lesion is thought to be in the interneuron connection between the Edinger-Westphal nucleus and the retinal ganglion cells in the midbrain [18].

Cataracts have been described uncommonly in association with both congenital and acquired syphilis.

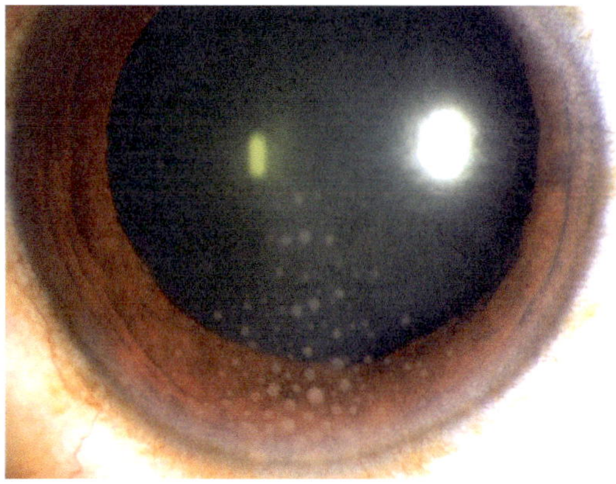

Fig. 4.1 Color slit lamp photograph of large "granulomatous" keratic precipitates in a patient with syphilitic uveitis (Reproduced with permission from Wender J, Eliott D, Jumper JM, Cunningham ET Jr. How to recognize ocular syphilis. Rev Ophthalmol, 2008, November, 124–130)

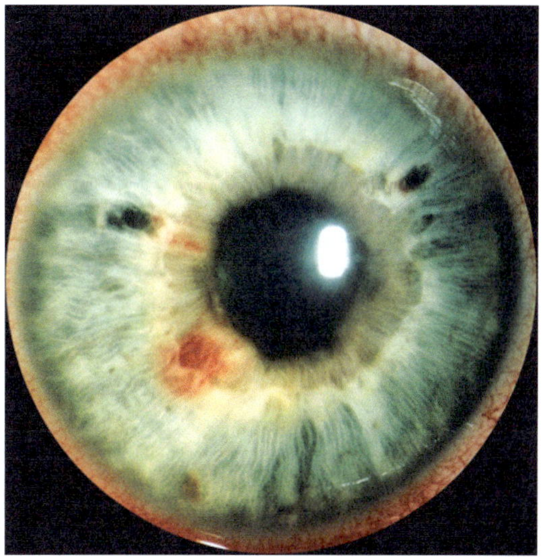

Fig. 4.2 Color slit lamp photograph of iris roseola in a patient with syphilitic uveitis. Two patent iridotomies are visible at 2 and 10 o'clock (Reproduced with permission from Wender J, Eliott D, Jumper JM, Cunningham ET Jr. How to recognize ocular syphilis. Rev Ophthalmol, 2008, November, 124–130)

4.4.2.3 Posterior Segment

Posterior segment complications appear to be particularly common in patients with syphilis [19]. Although the clinical presentation can be varied and a wide assortment of findings has been reported, there are posterior findings that, while not necessarily pathognomonic, are highly suggestive of syphilitic infection.

Isolated vitritis can occur in patients with syphilis; however, vitreous inflammation tends to occur more often in association with other posterior segment findings, most commonly retinitis [19, 20]. One report highlighted three cases of primary vitritis as the initial manifestation of syphilitic uveitis [21]. All the patients in the report were HIV positive.

While isolated optic disc edema has been reported as a presenting sign of syphilis [22, 23], optic disc swelling typically occurs in the setting of active uveitis (Fig. 4.3) [19, 20, 24].

Numerous descriptions and variations of retinitis have been reported in cases of syphilitic uveitis including wedge-shaped retinitis, ground-glass retinitis, and necrotizing retinitis [2, 11, 20, 25, 26]. Active syphilitic retinitis often contains both vasculitis and superficial precipitates or accumulations (Fig. 4.4), which together are quite suggestive of syphilis [26]. Similarly, acute syphilitic posterior placoid chorioretinitis (ASPPC), first described by Gass in 1990 [27], is a classic finding of syphilis (Fig. 4.5). In ASPPC, the lesions are typically yellow-white, placoid, circular, or oval and involve the macular or extramacular area. An active leading edge was often observed. Fluorescein angiography shows a hypofluorescent central lesion in the early-phase frames with progressive hyperfluorescence in the later frames, often observed with leopard spotting [2, 20, 27]. Spectral domain optical coherence tomography imaging shows characteristic outer retinal abnormalities, including disruption of the ellipsoid band, nodular thickening of the retinal pigment epithelium (RPE), loss of the outer segment/RPE junction, and in some cases loss of the external limiting membrane. Subretinal fluid was also observed, although was transient. Usually these findings reversed following appropriate treatment; however in some cases, the damage to the outer retinal anatomy was permanent and poor vision persisted [20, 28].

Localized exudative retinal detachments are relatively common in posterior syphilitic uveitis and have been widely reported [29–31]. Rhegmatogenous retinal detachments, in comparison, are much less common [32, 33]. Rhegmatogenous detachments typically occur early in the course of treatment, as the infection resolves, but prior to the resolution of inflammation,

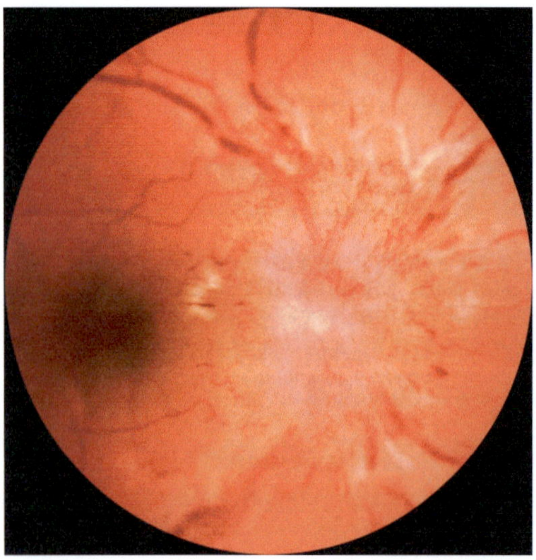

Fig. 4.3 Color fundus photograph of syphilitic papillitis in an HIV-positive patient (Reproduced with permission from Wender J, Eliott D, Jumper JM, Cunningham ET Jr. How to recognize ocular syphilis. Rev Ophthalmol, 2008, November, 124–130)

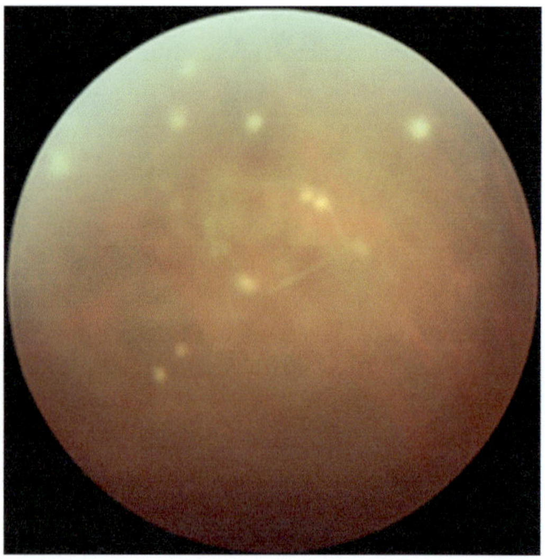

Fig. 4.4 Color fundus photograph of characteristic "ground-glass" retinitis associated with a serous retinal detachment, focal inflammatory accumulations, and retinal vasculitis in an HIV-positive patient with syphilitic uveitis (Reproduced with permission from Wender J, Eliott D, Jumper JM, Cunningham ET Jr. How to recognize ocular syphilis. Rev Ophthalmol, 2008, November, 124–130)

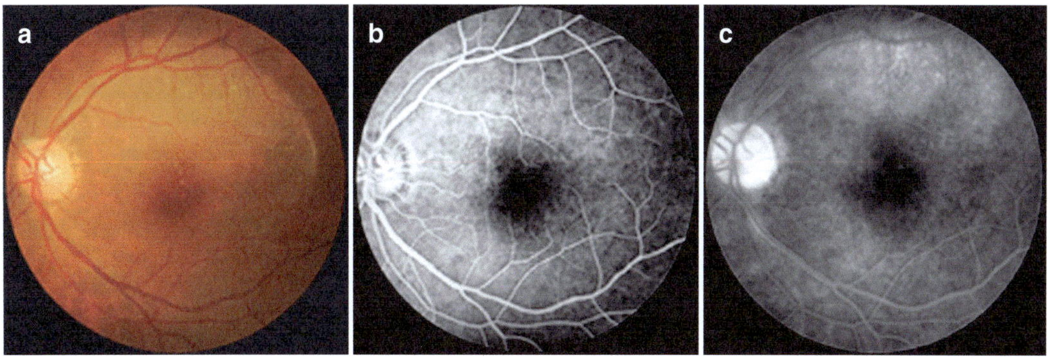

Fig. 4.5 Color fundus photograph (**a**) and serial fluorescein angiographic images (**b**, **c**) of acute syphilitic posterior placoid chorioretinopathy (ASPPC) showing a characteristic macular lesion and progressive hyperfluorescence (Reproduced with permission from Wender J, Eliott D, Jumper JM, Cunningham ET Jr. How to recognize ocular syphilis. Rev Ophthalmol, 2008, November, 124–130)

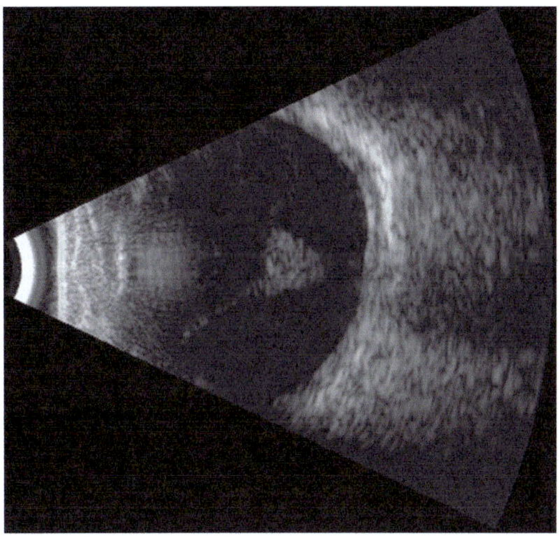

Fig. 4.6 B-scan ultrasonography showing a total rhegmatogenous retinal detachment in a patient with syphilitic panuveitis

and are thought to be due to contraction of the vitreous (Fig. 4.6) [33].

4.5 Diagnosis

Diagnosis of the "great imitator" requires a high level of clinical suspicion. The definitive method for diagnosis is direct visualization of *T. pallidum* using dark-field microscopy; however due to the technological difficulties of this test, it is rarely performed [34]. Serologic testing can be divided into two groups. First, the nontreponemal tests such as the venereal disease research laboratory (VDRL) and the rapid plasma reagin (RPR) tests detect antibodies to cardiolipin (lecithin) cholesterol antigen. The titers of the nontreponemal tests are often used as an indicator of both disease activity and of appropriate and complete treatment. In contrast, direct treponemal tests such as enzyme immunoassays (EIAs) and chemiluminescent immunoassays (CIAs) detect antibodies directed against treponemal antigens and so are used as more sensitive and specific indicators of past or current infection. These direct treponemal assays will remain reactive for years, despite adequate therapy [7].

Most practitioners today use both treponemal and nontreponemal tests to confirm syphilis infection in patients with syphilitic uveitis. The nontreponemal tests are inexpensive and often used for screening; however, they are not specific for syphilis, can produce false-positive results, and can be falsely negative in early stages of infection. If there is discordance between the treponemal and nontreponemal serologies, a confirmatory *Treponemal pallidum* particle agglutination (TP-PA) test can be used for syphilis diagnosis. In patients with confirmed syphilis infection, HIV testing is also warranted.

4.6 Differential Diagnosis

The differential diagnosis is quite broad for syphilitic uveitis, given its varied ocular manifestations. Nonulcerative stromal keratitis is often associated with congenital or acquired syphilis, but the differential includes tuberculosis, leprosy, sarcoidosis, lymphoma, Lyme disease, herpes simplex virus and herpes zoster virus, Epstein-Barr virus, mumps, human T-lymphotropic virus type 1, leishmaniasis, onchocerciasis, trypanosomiasis, Cogan's syndrome, or trauma such as contact lens overwear. In cases of syphilitic panuveitis, the differential diagnosis includes endogenous endophthalmitis, sarcoidosis, toxoplasmosis, tuberculosis, Lyme disease, Behçet's disease, and viral retinitis such as cytomegalovirus or acute retinal necrosis. The differential diagnosis for posterior placoid chorioretinopathy due to syphilis is similar to the differential for panuveitis, tuberculosis, Lyme disease, toxoplasmosis, and sarcoidosis, but also should include fungal infections, lymphoma, persistent placoid maculopathy, and metastasis.

4.7 Management

Patients with a new diagnosis of syphilis must first be reported in most countries and regions, patients with a new diagnosis of syphilis should be reported to the local health authorities. Penicillin G is the drug of choice for all stages of syphilis, although the specifics of the regimen are debated. In immunocompetent patients with early syphilis, defined as primary, secondary, or latent of less than 1 year's duration, a single intramuscular injection of 2.4 million units of benzathine penicillin G is considered adequate. Recommended treatment for patients with active chorioretinal disease is aqueous crystalline penicillin G (18–24 million units IV daily) or procaine penicillin (2.4 million units IM daily) with oral probenecid (500 mg four times daily) for 10–14 days. Response to treatment is verified by a fourfold decrease in titer by the same nontreponemal test. If there is confirmed neurosyphilis with positive cerebrospinal fluid, patients should be monitored at 6-month intervals with CSF studies until the cell count normalizes. In patients with concurrent HIV infection, the treatment regimen should be for 3 weeks rather than 10–14 days, and serologic testing should be performed at 6-month intervals for 2 years to monitor for treatment failure [11, 25].

The use of corticosteroids to help control the inflammation as a result of the syphilis infection is controversial. Topical corticosteroids should be used liberally; however, intravitreal steroid injections are generally avoided. Oral corticosteroids are also not routinely advised.

4.8 Prognosis

Although neurosyphilis and tertiary syphilis can be devastating, most new cases of syphilis are diagnosed in the primary or secondary stage of syphilis. When diagnosed in these earlier stages, the prognosis is usually quite good. Many of the systemic and ocular symptoms resolve without sequelae.

Conclusions

Syphilis infection is again on the rise globally. Although there are classic findings for syphilitic uveitis, syphilis is the "great imitator" and must be considered in nearly all cases of intraocular inflammation, particularly if a condition is not responding to usual treatment.

Core Messages

- Incidence of syphilis infection has risen following a nadir in 2000, particularly in men who have sex with men. HIV coinfection is common.
- Syphilis is known as the "great imitator," given its wide variety of ocular manifestations. Therefore, a high level of suspicion for *T. pallidum* infection must be maintained in new cases of uveitis, given that a high proportion of undiagnosed patients with syphilis present with uveitic symptoms.
- Diagnosis of syphilitic infection is made with serologic testing. Nontreponemal tests such as rapid plasma reagin (RPR) are used in conjunction with treponemal tests, such as the enzyme immunoassays

(EIAs) or chemiluminescent immunoassays (CIAs). If there is discordance between the treponemal and nontreponemal serologies, the *Treponema pallidum* particle agglutination (TP-PA) test is utilized for diagnosis. Response to treatment is monitored using the nontreponemal tests, which should seroconvert to negative following appropriate treatment.

- Treatment of syphilitic uveitis consists of aqueous crystalline penicillin G (18–24 million units IV daily) or procaine penicillin (2.4 million units IM daily) with oral probenecid (500 mg four times daily) for 10–14 days. If the patients are HIV positive, treatment should continue for 3 weeks. An alternative to this treatment is a single intramuscular injection of 2.4 million units of benzathine penicillin G weekly for three weeks. Within the United States, new cases of syphilis should be reported to the patient's respective State Department of Health.

Declaration of Interest
The authors report no conflicts of interest. The authors alone are responsible for the content and writing of the paper.

Acknowledgments Supported in part by the Pacific Vision Foundation and the San Francisco Retina Foundation.

References

1. Silverstein AM (1997) Changing trends in the etiologic diagnosis of uveitis. Doc Ophthalmol 94(1–2):25–37
2. Chao JR, Khurana RN, Fawzi AA et al (2006) Syphilis: reemergence of an old adversary. Ophthalmology 113:2074–2079
3. Centers for Disease Control and Prevention (2011) Sexually transmitted disease surveillance 2010. U.S. Department of Health and Human Services, Atlanta
4. Mathew RG, Goh BT, Westcott MC (2014) British ocular syphilis study (BOSS): 2-year national surveillance study of intraocular inflammation secondary to ocular syphilis. Invest Ophthalmol Vis Sci 55:5394–5400
5. Patton ME, Su JR, Nelson R, Weinstock H (2014) Primary and secondary syphilis – United States, 2005–2013. MMWR Morb Mortal Wkly Rep 63:402–406
6. Heffelfinger JD, Swing EB, Berman SM et al (2007) Trends in primary and secondary syphilis among men who have sex with men in the United States. Am J Public Health 97:1076–1083
7. Davis JL (2014) Ocular syphilis. Curr Opin Ophthalmol 25:513–518
8. Lefebvre M, Biron C, Guillouzouic A et al (2013) Syphilis in Nantes tertiary care hospital between 2000 and 2010: a case series of 36 hospitalized patients. Rev Med Interne 34:522–527
9. Halperin JJ (2010) A tale of two spirochetes: lyme disease and syphilis. Neurol Clin 28(1):277–291
10. LaFond RE, Lukehart SA (2006) Biological basis for syphilis. Clin Microbiol Rev 19(1):29–49
11. Tsai JH, Rao NA (2013) Spirochetal infections. In: Ryan SJ, Schachat AP, Sadda SR (eds) Retina, 5th edn. Saunders Elsevier, China. pp 1486–1489
12. Jeyakumar W, Chithra A, Shanmugasundararaj A (1989) Primary syphilis of the eyelid: case report. Genitourin Med 65(3):192–193
13. Casey R, Flowers CW Jr, Jones DD et al (1996) Anterior nodular scleritis secondary to syphilis. Arch Ophthalmol 114:1015–1016
14. Lee SB, Kim KS, Lee WK et al (2013) Ocular syphilic characterised by severe scleritis in a patient infected with HIV. Lancet Infect Dis 13:994
15. Hariprasad SM, Moon SJ, Allen RC, Wilhelmus KR (2002) Keratopathy from congenital syphilis. Cornea 21:608–609
16. Wilhemus KR, Jones DB (2006) Adult-onset syphilitic stromal keratitis. Am J Ophthalmol 141:319–321
17. Dinis da Gama R, Cidade M (2002) Interstitial keratitis as the initial expression of syphilitic reactivation. N Engl J Med 346:1799
18. Aziz TA, Holman RP (2010) The Argyll Robertson pupil. Am J Med 123:120–121
19. Browning DJ (2000) Posterior segment manifestations of active ocular syphilis, their response to a neurosyphilis regimen of penicillin therapy, and the influence of human immunodeficiency virus status on respons. Ophthalmology 107:2015–2023
20. Eandi CM, Neri P, Adelman RA et al (2012) Acute syphilitic posterior placoid chorioretinitis. Report of a case series and comprehensive review of the literature. Retina 32:1915–1941
21. Kuo IC, Kapusta MA, Rao NA (1998) Vitritis as the primary manifestation of ocular syphilis in patients with HIV infection. Am J Ophthalmol 125: 306–311
22. Weinstein JM, Lexow SS, Ho P, Spickards A (1981) Acute syphilitic optic neuritis. Arch Opthahlmol 99:1392–1395

23. Fonollosa A, Martinez-Indart L, Artaraz J, et al (2014) Clinical manifestations and outcomes of syphilis-associated uveitis in northern Spain. Ocul Immunol Inflamm. Epub ahead of print
24. Tucker JD, Li JZ, Robbins GK et al (2011) Ocular syphilis among HIV-infected patients: a systematic analysis of the literature. Sex Transm Infect 87: 4–8
25. Dugel PR, Thach AB (2004) Syphilitic uveitis. In: Yanoff M, Duker JS (eds) Ophthalmology, 2nd edn. Mosby, an affiliate of Elsevier, St. Louis, MO, USA. pp 1135–1138
26. Fu EX, Geraets RL, Dodds EM et al (2010) Superficial retinal precipitates in patients with syphilitic retinitis. Retina 30:1135–1143
27. Gass JD, Braunstein RA, Chenoweth RG (1990) Acute syphilitic posterior placoid chorioretinitis. Ophthalmology 97:1288–1297
28. Pichi F, Ciardella AP, Cunningham ET Jr et al (2014) Spectral domain optical coherence tomography findings in patients with acute syphilitic posterior placoid chorioretinopathy. Retina 34: 373–384
29. DeLuise VP, Clark SW 3rd, Smith JL (1982) Syphilitic retinal detachment and uveal effusion. Am J Ophthalmol 94:757–761
30. Jumper JM, Machemer R, Gallemore RP, Jaffe GJ (2000) Exudative retinal detachment and retinitis associated with acquired syphilitic uveitis. Retina 20:190–194
31. Diaz-Valle D, Allen DP, Sanchez AA et al (2005) Simultaneous bilateral exudative retinal detachment and peripheral necrotizing retinitis as presenting manifestations of concurrent HIV and syphilis infection. Ocul Immunol Inflamm 13:459–462
32. Williams JK, Kirsch LS, Russack V, Freeman WR (1996) Rhegmatogenous retinal detachments in HIV-positive patients with ocular syphilis. Ophthalmic Surg Lasers 27:699–705
33. Haug SJ, Takakura A, Jumper JM et al (2014) Rhegmatogenous retinal detachment in patients with acute syphilitic panuveitis. Ocul Immunol Inflamm 24:1–8 Epub ahead of print
34. CDC (2011) Discordant results from reverse sequence syphilis screening – five laboratories, United States, 2006–2010. MMWR Morb Mortal Wkly Rep 60(5):133–137

5 Lyme Disease

Pia Allegri and Carl P. Herbort Jr.

5.1 General Aspects of Lyme Disease

5.1.1 Epidemiology

Very few epidemiological data are available as yet. In the USA, incidence was estimated from 6 to 98 per 100,000 inhabitants, whereas in Europe up to 155 per 100,000 inhabitants are affected [1–3].

Many cases occur during spring and summer due to the more frequent exposure to wild areas or open-air life in these seasons [4]. Its frequency is increasing mainly due to the increase of wild animals (such as small mammals) which are the reservoir for ticks.

Age groups present two peaks of incidence: the first between 5 and 14 years of age and the second between 30 and 59 years [5–7].

P. Allegri (✉)
Ophthalmology Department, Uveitis Tertiary Referral Center, Rapallo Hospital, Via San Pietro, 8–Rapallo, Genova, Italy
e-mail: pallegri@asl4.liguria.it

C.P. Herbort Jr.
Montchoisi Ophthalmology Teaching Unit, Centre for Ophthalmic Specialised Care (COS), Rue Charles-Monnard, Lausanne, Switzerland
e-mail: carl.herb@bluewin.ch

5.1.2 Pathogenesis

Lyme borreliosis (LB) takes the name from the Connecticut town where it was first recognized in 1975 [2]. Lyme disease (LD) causative agents are flagellated, very adaptable bacteria of the *Spirochete* family called *Borrelia* of which 11 different genomic species are currently recognized, the most frequent human pathogen being *Borrelia burgdorferi*, discovered by the Swiss scientist Wilhelm Burgdofer in 1982. They can survive and multiply in animal reservoirs (small mammals, mice, voles, rodents, and birds).

The vector transmitting tick is *Ixodes ricinus* species complex [8–10].

Lyme borreliosis is known as a disorder that can mimic many other diseases, thus gaining the title of "new great imitator," syphilis (another spirochetal illness) being the "first great imitator" [11].

LD pathogenesis is as yet not well known, and symptoms are believed to be directly related to the association of infection and delayed hypersensitivity mechanism. Late or chronic disease pathogenesis is controversial because it is uncertain whether these cases represent treatment failures with persistence of *Borrelia* in the body or an autoimmune infectious-derived illness [12].

Clinical manifestations sometimes differ between the USA and Europe, the reason probably lying in relations to different *Borrelia* subtypes. In some cases, an additional tick-borne coinfection may be present 13–15].

S.-P. Chee, M. Khairallah (eds.), *Emerging Infectious Uveitis*, DOI 10.1007/978-3-319-23416-8_5

5.1.3 Systemic Manifestations

Skin *Erythema migrans* (EM) is a red macula or papula at the site of the tick bite (Fig. 5.1) enlarging in some days into a red patch. The following progressive central clearing of the lesion has a "ring-like" appearance (Fig. 5.2). EM is the first and only typical sign for a clinical diagnosis, but in any case, serological data confirmation is needed [16].

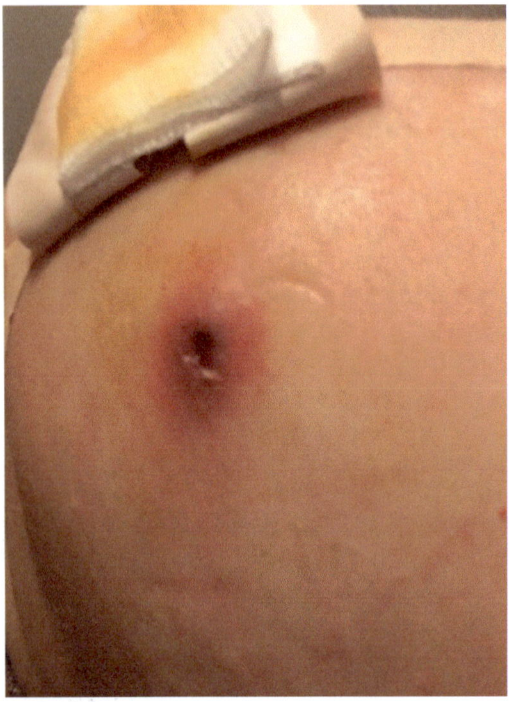

Fig. 5.1 Tick bite on a shoulder with central black spot

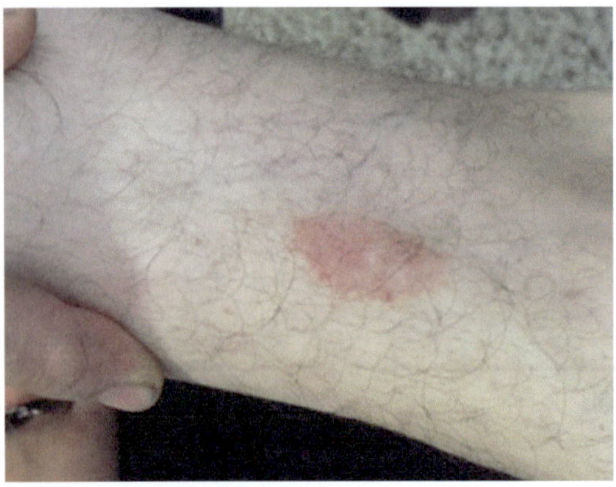

Fig. 5.2 Skin *erythema migrans*

Systemic symptoms of malaise, fatigue, headache, and joint or muscle pain are associated with EM in half of all patients [17].

Borrelial *lymphocytoma* and *acrodermatitis atrophicans* are other manifestations of LD, the skin being the most affected body tissue [18–23].

Nervous System Early neuroborreliosis symptoms are related to protracted aseptic meningitis (transient or persistent headache) and cranial nerve (mainly facial nerve with transient facial palsy) or peripheral nerve involvement (pain as a result of radiculoneuritis) [24, 25].

Cerebrospinal fluid (CSF) examination shows lymphocytic pleocytosis.

One tenth of European patients show disseminated encephalomyelitis symptoms resembling multiple sclerosis, whereas American-affected subjects more frequently report signs of encephalopathy (neuropsychiatric features) [26–33].

Heart Changing atrioventricular blocks as a result of conduction disturbances and arrhythmias are frequent but usually transient. If they persist, they can lead to chronic cardiomyopathy [34–41].

Joints Intermittent attacks of asymmetrical inflammation of one or more joints are typical of Lyme arthritis. The mono-/oligoarticular form is more frequent in American patients. 10 % of patients have long-standing arthritis with longer than 1-year duration. Increase of ESR and IgM, leukocytosis, and the presence of circulating immune complexes (CIC) and cryoglobulins are not specific serologic inflammatory features. Synovial fluid examination shows increased presence of polymorphonuclear leukocytes [42–44].

5.1.4 Stages of Lyme Disease

Untreated LD clinical manifestations occur in three stages:

1st stage corresponds to *erythema migrans* skin rash which appears 3–30 days after the tick bite.

2nd stage is related to multi-organ involvement with neurologic, cardiac, joint inflammatory involvement which appears weeks to months after the tick bite.

3rd stage is the stage of chronic arthritis and neurologic syndromes [45, 46].

5.2 Ocular Manifestations

In animal model studies, it was shown that *Borrelia* invades the eye very early after infection but may remain quiescent for a long time [47–50].

Several eye inflammatory signs and symptoms can appear, some months after the onset of systemic Lyme disease, and ocular chronic late manifestations are usually associated with other expressions of the disease such as arthritis [44].

Eyes can be affected: *primarily* as a result of the direct involvement of the ocular tissues (conjunctivitis, episcleritis, scleritis, or keratitis are the main signs, followed by anterior uveitis, retinal vasculitis, retinochoroiditis, and optic nerve inflammation, rarely panuveitis) or *secondarily* as a result of systemic manifestations (orbital myositis and palsies of cranial nerves) [50–53].

In children, symptoms and signs of intermediate uveitis are very frequent [54–60].

5.2.1 Symptoms

Severe photophobia, color vision disorders, or visual hallucinations and periocular pain are symptoms frequently reported by patients affected by corneal or neuro-ophthalmic involvement.

Blurred vision, floaters, and worsening of visual acuity are typical symptoms of vitreoretinal inflammatory involvement [60, 61].

During the flu-like illness of LD, a nonspecific follicular conjunctivitis may occur in 1/10 of patients, and it is frequently associated with lid or conjunctival chemosis and/or episcleritis. A patient – even if a child – with any of these manifestations should be questioned as to endemic area, tick bite, skin rash, and arthritis and should undergo serological testing [62, 63]. Children and people living or working in rural endemic areas are the most exposed.

5.2.2 Signs

Early-stage manifestations The first sign of ocular involvement is follicular conjunctivitis related to flu-like illness symptoms, followed some weeks later by nummular keratitis [63]. Superficial and interstitial keratitis can be localized in the limbus area and can produce corneal limbus ulcers (Fig. 5.3). Exposure keratitis related to the seventh peripheral nerve palsy is also described [64–66].

Borrelia-associated crystalline keratopathy is a rare reported manifestation [67].

Late-stage manifestations Episcleritis [68] (Fig. 5.4), iritis, anterior uveitis, vitritis (with "spider's web" aspect), intermediate uveitis, and

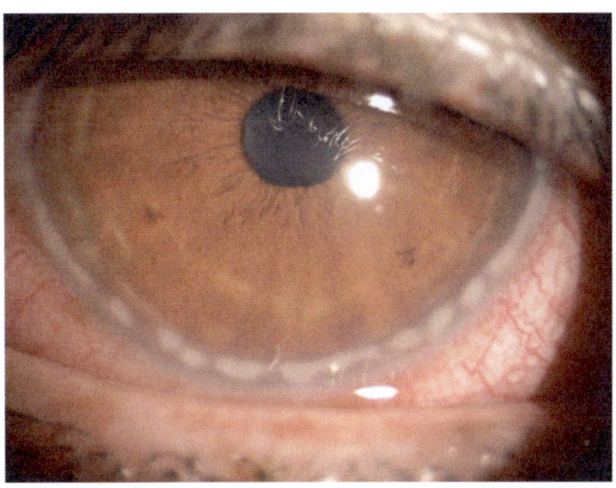

Fig. 5.3 360° borrelial limbal keratitis

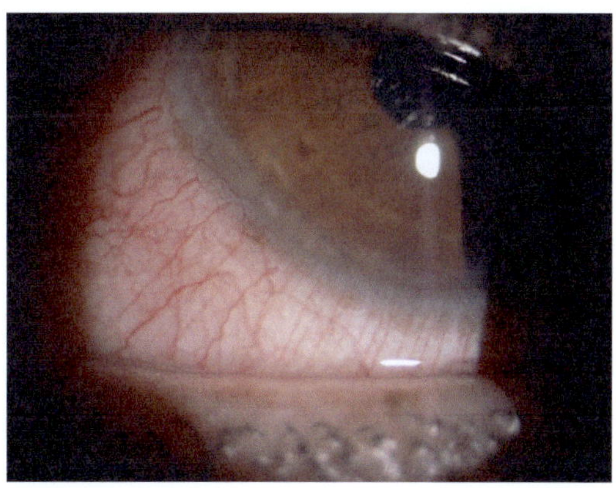

Fig. 5.4 Episcleritis and limbal keratitis

posterior involvement occur infrequently and usually appear in the late stages [69–71].

Uveitis is usually a late finding, and anterior uveitis is frequently associated with papillitis. It is characterized by granulomatous keratic precipitates or various degrees of flare and cells (Fig. 5.5); sometimes, posterior synechiae (usually in the inferior part of the iris) and iris nodules may be present [72, 73].

Intermediate uveitis typically affects children and presents as hyalitis and granulomatous vitritis ranging from traces to 4+ and spider's web aspect [60, 74] (Fig. 5.6).

Vitreous snowballs typically are yellow-white inflammatory aggregates and are found in the mid vitreous and inferior periphery. Snowbanks are exudates on the pars plana which, when present, are usually found inferiorly, but may also extend all around the retinal periphery; this finding is usually associated with severe forms of the disease and needs aggressive therapy [75] (Fig. 5.7). Retinal changes are represented by arteriolar winding and vascular sheathing mainly of peripheral veins, neovascularization, and retinal detachment [74, 75].

Posterior uveitis may show (1) a serous posterior pole detachment (if bilateral, it is difficult to distinguish from Vogt-Koyanagi-Harada syndrome) (Figs. 5.8, 5.9, 5.10, 5.11, and 5.12), (2) a peripheral multifocal choroiditis with an aspect similar to that of sarcoidosis (Figs. 5.13 and 5.14), and/or (3) cotton wool spots, typically followed

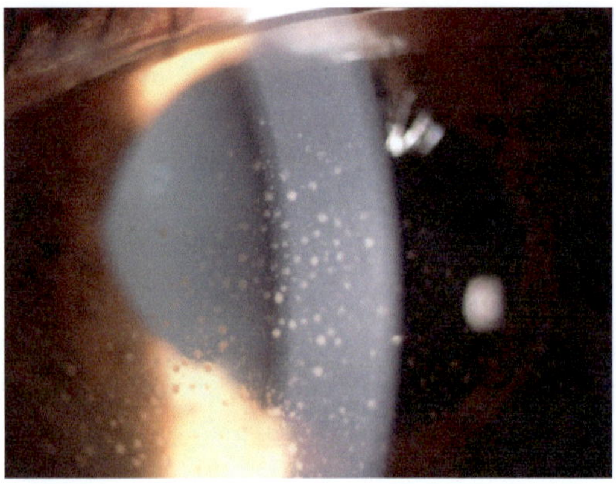

Fig. 5.5 Lyme disease typical granulomatous uveitis

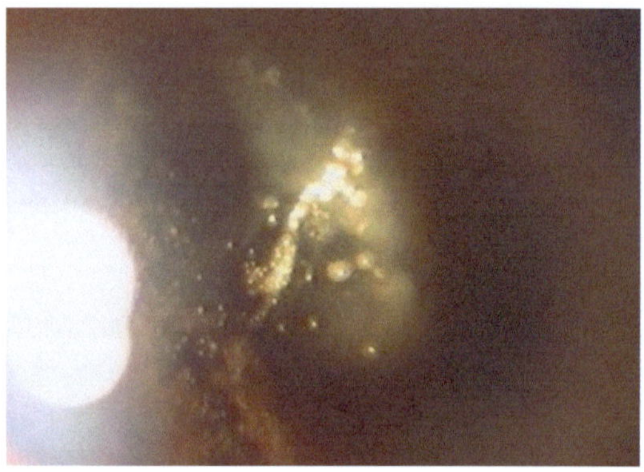

Fig. 5.6 Spider's web characteristic Lyme vitreous inflammation

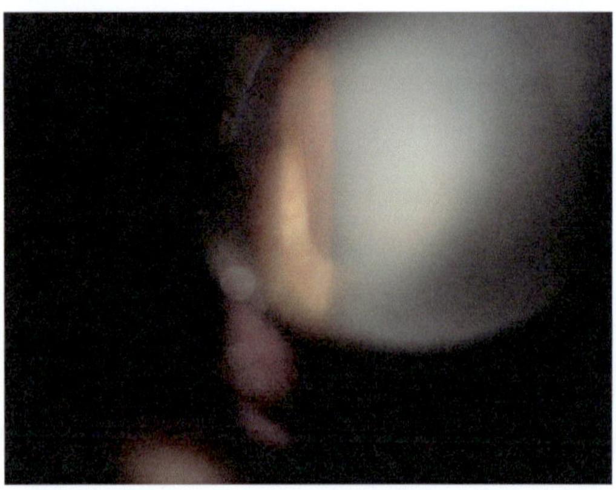

Fig. 5.7 Intermediate uveitis in a Lyme-affected child (7 years old) with a 360° snowbank at the level of the pars plana

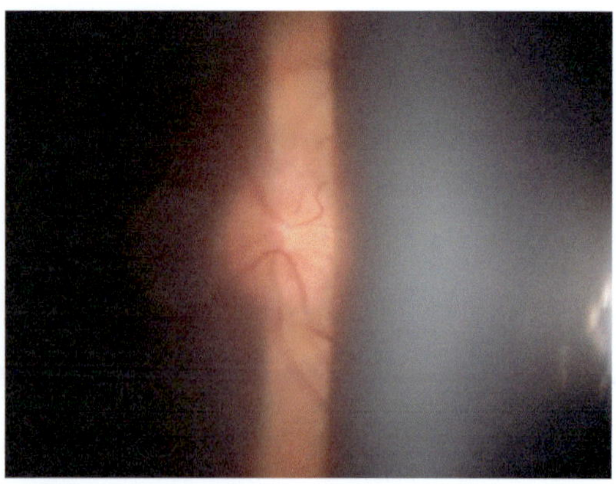

Fig. 5.8 Borrelial unilateral papillitis

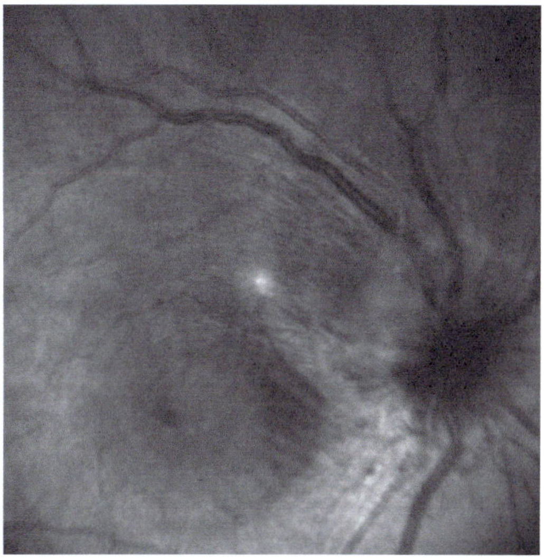

Fig. 5.9 Red-free retinography. Unilateral acute papillitis

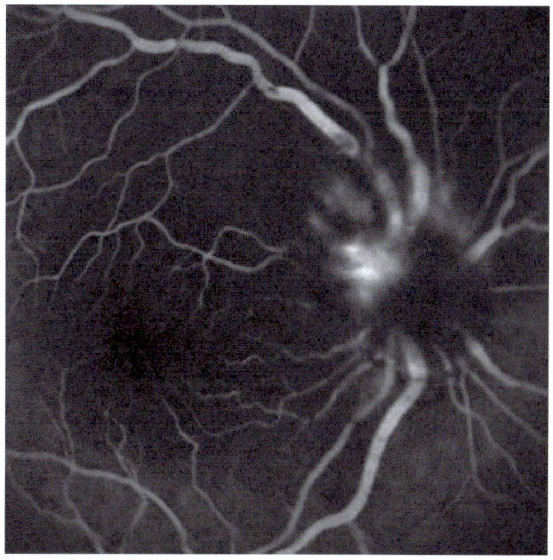

Fig. 5.10 Fluorescein angiography (FA) early angiogram of Lyme unilateral acute papillitis

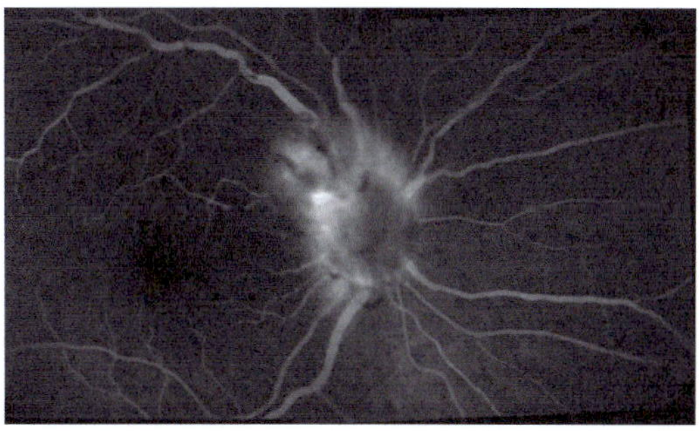

Fig. 5.11 FA late angiogram of unilateral acute papillitis showing intense leakage from the optic nerve

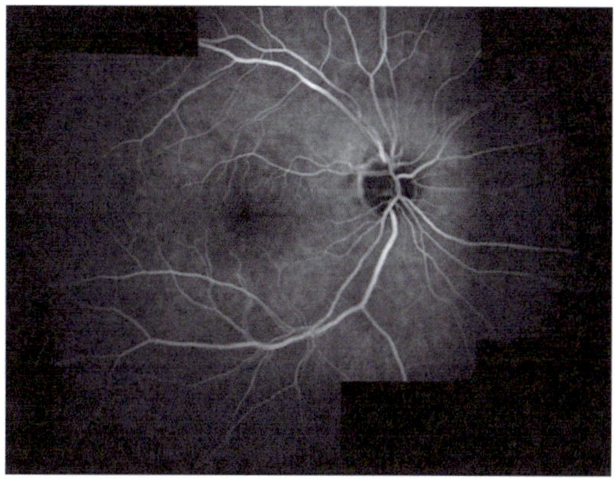

Fig. 5.12 FA shows full recovery after 1-month systemic therapy

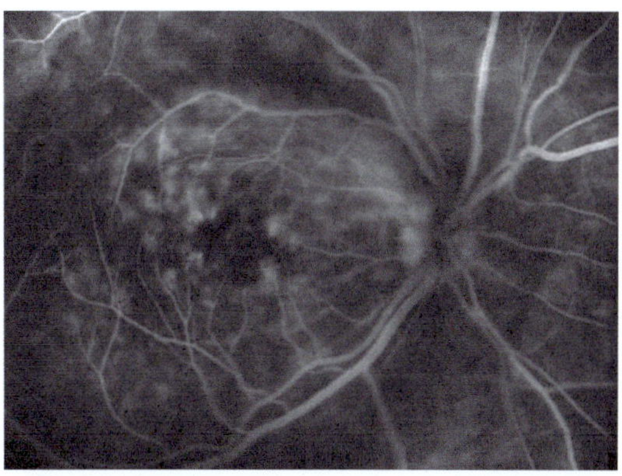

Fig. 5.13 FA shows RE posterior pole inflammatory serous detachment

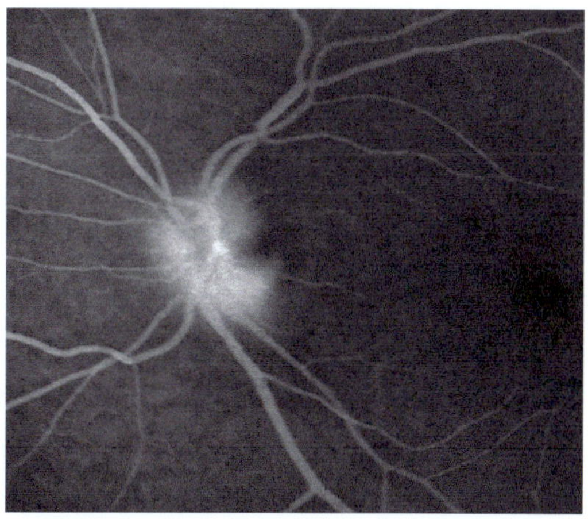

Fig. 5.14 FA shows LE papillitis (in the same patient)

by recurrent episodes of anterior uveitis [76, 77]. A distinct clinical entity related to LD posterior pole involvement is peripheral multifocal choroiditis with multiple small retinal lesions associated with intraocular inflammation [78, 79].

Retinal vasculitis is actually more frequent than in previous reports (Fig. 5.15) and involves both the arterial and the venous system and may result in vascular occlusion [61, 80, 81]. Occlusive vasculitis, mainly of retinal veins, has a similar appearance to syphilitic retinal vasculitis.

Panuveitis is rare but a blinding disease [82].

Fluorescein angiography in cases of neuroretinitis may show retinal edema and areas of cystoid patchy and peripapillary hyperfluorescence in the macula and peripapillary area; it shows also focal leakage as a sign of retinal vasculitis which can affect either veins or arteries [72, 78, 82] (Fig. 5.16 and Figs. 5.17, 5.18, 5.19, 5.20, 5.21, and 5.22).

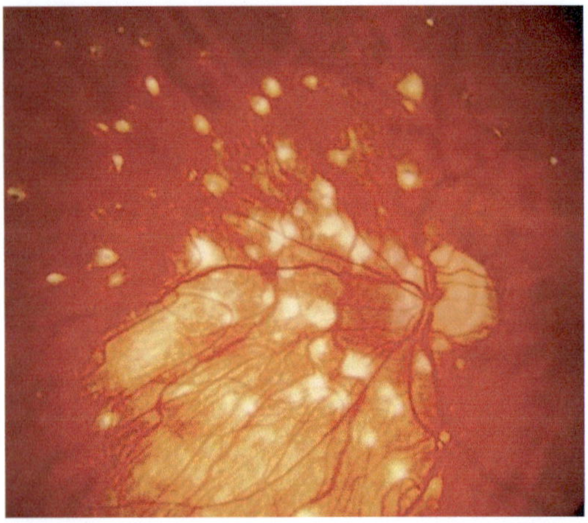

Fig. 5.15 Peripheral multifocal choroiditis resembling sarcoidosis

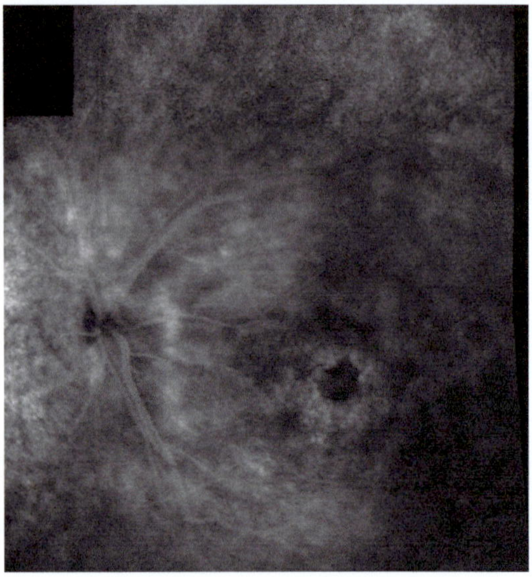

Fig. 5.16 FA late angiograms showing diffuse borrelial retinal vasculitis and cystoid macular edema

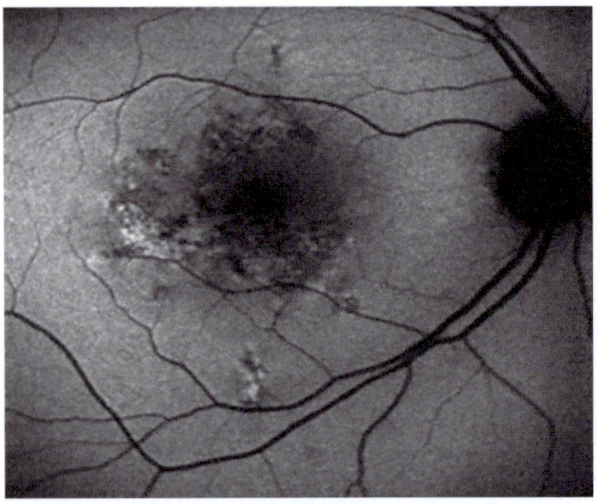

Fig. 5.17 RE autofluorescence patchy area at the posterior pole of RPE inflammation and mottled pigment

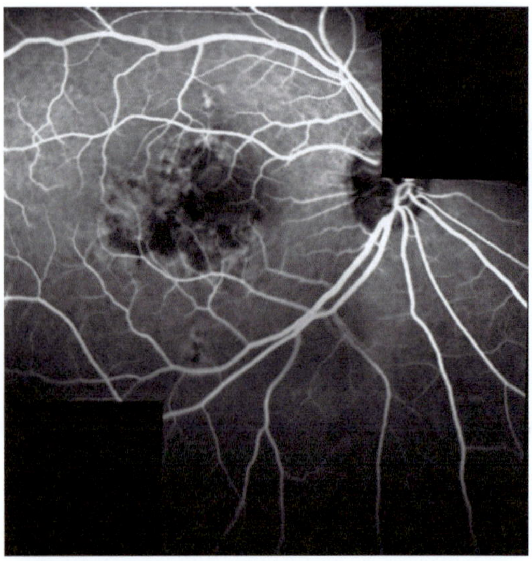

Fig. 5.18 RE FA epithelitis and mottled pigment

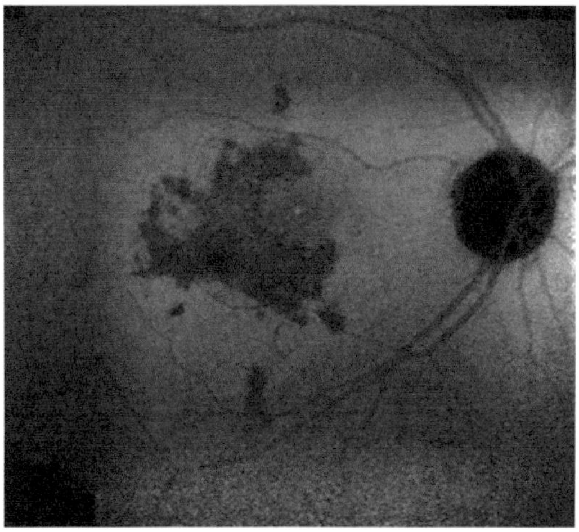

Fig. 5.19 RE ICG-A patchy area at the posterior pole of RPE inflammation or hypoperfusion

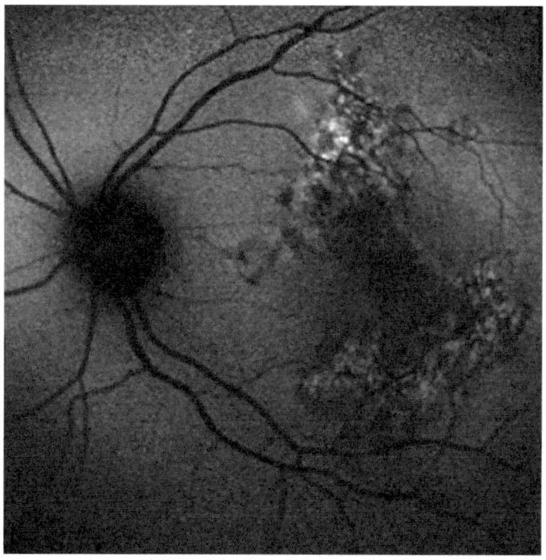

Fig. 5.20 LE autofluorescence showing the same aspect of RE

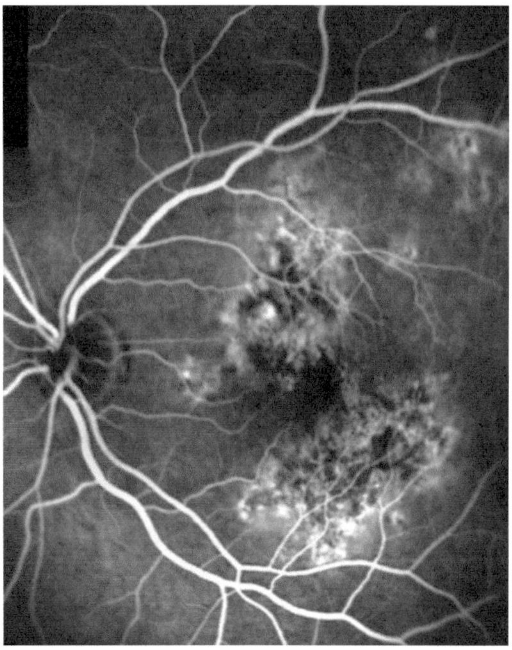

Fig. 5.21 RE FA epithelitis and mottled pigment

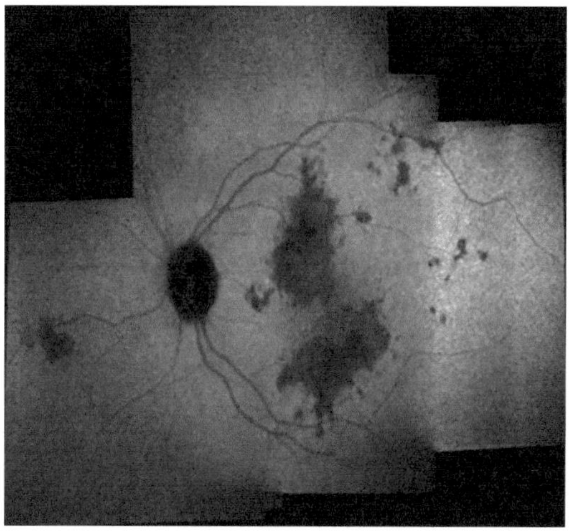

Fig. 5.22 RE ICG-A patchy area at the posterior pole of RPE inflammation or hypoperfusion

5.3 Neuro-ophthalmological Manifestations

Neuro-ophthalmological manifestations belong to the early stages of the disease probably due to the *Borrelia* blood-brain barrier passage and include multiple cranial nerve involvement (Bell's palsy), optic disc edema both inflammatory and intracranial hypertension derived, late optic atrophy, and neuroretinitis [83, 84]. Sometimes orbital involvement with myositis begins with diplopia mimicking neurological involvement [85].

Optic neuropathy is rare and is characterized by painless visual loss, unilateral or bilateral optic nerve head swelling, and ischemic optic neuropathy [86–88] (Fig. 5.23). If appearing as the first sign of the disease, it might be indistinguishable from the first neuritic attack of multiple sclerosis [89, 90].

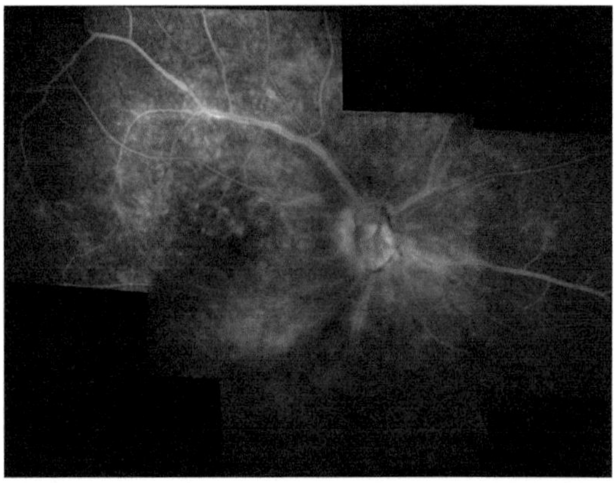

Fig. 5.23 FA showing Lyme disease typical retinal sectorial vasculitis

5.4 Diagnostic Investigations

LD diagnosis is difficult, and it is mainly based on medical history, physical examination, and Lyme infection serological tests. Ideally, detection of the causative agent via culture or PCR from infected tissues, blood, and synovial or cerebrospinal fluid should be performed; but this can only take place in specialized laboratories.

Lyme routine screening test, such as immunoblot tests (immunofluorescence, ELISA, hemagglutination), is still performed by searching specific antibodies. Hemagglutination test, although representing a helpful indication toward the correct diagnosis, cannot yield sure proof of Lyme borreliosis because of the presence of false positivity in high percentage [47, 91–94].

The 2nd International Conference on Serologic Diagnosis of LD (1995) recommended a two-step approach with at first IgM and IgG ELISA test followed by Western blotting; following these recommendations, IgM blot positive results (with two or three specific bands) are only considered if occurring during the first 4 weeks of infection; IgG blots are applicable at any time of the disease, but they must be considered positive only if they have at least five out of ten specific bands [47].

Some studies assessed the sensitivity and specificity of these major available tests and stated that both tests were sensitive means of support for the diagnosis of LD except for *erythema migrans* which is diagnostic by itself [48, 91]. Positive IgM and IgG may persist for years [93]. False-positive results are related to the cross-reactive antibodies mainly with other arthropod-derived infections and syphilis. Antibody titers to *Borrelia burgdorferi* decrease after antibiotic treatment [49, 95–98].

Borrelial DNA can be detected by PCR in the majority of the patients before antibiotic therapy [99].

Diagnostic criteria, mainly for ocular LD, are until now only exclusion criteria which are based on (1) clinical findings consistent with LD, (2) patient living in an endemic area, (3) positive serology, and (4) response to antibiotic treatment.

To obtain a correct diagnosis, the physician has to follow the indications of the Centers for Disease Control and Prevention and rely upon a specialized laboratory center provided with ELISA, Western Blot and PCR testing for Borrelia Infection. https://www.cdc.gov/lyme and LymeDisease.org.

5.5 Differential Diagnosis

Differential diagnosis is essential, mainly in cases of cross-reactions with syphilis and herpes viruses. As previously reported, LD is a multifaceted disorder which mimics a number of diseases, thus making the diagnosis very hard to be performed. Subjects suffering from retinal vasculitis and living in endemic LD areas have to be tested for Lyme Borreliosis [62].

In *early stages*, allergic conjunctivitis, keratoconus, meningioma, and CNS lymphoma have to be ruled out.

In *late stages*, paraneoplastic syndrome, multiple sclerosis, sarcoidosis, syphilis, and herpetic infections must be excluded [100].

5.6 Treatment

Prophylactic treatment within 3 days after the infected tick bite with one dose of 200 mg doxycycline was shown to be effective in preventing the disease in 87 % of subjects [23, 101, 102].

5.6.1 Prophylaxis and Vaccination

Recombinant vaccines have been developed, but they are not yet available on the market [103–108].

5.6.2 Therapeutic Protocol

There is no consensus regarding which therapeutic protocol should be used in the ocular involvement of LD. Specific and early antibiotic therapy is proven to treat all LD clinical manifestations [109, 110]. Difficulties can arise in the antibiotic choice for children or pregnant or breastfeeding women [111–119].

Specific treatment is shown in Table 5.1.

Children, pregnant, or breastfeeding women and people allergic to penicillin-derived drugs have to be given a 2–3 weeks course with erythromycin (500 mg/QID) [115–123].

Reinfections are usually treated in the same way as first infection [124].

It is proved that chronic persistent LB does not benefit from antibiotic therapies, even if prolonged for over 1 year and although intravenously administered [125–128].

Table 5.1 Suggested antibiotic treatment for ocular Lyme disease in adults and children

Adults	
Oral use	
Doxycycline	2 × 100 mg/day × 2–3 weeks
Amoxicillin	3 × 500–1000 mg/day × 2 weeks
Azithromycin	2 × 500 mg first day followed by 1 × 500 mg next 4 days (less effective than amoxicillin)
Cefuroxime axetil	2 × 500 mg/day × 2 weeks
Phenoymethylpenicillin	3 × 1–1.5 MU/day × 2 weeks
Intravenous treatment	
Ceftriaxone IV	2 g/day × 2–4 weeks or other third-generation cephalosporins (i.e., cefotaxime)
Penicillin G	20 MU/day × 2–4 weeks
Children	
Oral use	
Amoxicillin	3 × 25–50 mg/kg/day × 2 weeks
Azithromycin	2 × 20 mg/kg/day first day followed by 10 mg/kg/day next 4 days (less effective than amoxicillin)
Cefuroxime axetil	2 × 30–40 mg/kg/day × 2 weeks
Phenoymethylpenicillin	3 × 0.1–0.15 MU/Kg/day × 2 weeks
Intravenous treatment	
Ceftriaxone	50–100 mg/kg × 2–4 weeks or other third-generation cephalosporins (i.e., cefotaxime)
Penicillin G	0.25–0.5 MU/day × 2–4 weeks

When the nervous system is affected by Lyme disease, an aggressive intravenous antibiotic treatment is usually necessary although some patients develop persistent neurologic symptoms (multiple recurrences or long-lasting disease) [83].

Treatment failure is rare and sometimes bound to *Borrelia* persistence within the involved tissues with consequent tissue damage or postinfective autoimmune syndrome and sometimes associated with a late correct therapeutic approach related to a first wrong diagnosis in subjects with arthritis. Frequently, in facts, patients affected by systemic LD are misdiagnosed with many autoimmune diseases, i.e. multiple sclerosis, rheumatoid arthritis, juvenile idiopathic arthritis, fibromyalgia and erroneously treated, converting a treatable infectious disease into a chronic illness [127].

Local corticosteroids are used to treat conjunctivitis, episcleritis, scleritis, or anterior uveitis, and they are usually combined with cycloplegics.

Systemic corticosteroids are used to treat posterior severe involvement or neuro-ophthalmic complications.

Immune-suppressive treatment is usually contraindicated in this disease [55].

Core Messages

Main take-home message, following recent literature data and our personal experience, is that

- If the subject permanently or temporarily living in an endemic area was bitten by a tick and presents any ocular symptoms or signs, although with a negative serology, he/she has to be treated with a full antibiotic therapy [129–132].
- Ophthalmologists have to take into account in the differential diagnosis this emerging infectious entity, in people living or coming from endemic areas mainly, because LD first clinical presentation, at onset, can occur as an ocular manifestation.
- A careful history concerning a tick bite or erythema migrans appearance has to be conducted.
- Antibiotic treatment is beneficial at any stage of the disease, but most successful early in the course of the illness.

Conclusions

Lyme disease is a multifaceted body infection in continuous expansion; its ocular manifestations can involve many of the ocular structures and occur at any stage of the disease. An early diagnosis based on a careful history of a patient living in an endemic area and typical systemic or local (ocular) signs can prevent the evolution to a chronic difficult-to-treat condition.

References

1. Stanek G, Strie F (2003) Lyme Borreliosis. Lancet 362:1639–1647
2. Steere AC, Malawista SE, Snydman DR et al (1977) Lyme arthritis: an epidemic oligoarticular arthritis in children and adults in three connecticut communities. Arthritis Rheum 20:7–17
3. Burgdorfer W, Barbour AG, Hayes SF et al (1982) Lyme disease – a tick borne spirochetosis? Science 216:1317–1319
4. Lipsker D, Hansmann Y, Limbach F et al (2001) Disease expression of Lyme borreliosis in northeastern France. Eur J Clin Microbiol Infect Dis 20(4):225–230
5. Nahimana I, Gern L, Blanc DS et al (2004) Risk of *Borrelia burgdorferi* infection in western Switzerland following a tick bite. Eur J Clin Microbiol Infect Dis 23:603–608
6. Khairallah M, Chee SP, Rathinam SR et al (2010) Novel infectious agents causing uveitis. Int Ophthalmol 30(5):465–483
7. Rothermel H, Hedges TR 3rd, Steere AC (2001) Optic neuropathy in children with Lyme disease. Pediatrics 108(2):477–481
8. Stanek G, Wormser GP, Gray J et al (2012) Lyme borreliosis. Lancet 379:461–473
9. Stanek G, Reiter M (2011) The expanding Lyme Borrelia complex – clinical significance of genomic species? Clin Microbiol Infect 17(4):487–493
10. Stanek G (2009) Pandora's Box: pathogens in Ixodes ricinus ticks in Central Europe. Wien Klin Wochenschr 121(21–22):673–683

11. Zaidman GW (1993) The ocular manifestations of Lyme disease. Int Ophthalmol Clin 33(1):9–22
12. Steere AC, Grodzicki RL, Kornblatt AN et al (1983) The spirochetal etiology of Lyme disease. N Engl J Med 308:733–740
13. Krause PJ, Telford SR III, Spielman A et al (1996) Concurrent Lyme disease and Babesiosis: evidence for increased severity and duration of illness. JAMA 275:1657–1660
14. Swanson SJ, Neitzel D, Reed KD et al (2006) Coinfections acquired from ixodes ticks. Clin Microbiol Rev 19(4):708–727
15. Benach JL, Coleman JL, Habicht GS et al (1985) Serological evidence for simultaneous occurrences of Lyme disease and babesiosis. J Infect Dis 152(3):473–477
16. Boyé T (2007) What kind of clinical, epidemiological and biological data is essential for the diagnosis of Lyme borreliosis? Dermatological and ophthalmological courses of Lyme borreliosis. Médecine et maladies infectieuses 37:75–88
17. Malane MS, Grant-Kels JM, Feder H et al (1991) Diagnosis of Lyme disease based on dermatologic manifestations. Ann Intern Med 114:490–498
18. Müllegger R (2004) Dermatological manifestations of Lyme borreliosis. Eur J Dermatol 14:296–309
19. Strle F, Nelson JA, Ruzic-Sabljic et al. (1996) European Lyme borreliosis: 231 culture-confirmed cases involving patients with erythema migrans. Clin Infect Dis 23(1):61–65
20. Wienecke R, Zöling N, Neubert U et al (1994) Molecular Subtyping of *Borrelia burgdorferi* in erythema Migrans and Acrodermatitis Chronica Atrophicans. J Invest Dermatol 103:19–22
21. Elston DM (2010) Tick bites and skin rashes. Curr Opin Infect Dis 23(2):132–138
22. Asbrink E, Hovmark A (1990) Lyme borreliosis: aspects of tick-borne Borrelia burgdorferi infection from a dermatologic viewpoint. Semin Dermatol 9(4):277–291
23. Nadelman RB, Wormser GP (1998) Lyme borreliosis. Lancet 352:557–565
24. Créange A (2007) Clinical manifestations and epidemiological aspects leading to a diagnosis of Lyme borreliosis: neurological and psychiatric manifestations in the course of Lyme borreliosis. Med Mal Infect 37(7–8):532–539
25. Blanc F, GEBLY (2007) Neurologic and psychiatric manifestations of Lyme disease. Med Mal Infect 37(7–8):435–445
26. Pfister HW, Rupprecht TA (2006) Clinical aspects of neuroborreliosis and post-Lyme disease syndrome in adult patients. Int J Med Microbiol 296(40):11–16
27. Oksi J, Kalimo H, Marttila RJ et al (1996) Inflammatory brain changes in Lyme borreliosis. A report on three patients and review of literature. Brain 119(6):2143–2154
28. Halperin JJ (2014) Lyme disease: neurology, neurobiology, and behavior. Clin Infect Dis 58(9):1267–1272
29. Luft BJ, Steinman CR, Neimark HC et al (1992) Invasion of the central nervous system by Borrelia burgdorferi in acute disseminated infection. JAMA 267(10):1364–1367
30. Pachner AR, Steere AC (1985) The triad of neurologic manifestations of Lyme disease: meningitis, cranial neuritis, and radiculoneuritis. Neurology 35(1):47–53
31. Berglund J, Stjernberg L, Ornstein K et al (2002) 5-y Follow-up study of patients with neuroborreliosis. Scand J Infect Dis 34(6):421–425
32. Kameda G, Vieker S, Hartmann J et al (2012) Diastolic heart murmur, nocturnal back pain, and lumbar rigidity in a 7-year girl: an unusual manifestation of lyme disease in childhood. Case Rep Pediatr 976961. doi:10.1155/2012/976961 Epub 2012 Sep 29
33. Peltomaa M, Pyykkö I, Seppälä I et al (2002) Lyme borreliosis and facial paralysis – a prospective analysis of risk factors and outcome. Am J Otolaryngol 23(3):125–133
34. Dubrey SW, Mehta PA, O'Connell S (2011) Lyme disease and the heart in the UK. Br J Hosp Med (Lond) 72(11):621–625
35. Lamaison D (2007) Cardiac involvement in Lyme disease. Med Mal Infect 37(7–8):511–517
36. McAlister HF, Klementowicz PT, Andrews C et al (1989) Lyme carditis: an important cause of reversible heart block. Ann Intern Med 110(5):339–345
37. Haddad FA, Nadelman RB (2003) Lyme disease and the heart. Front Biosci 8:s769–s782
38. Bhattacharya IS, Dweck M, Francis M (2010) Lyme carditis: a reversible cause of complete atrioventricular block. J R Coll Physicians Edinb 40(2):121–122
39. Nagi KS, Joshi R, Thakur RK (1996) Cardiac manifestations of Lyme disease: a review. Can J Cardiol 12(5):503–506
40. Lo R, Menzies DJ, Archer H et al (2003) Complete heart block due to lyme carditis. J Invasive Cardio 115(6):367–369
41. Raveche ES, Schutzer SE, Fernandes H et al (2005) Evidence of Borrelia autoimmunity-induced component of Lyme carditis and arthritis. J Clin Microbiol 43(2):850–856
42. Haugeberg G, Hansen IJ, Skarpaas T et al (2014) Lyme arthritis in Southern Norway-an endemic area for Lyme borreliosis. BMC Infect Dis 14:185
43. Biesiada G, Czepiel J, Leśniak MR et al (2012) Lyme disease: review. Arch Med Sci 8(6):978–982
44. Weinstein A, Britchkov M (2002) Lyme arthritis and post-Lyme disease syndrome. Curr Opin Rheumatol 14(4):383–387
45. Lobraico J, Butler A, Petrini J et al (2014) New insights into stages of Lyme disease symptoms from a novel hospital-based registry. J Prim Care Community Health 5(4):284–287
46. Duray PH, Steere AC (1988) Clinical pathologic correlations of Lyme disease by stage. Ann NY Acad Sci 539:65–79

47. Centers for Disease Control and Prevention (1995) Recommendations for test performance and interpretation from the Second National Conference on Serologic Diagnosis of Lyme Disease. MMWR Morb Mortal Wkly Rep 44:590–591
48. Cameron DJ, Johnson LB, Maloney EL (2014) Evidence assessments and guideline recommendations in Lyme disease: the clinical management of known tick bites, erythema migrans rashes and persistent disease. Expert Rev Anti Infect Ther 12(9):1103–1135
49. Brouqui P, Bacellar F, Baranton G et al (2004) Guidelines for the diagnosis of tick-borne bacterial diseases in Europe. Clin Microbiol Infect 10(12):1108–1132
50. Carvounis PE, Mehta AP, Geist CE (2004) Orbital myositis associated with Borrelia burgdorferi (Lyme disease) infection. Ophthalmology 111(5):1023–1028
51. Guex-Crosier Y, Herbort CP (1992) Lyme disease in Switzerland: ocular involvement. Klin Monbl Augenheilk 200:545–546
52. Fatterpekar GM, Gottesman RI, Sacher M et al (2002) Orbital Lyme disease: MR imaging before and after treatment: case report. Am J Neuroradiol 23(4):657–659
53. Attia S, Khairallah M (2009) Spirocheatal uveitis: Lyme disease. In: Gupta A, Gupta V, CP H, Khairallah M (eds) Uveitis: text and imaging, vol 25, 1st edn. Jaypee, New Delhi, pp 600–605
54. Seidenberg KB, Leib ML (1990) Orbital myositis with Lyme disease. Am J Ophthalmol 109(1):13–16
55. Rothermel H, Hedges TR 3rd, Steere AC (2001) Optic neuropathy in children with Lyme disease. Pediatrics 108(2):477–478
56. Lesser RL (1995) Ocular manifestations of Lyme disease. Am J Med 98(4A):60–62
57. Bodaghi B (2007) Ocular manifestations of Lyme disease. Médecine et maladies infectieuses 37:518–522
58. Huppertz HI, Münchmeier D, Lieb W (1999) Ocular manifestations in children and adolescents with Lyme arthritis. BJO 83:1149–1152
59. Sauer A, Hansmann Y, Jaulhac B et al (2012) Ocular Lyme disease occurring during childhood: five case reports. J Fr Ophthalmol 35(1):17–22
60. Mattéi J, Pélissier P, Richard O et al (2011) Uveités de Lyme: à propos de 2 observations. Archives de Pédiatrie 18:49–53
61. Onyett H (2014) Lyme disease in Canada: Focus on children. Paediatr Child Health 19(7):379–388
62. Heinz C, Schoonbrood S, Heiligenhaus A (2014) Intermediate uveitis in children and young adults: differences in clinical course, associations and visual outcome. Br J Ophthalmol 98(8):1107–1111
63. Zaidman GW, Roy H (2014) Ophthalmic aspects of Lyme disease. Overview of Lyme disease. http://emedicine.medscape.com/article/1202521-overview. Accessed 16 Jan 2015
64. Mikkilä HO, Seppälä IJ, Viljanen MK et al (2000) The expanding clinical spectrum of ocular Lyme Borreliosis. Ophthalmology 107(3):581–587
65. Mombaerts IM, Maudgal PC, Knockaert DC (1991) Bilateral follicular conjunctivitis as a manifestation of Lyme disease. Am J Ophthalmol 112(1):96–97
66. Dietrich T, Geissdörfer W, Schlötzer-Schrehardt U et al (2008) Borrelia-associated crystalline keratopathy with intracorneal detection of Borrelia garinii by electron microscopy and PCT. Cornea 27(4):498–500
67. Orlin SE, Lauffer JL (1989) Lyme disease keratitis. Am J Ophthalmol 107(6):678–680
68. Baum J, Barza M, Weinstein P et al (1988) Bilateral keratitis as a manifestation of Lyme disease. Am J Ophthalmol 105(1):75–77
69. Kornmehl EW, Lesser RL, Jaros P et al (1989) Bilateral keratitis in Lyme disease. Ophthalmology 96(8):1194–1197
70. Zaidman GW (1990) Episcleritis and symblepharon associated with Lyme keratitis. Am J Ophthalmol 109(4):487–488
71. Krist D, Wenkel H (2002) Posterior scleritis associated with Borrelia burgdorferi (Lyme disease) infection. Ophthalmology 109(1):143–145
72. Boutros A, Rahn E, Nauheim R (1990) Iritis and papillitis as a primary presentation of Lyme disease. Ann Ophthalmol 22:24–25
73. Howlett JM, Booth AP (2012) Ocular inflammation as a manifestation of Lyme borreliosis. BMJ 345:e4721. doi:10.1136/bmj.e4721
74. Karma A, Seppälä I, Mikkilä H et al (1995) Diagnosis and clinical characteristics of ocular Lyme borreliosis. Am J Ophthalmol 119(2):127–135
75. Rothova A, Suttorp-Van Schulten MS (1995) Diagnosis and clinical characteristics of ocular Lyme borreliosis. Am J Ophthalmol 120(2):263–264
76. Rothova A, Kuiper H, Spanjaard L et al (1991) Spider web vitritis in Lyme borreliosis. Lancet 337(8739):490–491
77. Kuiper H, Koelman JH, Hager MJ (1989) Vitreous clouding associated with Lyme borreliosis. Am J Ophthalmol 108(4):453–454
78. Whitcup SM (2004) Lyme disease. In: Nussenblatt RB, Whitcup SM (eds) Uveitis. Fundamentals and clinical practice, 3rd edn. Mosby, Philadelphia, pp 170–174
79. Klaeger AJ, Herbort CP (2010) Cotton wool spots as possible indicators of retinal vascular pathology in ocular Lyme borreliosis. Int Ophthalmol 30:599–602
80. Lardenoye CW, Van der Lelij A, de Loos WS et al (1997) Peripheral multifocal chorioretinitis: a distinct clinical entity? Ophthalmology 104(11):1820–1826
81. Suttorp-Schulten MS, Luyendijk L, van Dam AP et al (1993) Birdshot chorioretinopathy and Lyme borreliosis. Am J Ophthalmol 115(2):149–153
82. Lightman DA, Brod RD (1991) Branch retinal artery occlusion associated with Lyme disease. Arch Ophthalmol 109(9):1198–1199
83. Lang GE, Schönherr U, Naumann GO (1991) Retinal vasculitis with proliferative retinopathy in a patient with evidence of Borrelia burgdorferi infection. Am J Ophthalmol 111(2):243–244

84. Kadz B, Putteman A, Verougstraete C et al (2005) Lyme disease from an ophthalmological point of view. J Fr Ophtalmol 28(2):218–223
85. Sorensen RW (1989) Lyme disease: neurologic manifestations. Compr Ther 15(7):16–22
86. Rupprecht TA, Koedel U, Fingerle V et al (2008) The pathogenesis of lyme neuroborreliosis: from infection to inflammation. Mol Med 14(3–4):205–212
87. Burkhard C, Gleichmann M, Wilhelm H (2001) Optic nerve lesion following neuroborreliosis: a case report. Eur J Ophthalmol 11(2):203–206
88. Pachner AR (2005) Defining the spectrum of Lyme disease: a difficult proposition. J Neuro Ophthalmol 25(2):67–68
89. Borchers AT, Keen CL, Huntley AC, Gershwin ME (2015) Lyme disease: A rigorous review of diagnostic criteria and treatment. J Autoimmun 57C:82–115
90. Träisk F, Lindquist L (2012) Optic nerve involvement in Lyme disease. Curr Opin Ophthalmol 23(6):485–490
91. Rothermel H, Hedges TR, Steere AC (2001) Optic neuropathy in children with Lyme disease. Pediatrics 108(2):477–481
92. Burkhard C, Gleichmann M, Wilhelm H (2001) Optic nerve lesion following neuroborreliosis: a case report. Eur J Ophthalmol 11(2):203–206
93. Jacobson DM (2003) Lyme disease and optic neuritis: long-term follow-up of seropositive patients. Neurology 60(5):881–882
94. Kalish RA, McHugh G, Granquist J et al (2001) Persistence of IgM or IgG antibody responses to Borrelia burgdorferi 10–20 years after active Lyme disease. Clin Infect Dis 33:780–785
95. Mogilyansky E, Loa CC, Adelson ME et al (2004) Comparison of Western immunoblotting and the C6 Lyme antibody test for laboratory detection of Lyme disease. Clin Diagn Lab Immunol 11:924–929
96. Steere AC, McHugh G, Daml N et al (2008) Prospective study of serologic tests for Lyme disease. Clin Infect Dis 47(2):188–195
97. Aguero-Rosenfeld ME, Wormser GP (2015) Lyme disease: diagnostic issues and controversies. Expert Rev Mol Diagn 15(1):1–4
98. Wilske B (2002) Microbiological diagnosis in Lyme borreliosis. Int J Med Microbiol 291(33):114–119
99. Liang FT, Steere AC, Marques AR et al (1999) Sensitive and specific serodiagnosis of Lyme disease by enzyme-linked immunosorbent assay with a peptide based on an immunodominant conserved region of Borrelia burgdorferi vlsE. J Clin Microbiol 37(12):3990–3996
100. Branda JA, Aguero-Rosenfeld ME, Ferraro MJ et al (2010) 2-tiered antibody testing for early and late Lyme disease using only an immunoglobulin G blot with the addition of a VlsE band as the second-tier test. Clin Infect Dis 50(1):20–26
101. Dessau RB, Fingerle V, Gray J et al (2014) The lymphocyte transformation test for the diagnosis of Lyme borreliosis has currently not been shown to be clinically useful. Clin Microbiol Infect 20(10):786–787
102. Halpern MD, Molins CR, Schriefer M et al (2014) Simple objective detection of human Lyme disease infection using immuno-PCR and a single recombinant hybrid antigen. Clin Vaccine Immunol 21(8):1094–1105
103. Guex-Crosier Y, Herbort CP (1994) Recurrent uveitis, cystoid macular edema and pericarditis in Lyme disease. Ocul Immunol Inflamm 2:11–13
104. Shapiro ED (2015) Repeat or persistent Lyme disease: persistence, recrudescence or reinfection with Borrelia burgdorferi? F1000Prime Rep 5:7–11
105. Leenders AC (2001) Single-dose doxycycline for the prevention of Lyme disease. N Engl J Med 345(18):1349
106. Bellovin SM (2001) Single-dose doxycycline for the prevention of Lyme disease. N Engl J Med 345(18):1349–1350
107. Hunfeld KP, Brade V (2006) Antimicrobial susceptibility of Borrelia burgdorferi sensu lato: what we know, what we don't know, and what we need to know. Wien Klin Wochenschr 118(21–22):659–668
108. Meurice F, Parenti D, Fu D et al (1997) Specific issues in the design and implementation of an efficacy trial for a Lyme disease vaccine. Clin Infect Dis 25(1):S71–S75
109. de Silva AM, Telford SR 3rd, Brunet LR et al (1996) Borrelia burgdorferi OspA is an arthropod-specific transmission-blocking Lyme disease vaccine. J Exp Med 183(1):271–275
110. Van Hoecke C, Fu D, De Grave D et al (1998) Clinical and immunological assessment of a candidate Lyme disease vaccine in healthy adults: antibody persistence and effect of a booster dose at month 12. Vaccine 16(17):1688–1692
111. Meltzer MI, Dennis DT, Orloski KA (1999) The cost effectiveness of vaccinating against Lyme disease. Emerg Infect Dis 5(3):321–328
112. Earnhart CG, Marconi RT (2007) An octavalent Lyme disease vaccine induces antibodies that recognize all incorporated OspC type-specific sequences. Hum Vaccin 3(6):281–289
113. Lathrop SL, Ball R, Haber P et al (2002) Adverse event reports following vaccination for Lyme disease: December 1998–July 2000. Vaccine 20(11–12):1603–1608
114. Stanek G, Strle F (2009) Lyme borreliosis: a European perspective on diagnosis and clinical management. Curr Opin Infect Dis 22(5):450–454
115. Strle F, Maraspin V, Lotric-Furlan S et al (1996) Azithromycin and doxycycline for treatment of Borrelia culture-positive erythema migrans. Infection 24(1):64–68
116. Winward KE, Smith JL, Culbertson WW et al (1989) Ocular Lyme borreliosis. Am J Ophthalmol 108(6):651–657
117. Steere AC, Gross D, Meyer AL et al (2001) Autoimmune mechanisms in antibiotic treatment-resistant lyme arthritis. J Autoimmun 16(3):263–268
118. Shapiro ED (2014) Clinical practice. Lyme disease. N Engl J Med 370(18):1724–1731

119. Karma A, Mikkilä H (1996) Ocular manifestations and treatment of Lyme disease. Curr Opin Ophthalmol 7(3):7–12
120. Maraspin V, Ružić-Sabljić E, Pleterski-Rigler D et al (2011) Pregnant women with erythema migrans and isolation of borreliae from blood: course and outcome after treatment with ceftriaxone. Diagn Microbiol Infect Dis 71(4):446–448
121. Smith GN, Gemmill I, Moore KM (2012) Management of tick bites and lyme disease during pregnancy. J Obstet Gynaecol Can 34(11):1087–1091
122. Liu TS, Crow RW (2013) Bilateral idiopathic optic neuritis in pregnancy. Semin Ophthalmol 28(1):46–49
123. Dotters-Katz SK, Kuller J, Heine RP (2013) Arthropod-borne bacterial diseases in pregnancy. Obstet Gynecol Surv 68(9):635–649
124. Strobino BA, Williams CL, Abid S et al (1993) Lyme disease and pregnancy outcome: a prospective study of two thousand prenatal patients. Am J Obstet Gynecol 169(2):367–374
125. Walsh CA, Mayer EW, Baxi LV (2007) Lyme disease in pregnancy: case report and review of the literature. Obstet Gynecol Surv 62(1):41–50
126. Suttorp-Schulten MS, Kuiper H, Kijlstra A et al (1993) Long-term effects of ceftriaxone treatment on intraocular Lyme borreliosis. Am J Ophthalmol 116(5):571–575
127. Wormser GP, Stanek G, Strle F et al (2005) Advances in the treatment and prevention of Lyme borreliosis. Wien Klin Wochenschr 117(11–12):381–384
128. Arnez M, Pleterski-Rigler D, Luznik-Bufon T et al (2002) Children with multiple erythema migrans: are there any pre-treatment symptoms and/or signs suggestive for central nervous system involvement? Wien Klin Wochenschr 114(13–14):524–529
129. Arnez M, Pleterski-Rigler D, Luznik-Bufon T et al (2002) Solitary erythema migrans in children: comparison of treatment with azithromycin and phenoxymethylpenicillin. Wien Klin Wochenschr 114(13–14):498–500
130. Breier F, Kunz G, Klade H et al (1996) Erythema migrans: three weeks treatment for prevention of late Lyme borreliosis. Infection 24(1):69–72
131. Lipsker D, Antoni-Bach N, Hansmann Y et al (2002) Long-term prognosis of patients treated for erythema migrans in France. Br J Dermatol 146(5):872–876
132. Strominger MB, Slamovits TL, Herskovitz S et al (1994) Transient worsening of optic neuropathy as a sequela of the Jarisch-Herxheimer reaction in the treatment of Lyme disease. J Neuroophthalmol 14(2):77–80

6 Cat-Scratch Disease

Andre L. Curi and Rim Kahloun

6.1 Introduction

Cat-scratch disease (CSD) is a worldwide distributed self-limited, systemic illness caused by the gram-negative bacillus, *Bartonella henselae*. An array of ocular manifestations, dominated by neuroretinitis and retinitis, has been described in association with CSD [1–3].

6.2 Epidemiology

CSD is a worldwide zoonotic infection. The prevalence of CSD disease in the USA is approximately 22,000 cases per year [4]. In the Netherlands the incidence of CSD was estimated to be 2000 cases per year [2]. The seroprevalence of *Bartonella henselae* in Brazil is approximately 10 % [5].

Children and young adults are reported to be at increased risk for systemic *B. henselae* infection, which appears to have a seasonal pattern, occurring predominantly in the fall and winter [3]. HIV positivity may be a risk factor for *Bartonella* infection [2].

A.L. Curi (✉)
Department of Ophthalmology, National Institute of Infectious Disease, INI - Fiocruz, Rio de Janeiro, Brazil
e-mail: andre.curi@ipec.fiocruz.br

R. Kahloun
Department of Ophthalmology, Faculty of Medicine, Fattouma Bourguiba University Hospital, University of Monastir, Monastir, Tunisia

Ocular involvement occurs in 5–10 % of patients with cat-scratch disease [6].

6.3 Pathophysiology

The principal mode of transmission is through a cat scratch or bite. It has been shown that approximately 30 % of the patients denied any bite or scratch, but almost all of the patients have history of close contact with cats [7]. The cat flea may participate in the transmission of the bacteria among cats and from cat to human.

CSD can present different immunological responses causing inflammatory response with histiocytes, lymphocytes, giant cells, and necrosis. In immunosuppressed patients, it tends to present a vasoproliferative response. A close relationship between the bacteria and vascular endothelium has been demonstrated in experimental models [8, 9].

The eye can be involved either with the primary inoculation complex, resulting in Parinaud's oculoglandular syndrome, or by hematogenous spread, leading to an array of ocular and neuro-ophthalmic manifestations.

6.4 Clinical Features

6.4.1 Systemic Disease

The systemic condition is characterized by fever associated with regional lymphadenopathy, gen-

S.-P. Chee, M. Khairallah (eds.), *Emerging Infectious Uveitis*, DOI 10.1007/978-3-319-23416-8_6

erally near the site of the scratch. Patients present a pustule or papule of three to ten days after inoculation. The systemic condition is subject to differential diagnosis against febrile diseases such as infectious mononucleosis and systemic toxoplasmosis. Roughly 70 % of patients with ocular diseases will present some kind of symptoms [7].

More serious systemic cases can occur, particularly within the immunocompromised population, including endocarditis, encephalitis, aseptic meningitis, pneumonia, osteomyelitis, and hepatosplenic disease [3].

6.4.2 Ocular Disease

The ocular symptoms are extremely variable. The disease was originally described as a granulomatous conjunctivitis associated with necrosis and preauricular lymphadenopathy called Parinaud's oculoglandular syndrome [10]. CSD has been occasionally associated with conjunctival involvement simulating rhabdomyosarcoma [11], orbital abscess [12], disciform keratitis [13, 14], peripheral ulcerative keratitis [15], and anterior uveitis [16, 17].

The classic manifestation of intraocular CSD is neuroretinitis. In a recent case series, CSD has been reported in 30.8 % of neuroretinitis cases [18]. The ocular condition is usually unilateral, but bilateral cases have also been reported. Visual symptoms usually follow the inoculation by approximately 4 weeks and the systemic symptoms by 2 to 3 weeks. The most common complaint is decreased vision, with visual acuity ranging from 20/20 to light perception. A relative afferent pupillary defect, dyschromatopsia, and a visual field defect are usually seen. Mild anterior chamber and vitreous inflammation is also common [19]. Fundus examination typically shows optic disc edema associated with exudates in the form of a partial or complete macular star (Fig. 6.1a). The optic disc edema occurs approximately 1 week prior to the development of stellate maculopathy, which therefore may be absent at the time of initial presentation. The optic nerve involvement leads to peripapillary retinal thickening and, frequently, an exudative retinal detachment [20]. Intraretinal hemorrhages or telangiectatic vessels may be seen [21]. Fluorescein angiography shows leakage from the optic disc with no evidence of capillary abnormality in the macular area [22] (Fig. 6.1b). Indocyanine green angiography also may show optic disc hyperfluorescence. Optical coherence tomography may be helpful in detecting exudative retinal detachment [23] (Fig. 6.1c).

Neuroretinitis usually has a self-limited course, with most patients recovering good visual acuity over a period of several weeks [19]. The macular star usually resolves in approximately 2 to 3 months, but it may be present for up to 1 year. A few patients may be left with mild pallor of the optic disc [24]. Retinal pigment epithelium changes also may develop after a resolution of a prominent macular star.

CSD may occasionally present with a large inflammatory mass or exudate of the optic nerve head [25].

Unifocal or multifocal white areas of inner retinitis or chorioretinitis, of 50–100 microns, typically juxtavascular in location, may accompany neuroretinitis or occur in the absence of obvious optic disc involvement [7, 19, 26–28] (Fig. 6.2). Such retinal lesions were found to be more common than neuroretinitis by some authors [27] (Fig. 6.3).

Branch retinal arteriolar occlusion [24, 26, 27, 29, 30] may be associated with an area of focal retinitis. A case of central retinal artery and vein occlusion has been reported [31].

Less common chorioretinal manifestations of CSD include large inflammatory retinal mass in the posterior pole [25], subretinal mass with or without associated abnormal vascular network [32], intermediate uveitis with retinal vasculitis[33], unilateral panuveitis with clinical and fluorescein angiographic features simulating Vogt-Koyanagi-Harada disease [34], isolated serous macular detachment [35], serous macular detachment simulating central serous chorioretinopathy [36], macular hole [37, 38], and vitreous hemorrhage [39].

Due to the relationship between *Bartonella* and vascular endothelium, chorioretinal vasoproliferative lesions are observed, which are more

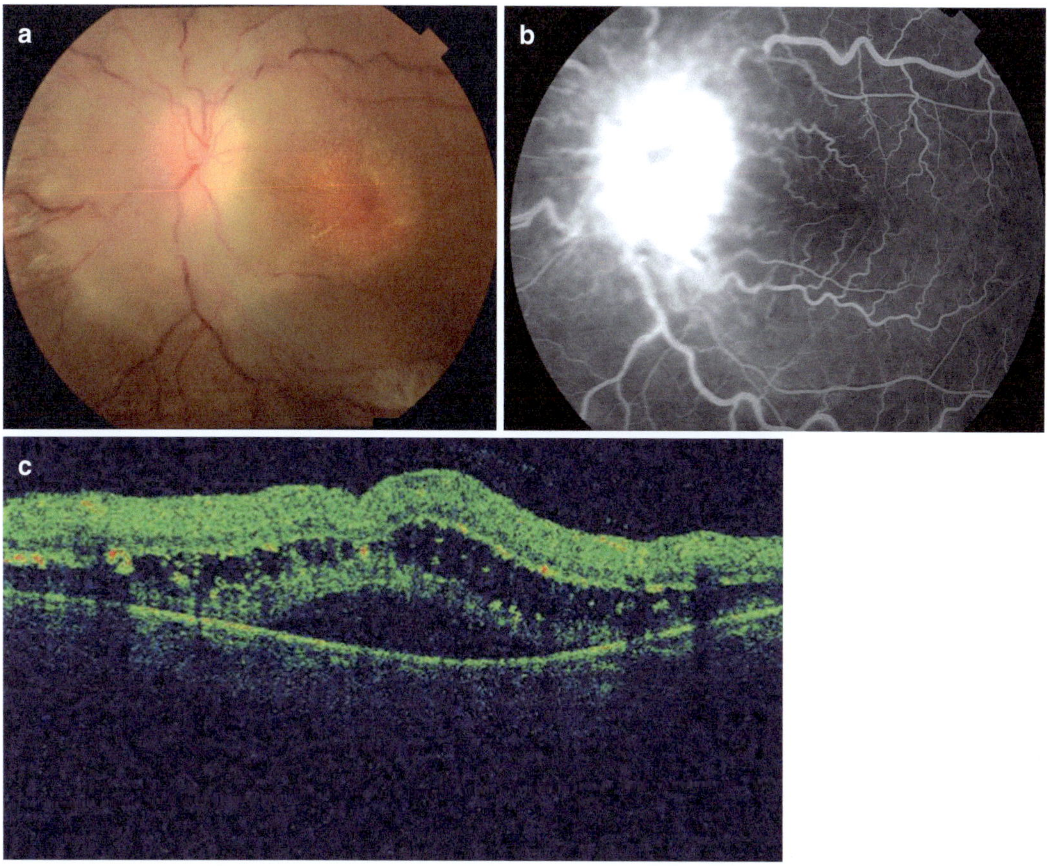

Fig. 6.1 (**a**) Fundus photograph of the left eye of a patient with cat-scratch disease shows optic disc edema with telangiectasis, a complete macular star, and a peripapillary serous retinal detachment. (**b**) Late-phase fluorescein angiogram shows optic disc hyperfluorescence with a normal macula. (**c**) Spectral domain optical coherence tomography shows macular serous detachment with cystoid macular edema

commonly found in immunosuppressed patients despite not being exclusive [31, 32].

6.5 Diagnosis

The diagnosis of CSD is based on epidemiological data, medical history, serology, polymerase chain reaction, and pathology. Despite the use of various data in diagnosing the disease, in practice it is the positive blood test that is considered as the decisive diagnostic information.

The epidemiological history is fundamental when diagnosis is suspected; therefore close contact with domestic animals is of prime significance. In a study conducted with patients with intraocular lesions of CSD, 100 % of the patients confirmed contact with a cat and roughly 65 % remembered having been scratched. In relation to the medical history, in a recent study, it was found that approximately 65 % of the patients with the ocular disease manifested some kind of systemic symptoms, findings also reported by Curi et al. [7].

Serology is the gold standard for diagnosis, with IgG for *B. henselae* positive indicating previous contact with the bacteria. In a population study, approximately 10 % of healthy individuals tested positive for *Bartonella* (IgG) [40, 41]. Recent or acute infection is diagnosed by IgG titers of greater than 1:256.

Polymerase chain reaction presents high specificity, but low sensitivity for cases of ocular disease [42, 43].

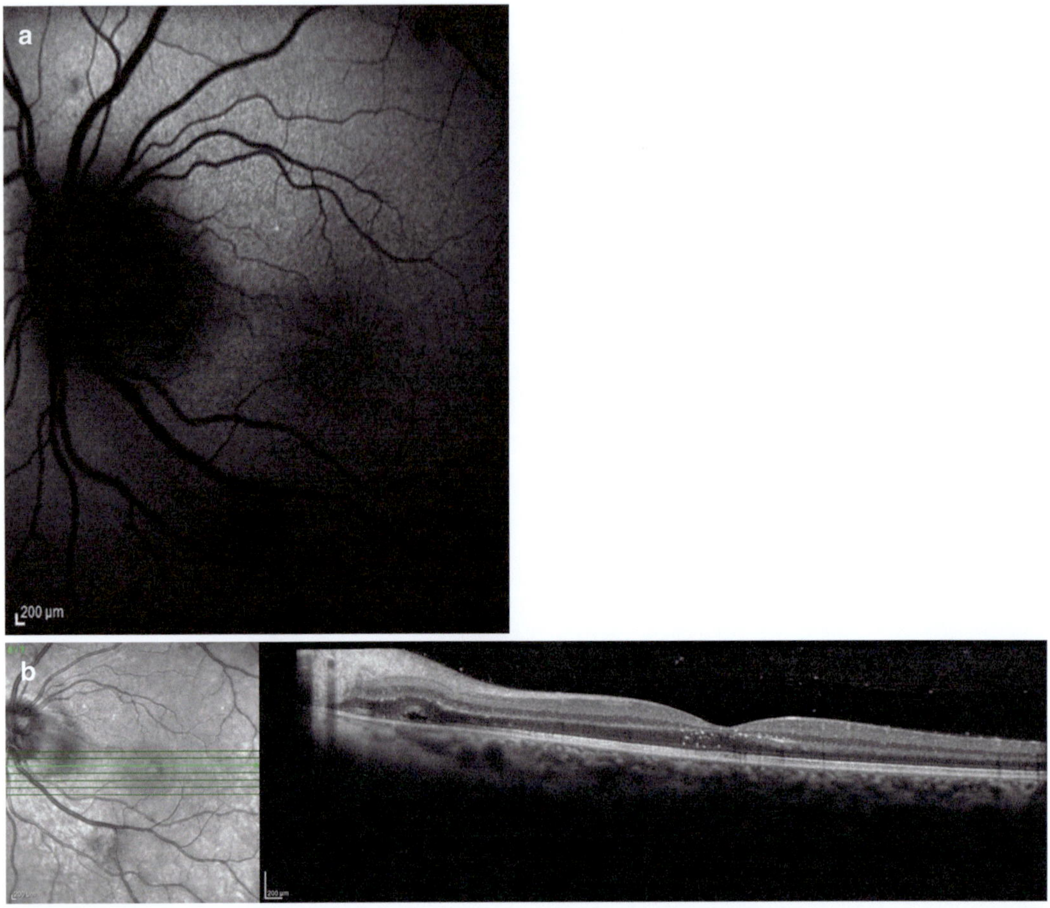

Fig. 6.2 (**a**) Fundus autofluorescence of the left eye of a patient with neuroretinitis related to cat-scratch disease shows peripapillary hypoautofluorescence and hypoautofluorescent striae in the macular area. (**b**) Optical coherence tomography shows peripapillary serous detachment with intraretinal macular hyperreflective dots related to macular hard exudates

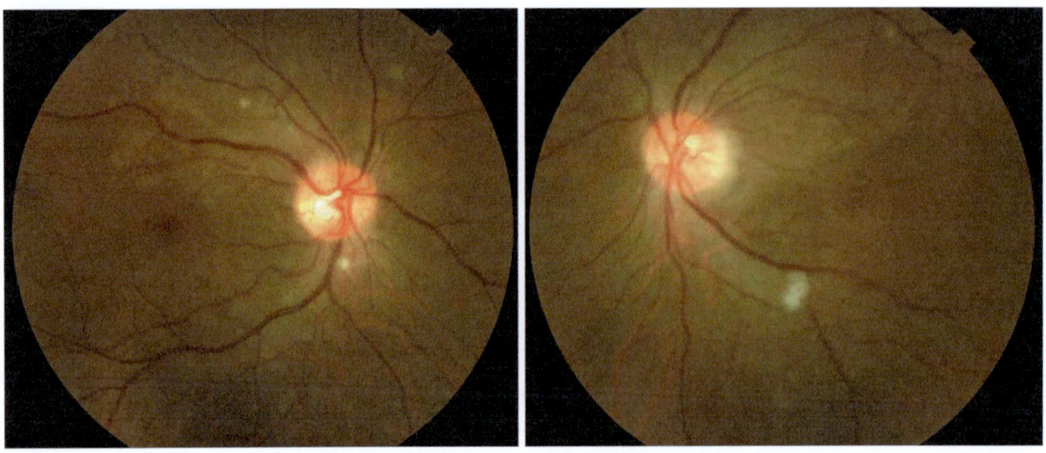

Fig. 6.3 Fundus photographs of a patient with cat-scratch disease show bilateral small retinal infiltrates without associated neuroretinitis

6.6 Differential Diagnosis

Differential diagnosis of retinitis and chorioretinitis associated with CSD includes toxoplasmosis retinochoroiditis, syphilis, rickettsiosis, Lyme disease, chikungunya, and Behçet disease.

Causes of neuroretinitis such as tuberculosis, sarcoidosis, toxoplasmosis, syphilis, varicella, herpes simplex, diffuse unilateral subacute neuroretinitis (DUSN), leptospirosis, and recurrent idiopathic neuroretinitis should always be considered as differential diagnosis of *Bartonella* neuroretinitis. Noninflammatory conditions that cause optic disc edema and macular star are also included in the differential diagnosis including diabetes, systemic hypertension, branch retinal vein occlusion, and anterior ischemic optic neuropathy [44].

The differential diagnosis of Parinaud's oculoglandular syndrome includes tularemia, syphilis, tuberculosis, sporotrichosis, lymphogranuloma venereum, pasteurellosis, Lyme disease, listerellosis, adenoviral infection, herpes simplex type 1 infection, mononucleosis, and rickettsioses [45, 46].

6.7 Management

Treatment of the ocular disease is still a subject of debate. Older works described CSD as a self-limited condition, but some benefits of antibiotic use have been observed.

Curi et al. found a significant number of patients with accentuated loss of visual acuity in presentation who showed improvement after antibiotic treatment.

Currently antibiotics are recommended to treat the secondary ocular symptoms of CSD: doxycycline100mg every 12 hours for 1 month. Other antibiotics have also been used with good response such as ciprofloxacin, azithromycin, rifampin, and trimethoprim-sulfamethoxazole [47]. In case of severe infection, doxycycline may be given intravenously or used in combination with rifampin, 300 mg orally twice daily. Children with CSD may be treated with azithromycin.

Among immunocompromised individuals, treatment is extended for 4 months [3]. In HIV seropositive patients, this timeframe is unknown, as relapse is possible after suspension of the antibiotic treatment. The CD4 count might be an important factor in the decision-making as regards the suspension of medication. Therefore, it is suggested that medication only be suspended when the CD4 count has increased, as occurs in other opportunist ocular diseases, such as cytomegalovirus retinitis and toxoplasmic retinochoroiditis.

Paradoxical response to treatment has been reported in ocular bartonellosis [48].

The role of systemic steroids in CSD is unknown and still debatable [49].

Prevention of CSD includes wash and disinfection of any wounds immediately after a cat scratch or bite and avoids contact with stray felines.

6.8 Prognosis

The prognosis of systemic disease is usually good in immunocompetent patients. In immunocompromised patients, even complications, prognosis is good provided appropriate and timely treatment [1, 3].

The prognosis of ocular disease is usually good with complete recovery of visual acuity in most patients. Few patients keep complaining of visual field loss for many months. In patients with neuroretinitis, macular exudates may take months to resolve. A few patients may be left with optic disc pallor or atrophy [24].

Core Messages

- Cat-scratch disease is a self-limited systemic illness caused by a gram-negative bacillus, *Bartonella henselae*, and characterized by regional lymphadenopathy with associated febrile illness.
- Neuroretinitis is the most typical ocular manifestation of cat-scratch disease, but

an array of other ocular changes may occur including Parinaud's oculoglandular syndrome, retinitis, chorioretinitis, and vascular changes.

- Diagnosis is primarily based on clinical findings and confirmed by serology and/or PCR.
- Treatment is based on antibiotics, mainly doxycycline.

References

1. Roe RH, Michael Jumper J, Fu AD, Johnson RN, Richard McDonald H, Cunningham ET (2008) Ocular bartonella infections. Int Ophthalmol Clin 48(3):93–105
2. Biancardi AL, Curi AL (2014) Cat scratch disease. Ocul Immunol Inflamm 22:148–154
3. Cunningham ET, Koehler JE (2000) Ocular bartonellosis. Am J Ophthalmol 130:340–349
4. Jackson LA, Perkins BA, Wenger JD (1993) Cat-scratch disease in the United States: an analysis of three national databases. Am J Public Health 83:1707–1711
5. da Costa PS, Brigatte ME, Greco DB (2005) Antibodies to Rickettsia rickettsii, Rickettsia typhi, Coxiella burnetii, Bartonella henselae, Bartonella quintana, and Ehrlichia chaffeensis among healthy population in Minas Gerais, Brazil. Mem Inst Oswaldo Cruz 100:853–859
6. Carithers HA (1985) Cat scratch disease: an overview based on a study of 1200 patients. Am J Dis Child 139:1124–1133
7. Curi AL, Machado D, Heringer G, Campos WR, Lamas C, Rozental T, Gutierres A, Orefice F, Lemos E (2010) Cat-scratch disease: ocular manifestations and visual outcome. Int Ophthalmol 30:533–558
8. Dehio C (2003) Recent progress in understanding Bartonella-induced vascular proliferation. Curr Opin Microbiol 6:61–65
9. Kirb JE (2004) In vitro modelo f Bartonela hanselae induced angiogenesis. Infect Immun 72:7315–7317
10. Cassady JV, Culbertson CS (1953) Cat-scratch disease and Parinaud's oculoglandular syndrome. Arch Ophthalmol 50:68–74
11. Marr BP, Shields CL, Shields JA, Eagle RC Jr (2003) Conjunctival cat-scratch disease simulating rhabdomyosarcoma. J Pediatr Ophthalmol Strabismus 40:302–303
12. Mirakhur B, Shah SS, Ratner AJ, Goldstein SM, Bell LM, Kim JO (2003) Cat scratch disease presenting as orbital abscess and osteomyelitis. J Clin Microbiol 41:3991–3993
13. Gabler B, Linde HJ, Reischl U, Lohmann CP (2000) Disciformkeratatis caused by Bartonellahenselae infection: detection of a rare ocular complication of cat-scratch disease with PCR. Klin Monbl Augenheilkd 217:299–302
14. Lohmann CP, Gabler B, Kroher G, Spiegel D, Linde HJ, Reischl U (2000) Disciforme keratitis caused by Bartonellahenselae: an unusual ocular complication in cat scratch disease. Eur J Ophthalmol 10:257–258
15. Prasher P, Di Pascuale M, Cavanagh HD (2008) Bilateral chronic peripheral ulcerative keratitis secondary to cat-scratch disease. Eye Contact Lens 34:191–193
16. Martínez-Osorio H, Calonge M, Torres J, González F (2005) Cat-scratch disease (ocular bartonellosis) presenting as bilateral recurrent iridocyclitis. Clin Infect Dis 40:e43–e45
17. ur Rehman S, Metcalfe TW, Barnham M (1998) Anterior uveitis associated with cat scratch disease. Br J Ophthalmol 82:587–588
18. Kahloun R, Khairallah-Ksiaa I, Abroug N, Mahmoud A, Ben Yahia S, Zaouali S, Jelliti B, Khairallah M (2015) Final diagnosis in patients referred with a diagnosis of neuroretinitis. Neuroophthalmology 39(6):266–270
19. Reed JB, Scales DK, Wong MT, Lattuada CP Jr, Dolan MJ, Schwab IR (1998) Bartonella henselae neuroretinitis in cat scratch disease. Diagnosis, management, and sequelae. Ophthalmology 105:459–466
20. Wade NK, Levi L, Jones MR, Bhisitkul R, Fine L, Cunningham ET Jr (2000) Optic disk edema associated with peripapillary serous retinal detachment: an early sign of systemic Bartonella henselae infection. Am J Ophthalmol 130:327–334
21. Bar S, Segal M, Shapira R, Savir H (1990) Neuroretinitis associated with cat scratch disease. Am J Ophthalmol 110:703–705
22. Lombardo J (1999) Cat-scratch neuroretinitis. J Am Optom Assoc 70:525–530
23. Finger ML, Borruat FX (2014) Dynamics of intraretinal fluid accumulation evidenced by SD-OCT in a case of cat scratch neuroretinitis. Eye (Lond) 28:770–771
24. Ormerod LD, Dailey JP (1999) Ocular manifestations of cat scratch disease. Curr Opin Ophthalmol 10:209–216
25. Cunningham ET Jr, McDonald HR, Schatz H, Johnson RN, Ai E, Grand MG (1997) Inflammatory mass of the optic nerve head associated with systemic Bartonella henselae infection. Arch Ophthalmol 115:1596–1597
26. Ormerod LD, Skolnick KA, Menosky MM, Pavan PR, Pon DM (1998) Retinal and choroidal manifestations of cat scratch disease. Ophthalmology 105:1024–1031
27. Solley WA, Martin DF, Newman NJ, King R, Callanan DG, Zacchei T, Wallace RT, Parks DJ, Bridges W, Sternberg P Jr (1999) Cat-scratch disease-posterior segment manifestations. Ophthalmology 106:1546–1553

28. Empeslidis T, Tsaousis KT, Konidaris V, Pradeep A, Deane J (2014) Multifocal chorioretinitis caused by Bartonella henselae: imaging findings of spectral domain optical coherence tomography during treatment with trimethoprim-sulfamethoxazole. Eye (Lond) 28:907–909
29. Zacchei AC, Newman NJ, Sternberg P (1995) Serous retinal detachment of the macula associated with cat scratch disease. Am J Ophthalmol 120:796–797
30. Cohen SM, Davis JL, Gass JDM (1995) Branch retinal arterial occlusions in multifocal retinitis with optic nerve edema. Arch Ophthalmol 113:1271–1276
31. Gray AV, Michels KS, Lauer AK, Samples JR (2004) Bartonella henselae infection associated with neuroretinitis, central retinal artery and vein occlusion, neovascular glaucoma, and severe vision loss. Am J Ophthalmol 137:187–189
32. Curi AL, Machado DO, Heringer G, Campos WR, Orefice F (2006) Ocular manifestation of cat-scratch disease in HIV positive patients. Am J Ophthalmol 14:400–401
33. Soheilian M, Markomichelakis N, Foster CS (1996) Intermediate uveitis and retinal vasculitis as manifestations of cat scratch disease. Am J Ophthalmol 122:58264
34. Khurana RN, Albini T, Green RL, Rao NA, Lim JI (2004) Bartonellahenselae infection presenting as a unilateral panuveitis simulating Vogt-Koyanagi-Harada syndrome. Am J Ophthalmol 138:1063–1065
35. Asensio-Sánchez VM, Rodríguez-Delgado B, García-Herrero E, Cabo-Vaquera V, García-Loygorri C (2006) Serous macular detachment as an atypical sign in cat scratch disease. Arch Soc Esp Oftalmol 81:717–719
36. Matsuo T, Kato M (2002) Submacular exudates with serous retinal detachment caused by cat scratch disease. Ocul Immunol Inflamm 10:147–150
37. Albini TA, Lakhanpal RR, Foroozan R, Holz ER (2005) Macular hole in cat scratch disease. Am J Ophthalmol 140:149–151
38. Alterman MA, Young BK, Eggenberger ER, Kaufman DI (2013) Macular hole: a rare complication of ocular bartonellosis. J Neuroophthalmol 33:153–154
39. Degueldre F, Bonnet S (2002) Cause of unusual unilateral vitreous hemorrhage: neuroretinitis of cat-scratch disease. Presentation of a case. Bull Soc Belge Ophtalmol 285:37–40
40. Dalton MJ, Robinson LE, Cooper J, Regnery RL, Olson JG, Childs JE (1995) The use of Bartonella antigens for serologic diagnosis of cat-scratch disease at a national referral center. Arch Intern Med 155:1670–1676
41. Barka NE, Hadfield T, Patnaik M, Schwartzman WA, Peter JB (1993) EIA for detection of Rochalimaeahenselae-reactive IgG, IgM, and IgA antibodies in patients with suspected cat-scratch disease (letter). J Infect Dis 167:1503
42. Mitchell BM, Font RL (2011) Molecular detection of Bartonella henselae for the diagnosis of cat scratch disease and bacillary angiomatosis of the conjunctiva. Cornea 30:807–814
43. Font RL, Del Valle M, Mitchell BM, Boniuk M (2011) Cat-scratch uveitis confirmed by histological, serological, and molecular diagnoses. Cornea 30:468–471
44. Khairallah M, Curi ALL, Jenzeri S, Messaoud R (2009) Cat-scratch disease. In: Gupta A, Gupta V, Herbort C, Khairallah M (eds) Uveitis text and imaging, 1st edn. Jaypee Brothers Medical Publishers, New Delhi
45. Abroug N, Khairallah-Ksiaa I, Kahloun R, Khochtali S, Zaouali S, Khairallah M (2015) Parinaud's oculoglandular syndrome revealing subclinical Rickettsia conorii infection. Int Ophthalmol 35:717–719
46. CharbelIssa P, Eis-Hu¨binger AM, Klatt K, Holz FG, Loeffler KU (2008) Oculoglandular syndrome associated with reactivated Epstein-Barr-virus infection. Br J Ophthalmol 92:740–855
47. Margileth AM (1992) Antibiotic therapy for cat-scratch disease: clinical study of therapeutic outcome in 268 patients and a review of the literature. Pediatr Infect Dis J 11:474–478
48. Zimran E, Shilo S, Florescu T, Dotan S, Balag S, Mevorach D, Shibolet O, Amer R (2012) Paradoxical response in ocular bartonellosis. J Ophthalmic Inflamm Infect 2:53–56
49. Rolain JM, Brouqui P, Koehler JE, Maguina C, Dolan MJ, Raoult D (2004) Recommendations for treatment of human infections caused by Bartonella species. Antimicrob Agents Chemother 48:1921–1933

7 Tuberculosis

Amod Gupta and Reema Bansal

7.1 Introduction

Tuberculosis is a major public health problem worldwide and has been recognized as one of the common causes of infectious uveitis in developing countries [1]. Intraocular tuberculosis (TB) is one of the rare forms of extrapulmonary TB. It usually occurs without concomitant pulmonary or other systemic TB. Any part of the eye can get affected by *Mycobacterium tuberculosis* (MTB). It has protean manifestations, and the diagnosis is often presumed by a set of clinical signs and corroborative laboratory evidence.

7.2 Epidemiology

Reports from different regions of the world indicate that the prevalence of ocular TB ranges from 0.39 % (South India) to 10.5 % (Saudi Arabia) [2–10]. In developing countries, the prevalence of intraocular TB among uveitis patients is about 10 % [11] and less than 1 % in the USA [12]. Different regions within the same country have also shown variations [13]. While it is reported to be 0.39 % in South India [2], a study from North India has shown prevalence of 9.86 % [3]. Recently, ocular TB has been found to be more common in Los Angeles (six patients with probable or definite TB out of 142 consecutive uveitis patients) [14] than in Chicago (14 patients with ocular TB out of 3606 uveitis patients in a 16-year period) [15]. Recently, there is a growing evidence of ocular TB from countries with low or intermediate burden of TB [15–21].

7.3 Pathophysiology

In extrapulmonary TB, the tubercle bacilli, after inhalation into the lungs, are believed to disseminate into the distant organs via hematogenous or lymphatic route. The active infection of extrapulmonary tissues may occur during primary infection or upon reactivation of the latent infection. As the intraocular tissues remain difficult to be biopsied, the exact mechanism of intraocular TB remains unclear. However, a significant understanding of the pathogenesis has been recently provided in a few experimental studies. Rao et al. offered an excellent model of ocular TB to address its pathogenesis. They exposed the guinea pig lungs to MTB via an aerosol delivery of the organisms that led to its hematogenous dissemination [22]. All animals developed pulmonary lesions, with dissemination to the spleen. Of six animals receiving no antitubercular therapy (ATT), ocular lesions developed in 42 % eyes. The granulomatous reaction seen on histological analysis of lungs and ocular tissues was similar to that seen in humans with TB. In the second group of four guinea pigs receiving ATT 14 days after

A. Gupta (✉) • R. Bansal
Advanced Eye Centre, PGIMER, Chandigarh, India

S.-P. Chee, M. Khairallah (eds.), *Emerging Infectious Uveitis*, DOI 10.1007/978-3-319-23416-8_7

infection, none showed granulomatous inflammation, suggesting the role of systemic anti-TB drugs in preventing ocular TB. The similarity between guinea pig model of TB and humans with TB was also reflected by development of pulmonary TB in all animals and ocular TB in some of them.

Vascular endothelial growth factor (VEGF) has been used as a biomarker for active TB disease. In another animal model of ocular TB following aerosol delivery of MTB in guinea pigs, Thayil et al. demonstrated microbiological, histological, and clinical features of intraocular TB infection [23]. The retinal pigment epithelium (RPE) and photoreceptors demonstrated VEGF expression, and choroidal granulomas showed reduced oxygen tension. The authors hypothesized that VEGF upregulation in lungs and RPE occurred through inflammatory mediators of MTB infection and/or local inflammation causing tissue hypoxia. Their results suggested a hematogenous route of intraocular infection rather than direct inoculation.

The presence of MTB genome within the retinal pigment epithelium (RPE) cells was first demonstrated by Rao et al. in an enucleated globe with panuveitis [24]. The authors suggested a preferential localization of the MTB within the RPE, providing the site for reactivation that may manifest clinically as choroiditis.

Nazari et al. investigated the mechanism of MTB phagocytosis and its growth in the RPE compared to macrophages [25]. They suggested that MTB is readily phagocytized by the RPE in a manner similar to macrophages, but the viability of RPE is not affected by the intracellular MTB. They control the bacillary growth (better than the macrophages) and, hence, can act as reservoirs for intraocular MTB infection.

7.4 Clinical Features

7.4.1 Systemic Disease

Ocular involvement in patients with active pulmonary TB is extremely rare (1.4–6.8 %) [26–28]. Majority of ocular TB cases occur as isolated disease, with very few associated with extraocular TB. In a study on consecutive patients with a diagnosis of ocular TB at a center in Italy, 45 patients had isolated ocular TB, and 17 had ocular TB with extraocular TB [29]. In Spain, 18 % of patients with culture-proven systemic TB had intraocular TB [30]. We found a very low rate (3 %) of systemic TB in our series of patients with presumed intraocular TB [31].

7.4.2 Ocular Disease

Men and women are equally affected in any age. There is a lack of consensus on clinical diagnostic criteria for intraocular TB [32, 33]. The clinical spectrum of intraocular TB is highly variable and may mimic features of other uveitides. While granulomatous anterior uveitis is common in intraocular TB, the presence of mutton-fat keratic precipitates needs exclusion of other known causes such as viral uveitis, sarcoidosis, Vogt-Koyanagi-Harada (VKH) disease, sympathetic ophthalmia, or syphilis.

7.4.2.1 Ocular Surface Disease

The primary eyelid TB is a rare condition, and it occurs usually secondarily to orbital involvement. It can manifest as a chronic painless swelling, discharging sinus, chalazion, or an atypical lid swelling after blepharoplasty [34–37]. Orbital TB may involve the lacrimal gland as dacryoadenitis [38, 39], soft tissue as tuberculoma or cold abscess with or without bony involvement, and periosteum as classic periostitis or may spread from paranasal sinuses [40–42]. It may masquerade as an orbital malignancy in the presence of proptosis [43].

Conjunctival involvement in TB may manifest as chronic conjunctivitis (ulceration, epibulbar mass, papillary lesion) [44], allergic conjunctivitis in a child [45], chronic conjunctivitis with neighboring cutaneous TB [46, 47], or a tuberculoma [48]. Corneal involvement may manifest as phlyctenular keratoconjunctivitis [49] and chronic red eye [50]. Involvement of sclera may occur as nodular episcleritis [51], sclerouveitis masquerading as ocular tumor [52], or posterior scleritis [53]. Infective scleritis in immunosuppressed patients may occur as a result of reactivation of latent MTB [54].

7.4.2.2 Anterior Uveitis

Anterior uveitis in intraocular TB is usually granulomatous with mutton-fat keratic precipitates (Fig. 7.1) [55–62]. It may be unilateral or bilateral. Iris nodules are less frequent, which are seen on pupillary border or iris surface. Chronic recurrent inflammation produces posterior synechiae, which are usually broad based, and has been found to be strong clinical predictors of TB uveitis, as compared to other etiologies [16, 62, 63]. Other rare features may include acute anterior uveitis [64] and hypopyon [65, 66].

7.4.2.3 Intermediate Uveitis

It presents with vitritis, snowballs, peripheral retinal phlebitis, and peripheral vascular sheathing. Cystoid macular edema is the cause of visual loss. In a study from high-endemic setting, TB was found the commonest etiology in a series of intermediate uveitis patients [67]. It may sometimes present as chronic, low-grade vitritis with phlebitis. In Singapore, a country with intermediate TB burden, significant vitritis and phlebitis were more commonly associated with latent TB infection [16].

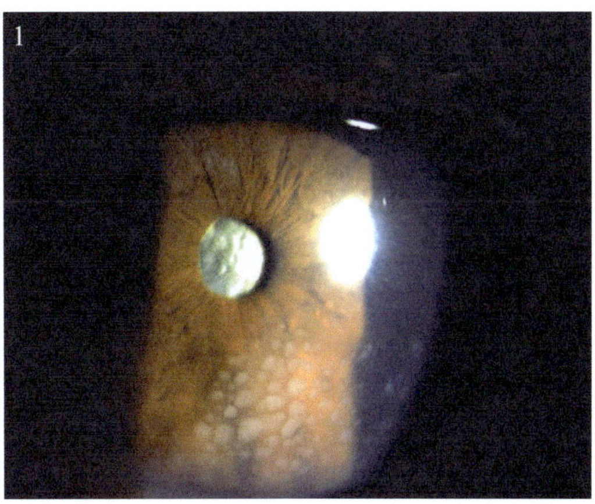

Fig. 7.1 Slit lamp photograph of the left eye of a 45-year-old female with tubercular anterior uveitis showing mutton-fat keratic precipitates

7.4.2.4 Posterior Uveitis

Choroidal TB

This is the commonest form of uveitis associated with TB [12, 31, 62, 68–70]. Choroidal tubercles were the earliest sign described in ocular TB in children with miliary tuberculosis [71]. They may be solitary or multiple in numbers and are usually diagnostic of disseminated TB, indicating a hematogenous spread of tubercle bacilli [72–78]. On fundus fluorescein angiography (FFA), they show an initial hypofluorescence followed by a late hyperfluorescence, with a peritubercular hyperfluorescence, suggesting active focal infection and inflammation [79]. They heal with atrophic scars and variable pigmentation. Optical coherence tomography (OCT) shows a raised RPE-choriocapillaris complex in the initial active stage with normal overlying retina and flattening of this region with scarring underneath [80]. While tubercles are small in size (0.2 mm–3 mm) and larger in numbers, a tuberculoma is larger in size (4 mm–14 mm) and appears predominantly in the posterior pole as a subretinal granuloma with surrounding exudative retinal detachment [81–84]. Caseation results from rapid bacillary growth within the granuloma and can be seen histopathologically in these abscesses [85]. A subretinal abscess may have overlying hemorrhages and develop retinal angiomatosis proliferans [86]. Larger tuberculomas may masquerade as ocular tumors [87]. The OCT shows retinal elevation with subretinal fluid that resolves with ATT and oral corticosteroids [88].

Multifocal serpiginoid choroiditis (MSC, previously called serpiginous-like choroiditis) is highly specific of tubercular uveitis [62]. It may be unilateral or bilateral and frequently affects young healthy males. Vitritis is often present. The lesions are multifocal and noncontiguous to optic disc and spread in a serpiginous pattern. They usually involve both the posterior pole and peripheral fundus and respond very well to ATT and oral corticosteroids (Fig. 7.2) [89, 90]. Despite initial aggressive inflammation involving the macula, the fovea is spared, and the patients maintain a good final visual acuity. On

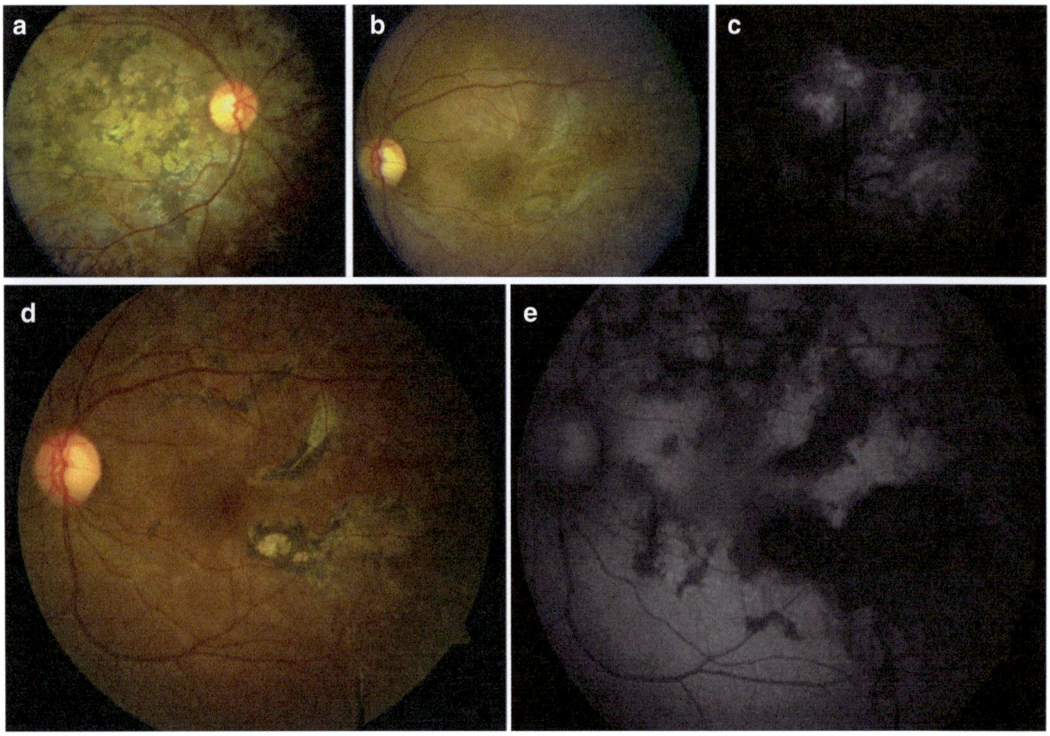

Fig. 7.2 Fundus photographs of a 31-year-old female with healed lesions of multifocal serpiginoid choroiditis in the right eye (**a**) and active lesions in the left eye (**b**) that showed hyperfluorescence in the late phase of fluorescein angiography (**c**). The QuantiFERON-TB Gold (QFT) test was positive. Following treatment with oral corticosteroids and antitubercular therapy, the left eye showed healed lesions at 21 months (**d**) that were hypoautofluorescent (**e**)

healing, the scars show significant pigmentation. It bears significant differences from the classic serpiginous choroiditis (SC), which affects elderly patients that has juxtapapillary, large, solitary lesions with minimal or no vitritis [91, 92]. The classic SC shows relentless progression and recurrent episodes despite corticosteroids and immunosuppressive agents and causes significant visual morbidity. In MSC, anterior segment inflammation and retinal vasculitis are rare [89, 93]. On FFA, the active lesions exhibit hypofluorescence in an early phase and progressively become hyperfluorescent in late phases, and the healed lesions (scars) show window defects [89, 94]. On indocyanine green angiography (ICGA), the lesions appear hypofluorescent in early, intermediate, and late phases [89, 94, 95]. The lesions show a characteristic pattern on fundus autofluorescence (FAF) imaging as they evolve from an acute stage to the healed stage, and this modality can be reliably used for clinical monitoring of the patients [94, 96]. The multimodal imaging with OCT reveals outer retinal morphological changes in the form of RPE-photoreceptor disruption in acute stages, followed by their atrophy as the lesions heal [97].

Retinal Vasculitis

It affects males more commonly than the females. It usually occurs without any systemic association. Previously called Eales' disease, its association with MTB has been reported by several studies [98–100]. It may be unilateral or bilateral and focal or diffuse, involving veins more commonly than the arteries. Perivascular infiltrates are seen as cuffing and are frequently associated with retinal hemorrhages. Vitritis is almost always present [101]. Snowball opacities, neuroretinitis, cystoid macular edema (CME), and branch retinal vein/artery occlusion are commonly associated with tubercular retinal vasculitis. The FFA shows staining and leakage from the vessel walls (which may be focal or diffuse), CME, optic disc staining, and typical occlusive nature of the vasculitis in the form of peripheral capillary nonperfusion (Fig. 7.3). Rosen et al. found ischemic retinal vasculitis as the most common form of uveitis in their series with a marked tendency to neovascularization [50]. Vitreous hemorrhage, neovascularization of the optic disc or elsewhere in the retina, and tractional retinal detachment result from untreated occlusive disease. Advanced cases may present with combined retinal detachment and iris or angle neovascularization.

It is frequently accompanied by choroiditis, which may be healed or active. The presence of retinal vasculitis with perivascular choroiditis scars has been found to be highly specific for TB in endemic countries [62, 102]. Central retinal vein occlusion (ischemic) and frosted branch angiitis are rare presentations [103, 104]. Active retinal vasculitis responds well to oral corticosteroids and ATT [31]. Laser photocoagulation and vitrectomy are required for neovascular sequelae.

Endophthalmitis and Panophthalmitis

These are atypical presentations in ocular TB and may mimic as ocular tumors [65, 66, 87, 105–108]. Diagnosis in these cases is confirmed by microbiological/histopathological evidence of MTB.

Optic Nerve Involvement

Involvement of optic nerve in ocular TB can result from direct infection or a hypersensitivity reaction and can present as optic disc tubercle, neuroretinitis, optic neuritis, retrobulbar neuritis, and papillitis [109–111].

7.5 Diagnosis

In the absence of a gold standard laboratory test demonstrating MTB in intraocular tissues, the diagnosis of intraocular TB presents a unique challenge and is restricted to a presumptive diagnosis by the clinical signs and corroborative evidence. Further, the lack of uniform diagnostic criteria adds to difficulties in diagnosing intraocular TB. Recently, Gupta et al. proposed a new classification system, based on clinical signs and diagnostic tests, for diagnosing intraocular TB as confirmed, probable, or possible intraocular TB [70]. According to this classification, a patient with a clinical sign(s) suggestive of ocular TB and microbiological confirmation of MTB from ocular fluids/tissues is diagnosed to have "confirmed ocular TB." A patient with suggestive clinical sign(s), exposure to TB/immunological evidence of TB, along with clinical/radiological/microbiological evidence of TB infection in extraocular sites would be diagnosed as "probable ocular TB." "Possible ocular TB" is diagnosed in the presence of a clinical sign of ocular TB, either with exposure to TB/immunological evidence of TBs or with clinical/radiological evidence of extraocular TB.

7.6 Indirect Evidence

Besides the clinical signs, corroborative evidence is provided by a positive tuberculin skin test (TST), or a positive interferon gamma release assays (IGRA), or radiological findings suggesting old or active TB on a chest X ray, or evidence of manifest TB elsewhere, exclusion of other causes of uveitis, and a positive response to ATT. The TST has been used since long for diagnosing and treating ocular TB due to its low cost and wide availability. The association of latent TB (as diagnosed by a positive TST) and uveitis has been shown in an endemic setting in the form of a favorable therapeutic response to ATT [31]. It, however, has its own limitations such as inability to distinguish between latent and manifest TB or between tuberculous and nontuberculous mycobacteria, false-positive (due to prior BCG vaccination or infection by atypical mycobacteria) or false-negative (immunocompromised state such as HIV infection) results, errors in conducting or interpreting the result, and need for a double visit by the patient. In a series of definite

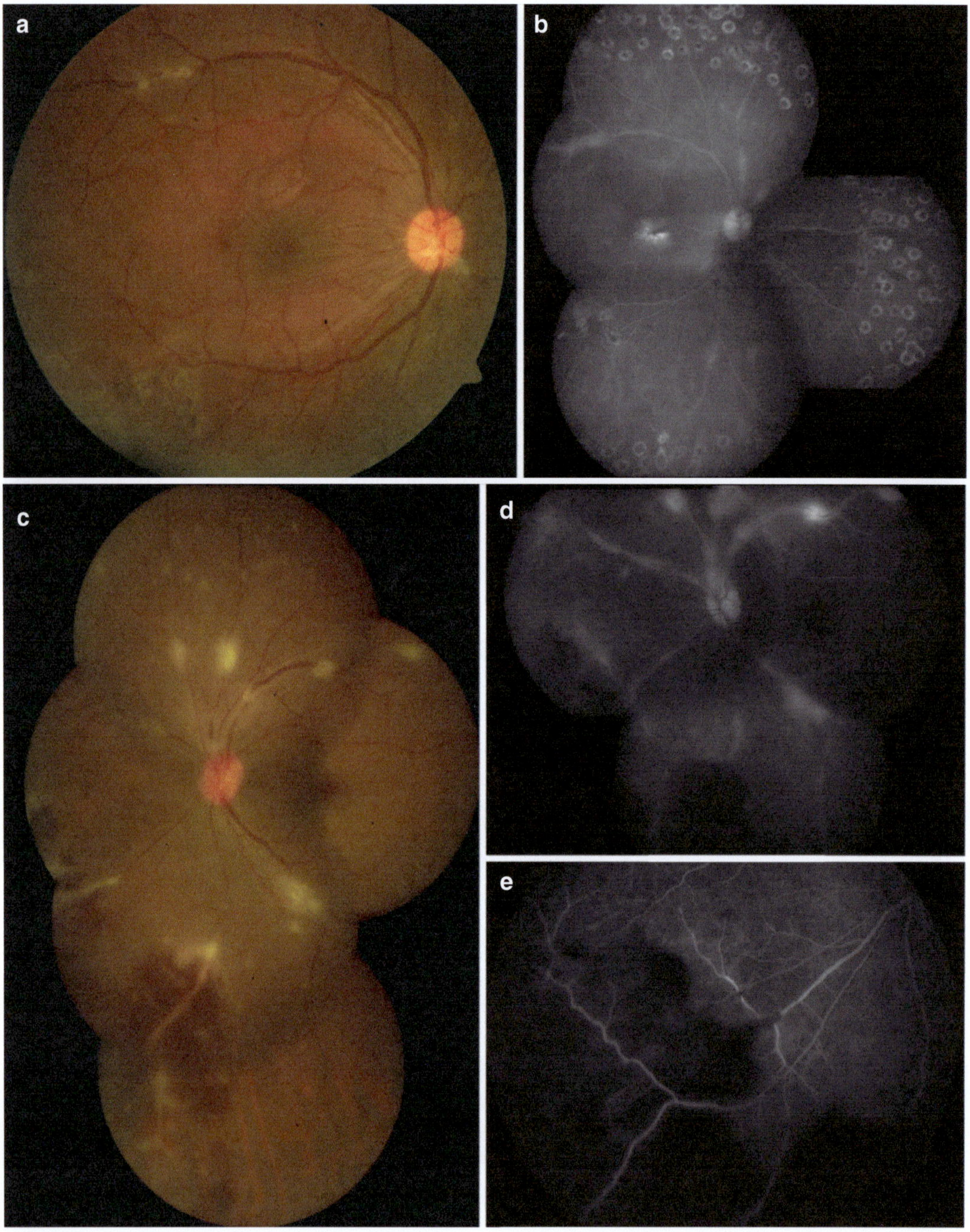

Fig. 7.3 Right eye fundus photograph (**a**) and fluorescein angiogram (**b**) of a 22-year-old male (having undergone pars plana vitrectomy and laser photocoagulation for vitreous hemorrhage in the past) with active retinal vasculitis and cystoid macular edema. The left eye also had active retinal vasculitis (**c**, **d**) with peripheral areas of capillary non-perfusion seen on fluorescein angiography (**e**). The tuberculin skin test was 17 × 18 mm. He received oral corticosteroids and antitubercular therapy, along with laser photocoagulation in left eye. At 16 months, both the eyes were quiescent (**f**, **g**)

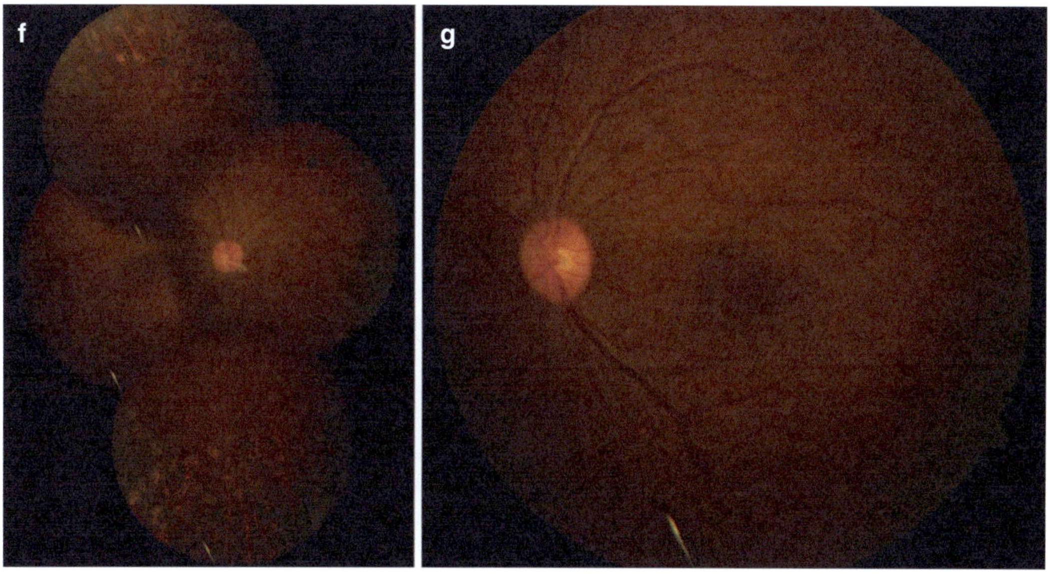

Fig. 7.3 (continued)

ocular TB cases, 40 % patients did not have a positive TST [112].

The more recent IGRAs have improved the specificity of a previous exposure to MTB, as they are not influenced by BCG vaccination or nontuberculous mycobacteria. Both TST and IGRAs indirectly detect an immune response to recent or prior exposure to MTB. The genomic region of MTB complex encodes several antigens that elicit a severe immunogenic response involving helper T cells, which can be measured in vitro through quantification of interferon gamma or interferon gamma-producing T cells by the IGRAs. But they also, like the TST, lack the ability to differentiate latent from manifest TB. QuantiFERON-TB Gold (QFT) In-Tube (Cellestis Inc., Carnegie, Australia) has been proved only slightly superior to TST in diagnosing TB uveitis [112]. On the other hand, Gineys et al. have used its cutoff value as a measure to identify cases of TB-related ocular inflammation that can benefit from ATT [113]. In a more recent prospective study on patients with TB-associated uveitis, T-SPOT.TB (Oxford Immunotec, Oxford, United Kingdom) test was found less sensitive but more specific than TST in populations with high prevalence of TB-associated uveitis, and hence, the authors concluded that TST should be the first-choice test in this population, while in low TB-prevalence populations, T-SPOT.TB test should be preferred to TST [114].

A recent survey among specialists dealing with different forms of TB (uveitis experts, pulmonologists, and rheumatologists) in India reported that the use of QFT Gold test in clinical practice was limited by its increased cost and limited data from India related to interpretation of the result [115].

Radiological evidence is usually sought in the chest X ray, as lungs are the primary sites of TB infection. Any evidence of present or previous TB on chest X ray increases the probability of uveitis being tubercular in origin, but this is rare as majority of intraocular TB cases occur in the absence of pulmonary TB. The reliability on chest X ray findings reduces further as some patients with primary TB may have a normal chest X ray [116]. Such patients need CT scan of the chest as a useful alternative [117]. In a series of definite ocular TB cases, 57 % had negative chest radiograph results [118]. Although usually inconclusive, chest X rays still form an integral part of the baseline laboratory workup of a patient with suspected TB uveitis.

When the above conventional radiological tests are negative, positron emission tomography-computed tomography (PET-CT) is useful in establishing TB as the cause of uveitis by demonstrating uptake of fluorodeoxyglucose (FDG) in metabolically active TB lesions [119, 120]. In patients with presumed ocular TB, Doycheva et al. demonstrated positive PET-CT findings in extraocular sites (mediastinal or hilar lymph nodes) in 45 % patients, which were diagnosed and treated accordingly [119]. While some patients may not demonstrate any systemic uptake at all, others may show an increased FDG uptake in various extraocular sites (pulmonary, extrapulmonary, or disseminated) suggesting a more widespread disease than presumed by the ophthalmologist [121]. There is, however, an insufficient evidence to suggest the use of PET-CT as a routine imaging modality in tubercular uveitis due to its high cost and limited reports of its use in uveitis diagnosis and management.

7.7 Direct Evidence

Demonstration of MTB in intraocular specimens (fluid or tissue) provides a direct and definitive evidence of intraocular TB. Smear positivity for acid-fast bacilli is extremely rare from ocular samples, due to low yield of fluid volume (aqueous/vitreous) as well as paucibacillary nature of intraocular TB [112]. Laborious and delayed culture reports often show no growth from ocular samples. Moreover, the risk of damage to ocular structures while sampling intraocular tissue/fluid adds limitations to performing histopathological diagnosis. Destructive interventions like evisceration or whole globe enucleation may require to be undertaken in cases of ocular TB masquerading as purulent ocular infections or tumors [85, 87] or those showing progressive worsening despite systemic corticosteroid treatment [24]. Although histopathological evidence forms the gold standard for diagnosing intraocular TB, it is never used as a first-line investigative tool.

Polymerase chain reaction (PCR) has long been reported in tubercular uveitis [101, 122–124]. While conventional PCR showed a low sensitivity and high specificity, multi-targeted PCR has emerged as a novel method by detecting different MTB genomes in intraocular samples and has shown an improved sensitivity [125]. Quantitative PCR (qPCR) is a fast method with minimum risk of cross contamination, which additionally quantifies the bacterial load in the tested sample [24, 126]. However, these tests require laboratories with good research facilities and, hence, remain limited only to resourceful settings. Further, poor correlation between qPCR and AFB results has been reported by Wroblewski et al., in which two out of three qPCR-positive patients did not show AFB in tissue sections [118]. One patient with positive AFB results had negative PCR results. Negative PCR results cannot exclude the diagnosis due to low sensitivity. Also, while performing these tests, the limited role of PCR technology in ocular TB should be kept in mind as suggested in paucibacillary form of cutaneous TB [127].

7.8 Newer Diagnostic Tools and Drug Resistance

The diagnostic armamentarium of intraocular TB has seen significant recent advances. While drug resistance has been a major health problem in pulmonary and extrapulmonary TB, it has been recently detected in intraocular TB [128–130]. The Xpert MTB/RIF assay (Cepheid, Sunnyvale, California) was approved by the WHO in 2010 for diagnosis of pulmonary TB [131]. It detects MTB DNA and simultaneously tests its susceptibility to rifampicin (RIF). The other advantages include quick results and elimination of cross contamination. High sensitivities and specificities have been reported from pulmonary and extrapulmonary samples [132–134]. The line probe assay [GenoType MTBDRplus (Hain Lifescience, GmbH, Nehren, Germany)] simultaneously detects MTB DNA as well as RIF and isoniazid (INH) resistance and produces results within about 5 h [135, 136]. In our experience, while both tests had low sensitivities (40 % and 60 %, respectively) for detecting MTB genome in a series of patients with MSC, they detected multidrug-resistant (MDR) tubercular uveitis in patients showing poor response to conventional four-drug ATT [130]. Early detection of MDR in intraocular TB is of immense relevance to prevent ocular morbidity, particularly in cases showing poor initial response, paradoxical worsening, or with atypical presentation. However, these rapid molecular tests have cost issues and need skill and specialized infrastructure, making their suitability restricted to tertiary care centers.

7.9 Management

There are no specific guidelines on the treatment protocol of intraocular TB [33]. There is a wide heterogeneity among uveitis specialists worldwide in the approach to diagnosis and management of ocular TB [32]. As an empirical treatment, ATT has been shown to be highly effective in reducing recurrence of uveitis when given with anti-inflammatory therapy in patients with presumed tubercular uveitis in endemic as well as low-endemic countries [31, 137, 138]. While corticosteroids are administered along with ATT and tapered as per the clinician's discretion depending upon the clinical response, ATT is administered for a prolonged duration in ocular TB, as recommended for any extrapulmonary site that is slow to respond to therapy [139]. Duration of more than minimum 9 months has been associated with an 11-fold reduction of recurrence of uveitis in a retrospective study [138]. Exclusion of other systemic disease or history of exposure to TB in non-endemic regions have been suggested as important factors in considering ATT in patients with relevant clinical presentation [138, 140]. Despite these suggestions, a simple algorithm still remains to be proposed for treating ocular TB. The conventional four-drug ATT comprises of isoniazid, rifampicin, ethambutol, and pyrazinamide for initial 2 months, followed by isoniazid and rifampicin for another 9–10 months, along with pyridoxine supplementation. Since most patients benefit from empiric ATT when started timely, an underdiagnosis would cause visual morbidity in an otherwise treatable uveitic entity. On the other hand, a judicious combination of clinical presentation and laboratory results is required to avoid overtreatment, as the ATT is expensive and potentially toxic. Besides potential drug toxicities, ATT may cause paradoxical response that is well known in pulmonary and extrapulmonary TB. Worsening of inflammation or the development of new lesions has been well documented in the eye after initiating ATT for ocular TB [141–145]. Although addition or rise of corticosteroids resolves this phenomenon, its occurrence in the eye may complicate judgment by raising several concerns such as poor compliance, drug resistance, disease relapse, or a nontubercular etiology.

In cases where rifampicin resistance is detected, the diagnosis is revised to MDR ocular TB, and the treatment comprises of levofloxacin 750 mg/day, ethionamide 750 mg/day, cycloserine 750 mg/day, streptomycin injection 1000 mg/day (intramuscular), and pyrazinamide 1500 mg/day for initial 5 months, followed by levofloxacin 750 mg/day, ethionamide 750 mg/day, and cycloserine 750 mg/day for another 18 months, under the supervision of a hepatologist with regular monitoring of liver and renal function tests.

7.10 Prognosis

A timely diagnosis of ocular TB and initiation of ATT with corticosteroids is associated with a favorable outcome in terms of reduced rate of recurrences [31, 137, 138].

Conclusion

The diagnosis of intraocular TB is challenged by a number of factors such as a wide variation in clinical manifestations, the absence of concurrent systemic TB, low sensitivity and specificity of laboratory tests, paucibacillary nature of ocular TB, and difficulty in obtaining adequate intraocular sample for histopathological diagnosis. The issues related to ATT such as lack of treatment guidelines, long duration of therapy, side effects, paradoxical worsening, recurrence of inflammation, and emergence of drug resistance further complicate the course in management of intraocular TB.

Core Messages

- Intraocular TB has a wide clinical spectrum worldwide. However, broad-based posterior synechiae, retinal vasculitis, and multifocal serpiginoid choroiditis have been recognized as highly specific for intraocular TB in an endemic country.
- Intraocular TB is being increasingly reported from non-endemic countries, too, predominantly in recent migrants from endemic areas.
- Recent experimental studies have shown significant advancements in the understanding of the pathogenesis of intraocular TB.
- A newer classification system has been proposed for intraocular TB (with "confirmed," "probable," and "possible" as three diagnostic groups), which needs to be validated in future studies.
- Specific clinical signs, immunological evidence of TB infection, documented exposure to TB, radiological evidence of TB infection, clinical evidence of extraocular TB, and microbiological/histopathological evidence of MTB are the criteria recommended for classifying intraocular TB.
- Antitubercular therapy with corticosteroids is highly effective in majority of cases.
- A high index of suspicion for multidrug resistant intraocular TB should be kept in mind for cases not responding to conventional therapy.
- Patients should be strictly monitored for any potential drug toxicities by an internist.

References

1. Rathinam SR, Cunningham ET Jr (2000) Infectious causes of uveitis in the developing world. Int Ophthalmol Clin 40(2):137–152
2. Biswas J, Narain S, Das D, Ganesh SK (1996) Pattern of uveitis in a referral uveitis clinic in India. Int Ophthalmol 20:223–228
3. Singh R, Gupta V, Gupta A (2004) Pattern of uveitis in a referral eye clinic in North India. Ind J Ophthalmol 52:121–125
4. Wakabayashi T, Morimura Y, Miyamoto Y, Okada AA (2003) Changing patterns of intraocular inflammatory disease in Japan. Ocul Immunol Inflamm 11:277–286
5. Henderly DE, Genstler AJ, Smith RE, Rao NA (1987) Changing patterns of uveitis. Am J Ophthalmol 103:131–136
6. Islam SM, Tabbara KF (2002) Causes of uveitis at the eye center in Saudi Arabia: a retrospective review. Ophthalmic Epidemiol 9:239–249
7. Nechaeva OB, Burylova EA (2009) The ocular tuberculosis epidemic situation in the Sverdlovsk region. Probl Tuberk Bolezn Legk 7:14–19
8. Abrahams IW, Jiang YQ (1986) Ophthalmology in China: endogenous uveitis in a Chinese ophthalmological clinic. Arch Ophthalmol 104:444–446
9. Mercanti A, Parolini B, Bonora A, Lequaglie Q, Tomazzoli L (2001) Epidemiology of endogenous uveitis in northeastern Italy: analysis of 655 new cases. Acta Ophthalmol Scand 79:64–68
10. Al-Mezaine HS, Kangave D, Abu El-Asrar AM (2010) Patterns of uveitis in patients admitted to a university hospital in Riyadh, Saudi Arabia. Ocular Immunol Inflamm 18:424–431
11. Gupta V, Gupta A, Rao NA (2007) Intraocular tuberculosis-an update. Surv Ophthalmol 52(6):561–587
12. Henderly DE, Genstler AJ, Smith RE, Rao NA (1987) Changing patterns of uveitis. Am J Ophthalmol 103:131–136
13. Rathinam SR, Namperumalasamy P (2007) Global variation and pattern changes in epidemiology of uveitis. Ind J Ophthalmol 55:173–183
14. Hong BK, Khanamiri HN, Bababeygy SR, Rao NA (2014) The utility of routine tuberculosis screening in county hospital patients with uveitis. Br J Ophthalmol 98:1091–1095
15. Patel SS, Saraiya NV, Tessler HH, Goldstein DA (2013) Mycobacterial ocular inflammation: delay in diagnosis and other factors impacting morbidity. JAMA Ophthalmol 131:752–758
16. Ang M, Hedayatfar A, Zhang R, Chee S-P (2012) Clinical signs of uveitis associated with latent tuberculosis. Clin Exp Ophthalmol 40(7):689–696
17. Nora RLD, van Velthoven MEJ, Ten Dam-van Loon NH, Misotten T, Bakker M, van Hagen MP et al (2014) Clinical manifestations of patients with intraocular inflammation and positive QuantiFERON-TB gold in-tube test in a country nonendemic for tuberculosis. Am J Ophthalmol 157(4):754–761

18. Vos AG, Wassenberg MWM, de Hoog J, Oosterheert JJ (2013) Diagnosis and treatment of tuberculous uveitis in a low endemic setting. Int J Infect Dis 17(11):e993–e999
19. Gan WL, Jones NP (2013) Serpiginous-like choroiditis as a marker for tuberculosis in a non-endemic area. Br J Ophthalmol 97:644–647
20. Sanghvi C, Bell C, Woodhead M, Hardy C, Jones N (2011) Presumed tuberculous uveitis: diagnosis, management and outcome. Eye 25:475–480
21. Manousaridis K, Ong E, Stenton C, Gupta R, Browning AC, Pandit R (2013) Clinical presentation, treatment, and outcomes in presumed intraocular tuberculosis: experience from Newcastle upon Tyne, UK. Eye 27:480–486
22. Rao NA, Albini TA, Kumaradas M, Pinn ML, Fraiq MM, Karakousis PC (2009) Experimental ocular tuberculosis in guinea pigs. Arch Ophthalmol 127:1162–1166
23. Thayil SM, Albini TA, Nazari H et al (2011) Local ischemia and increased expression of vascular endothelial growth factor following ocular dissemination of Mycobacterium tuberculosis. PLoS One 6:e28383
24. Rao NA, Saraswathy S, Smith RE (2006) Tuberculous uveitis: distribution of Mycobacterium tuberculosis in the retinal pigment epithelium. Arch Ophthalmol 124:1777–1779
25. Nazari H, Karakousis PC, Rao NA (2014) Replication of Mycobacterium tuberculosis in retinal pigment epithelium. JAMA Ophthalmol 132(6):724–729. doi:10.1001/jamaophthalmol.2014.270
26. Biswas J, Badrinath SS (1995–1996) Ocular morbidity in patients with active systemic tuberculosis. Int Ophthalmol 19(5):293–298
27. Donahue HC (1967) Ophthalmologic experience in tuberculous sanatorium. Am J Ophthalmol 64(4):742–748
28. Lara LP, Ocampo V Jr (2013) Prevalence of presumed ocular tuberculosis among pulmonary tuberculosis patients in a tertiary hospital in the Philippines. J Ophthalmic Inflamm Infect 3(1):1. doi:10.1186/1869-5760-3-1
29. Tognon MS, Fiscon M, Mirabelli P, Graziani G, Peracchi M, Sattin A, Marinello S, Vianello F, Sgarabotto D (2014) Tuberculosis of the eye in Italy: a forgotten extrapulmonary localization. Infection 42(2):335–342
30. Bouza E, Merino P, Muñnoz P et al (1997) Ocular tuberculosis. A prospective study in a general hospital. Medicine (Baltimore) 76:53–61
31. Bansal R, Gupta A, Gupta V, Dogra MR, Bambery P, Arora SK (2008) Role of anti-tubercular therapy in uveitis with latent/manifest tuberculosis. Am J Ophthalmol 146:772–779
32. Lou SM, Montgomery PA, Larkin KL, Winthrop K, Zierhut M, Rosenbaum JT et al (2015) Diagnosis and treatment for ocular tuberculosis among uveitis specialists: The international perspective. Ocul Immunol Inflamm 23(1):32–39
33. Lou SM, Larkin KL, Winthrop K, Rosenbaum JT, Members of Uveitis Specialists Study Group (2015) Lack of consensus in the diagnosis and treatment for ocular tuberculosis among uveitis specialists. Ocul Immunol Inflamm 23(1):25–31
34. Narsani AK, Jatoi SM, Dabir SA (2007) Isolated eyelid tuberculosis. J LUMHS 6:37–39
35. Aoki M, Kawana S (2002) Bilateral chalazia of the lower eyelids associated with pulmonary tuberculosis. Acta Derm Venereol 82:386–387
36. Mittal R, Tripathi D, Sharma S, Balne PK (2013) Tuberculosis of eyelid presenting as a chalazion. Ophthalmology 120:1103e3–1103e4
37. Mauriello JA Jr (2003) Atypical bacterial infection of the periocular region after periocular and facial surgery. Ophthal Plast Reconstr Surg 19:182–188
38. van Assen S, Lutterman JA (2002) Tuberculous dacryoadenitis: a rare manifestation of tuberculosis. Neth J Med 60:327–329
39. Chakraborti C, Biswas R, Mondal M, Mukhopadhya U, Datta J (2011) Tuberculous dacryoadenitis in a child. Nepal J Ophthalmol 3:210–213
40. Sen DK (1980) Tuberculosis of the orbit and lacrimal gland: a clinical study of 14 cases. J Pediatr Ophthalmol Strabismus 17:232–238
41. Mohammad A, El-Nasser A, Al-Hussaini MK, Karoosh SS, Abd El-Moneim MT, Carey BJ, Karcioglu ZA (1992) Tuberculosis of the orbit and lacrimal gland. Orbit 11:199–204
42. Madqe SN, Prabhakaran VC, Shome D, Kim U, Honavar S, Selva D (2008) Orbital tuberculosis: a review of literature. Orbit 27:267–277
43. Chin PK, Jacobs MB, Hing SJ (1997) Orbital tuberculoma masquerading as an orbital malignancy. Aust N Z J Ophthalmol 25:67–69
44. Chaurasia S, Ramappa M, Murthy SI, Vemuganti GK, Fernandes M, Sharma S, Sangwan V (2014) Chronic conjunctivitis due to Mycobacterium tuberculosis. Int Ophthalmol 34(3):655–660
45. Rose JS, Arthur A, Raju R, Thomas M (2011) Primary conjunctival tuberculosis in a 14 year old girl. Indian J Tuberc 58(1):32–34
46. Cook CD, Hainsworth M (1990) Tuberculosis of the conjunctiva occurring in association with a neighbouring lupus vulgaris lesion. Br J Ophthalmol 74(5):315–316
47. Pommier S, Chazalon E, Morand JJ, Meyer F (2008) Chronic cicatrizing conjunctivitis in a patient with hemifacial cutaneous tuberculosis. Br J Ophthalmol 92(5):616, 712–616, 713
48. Singh I, Chaudhary U, Arora B (1989) Tuberculoma of the conjunctiva. J Indian Med Assoc 87(11):265–266
49. Rohatgi J, Dhaliwal U (2000) Phlyctenular eye disease: a reappraisal. Jpn J Ophthalmol 44(2):146–150
50. Jennings A, Bilous M, Asimakis P, Maloof AJ (2006) Mycobacterium tuberculosis presenting as chronic red eye. Cornea 25(9):1118–1120

51. Bathula BP, Pappu S, Epari SR, Palaparti JB, Jose J, Ponnamalla PK (2012) Tubercular nodular episcleritis. Indian J Chest Dis Allied Sci 54(2):135–136
52. Damodaran K, George AE, Goel S, Khetan V, Noronha V, Biswas J (2012) Tubercular sclerouveitis masquerading as an ocular tumor: a case report. Ocul Immunol Inflamm 20(5):368–371
53. Gupta A, Gupta V, Pandav SS, Gupta A (2003) Posterior scleritis associated with systemic tuberculosis. Indian J Ophthalmol 51(4):347–349
54. Biswas J, Aparna AC, Annamalai R, Vaijayanthi K, Bagyalakshmi R (2012) Tuberculous scleritis in a patient with rheumatoid arthritis. Ocul Immunol Inflamm 20(1):49–52
55. Helm CJ, Holland GN (1993) Ocular tuberculosis. Surv Ophthalmol 38(3):229–256
56. Rosen PH, Spalton DJ, Graham EM (1990) Intraocular tuberculosis. Eye Lond Engl 4(Pt 3):486–492
57. Cutrufello NJ, Karakousis PC, Fishler J, Albini TA (2010) Intraocular tuberculosis. Ocul Immunol Inflamm 18(4):281–291
58. Alvarez GG, Roth VR, Hodge W (2009) Ocular tuberculosis: diagnostic and treatment challenges. Int J Infect Dis IJID Off Publ Int Soc Infect Dis 13(4):432–435
59. Bodaghi B, LeHoang P (2000) Ocular tuberculosis. Curr Opin Ophthalmol 11(6):443–448
60. Cunningham ET, Rathinam SR, Albini TA, Chee S-P, Zierhut M (2015) Tuberculous uveitis. Ocul Immunol Inflamm 23(1):2–6
61. Tabbara KF (2007) Tuberculosis. Curr Opin Ophthalmol 18(6):493–501
62. Gupta A, Bansal R, Gupta V, Sharma A, Bambery P (2010) Ocular signs predictive of tubercular uveitis. Am J Ophthalmol 149(4):562–570
63. Lara LPR, Ocampo V (2013) Prevalence of presumed ocular tuberculosis among pulmonary tuberculosis patients in a tertiary hospital in the Philippines. J Ophthalmic Inflamm Infect 3(1):1
64. Karaconji T, Maconochie Z, McCluskey P (2013) Acute anterior uveitis in Sydney. Ocul Immunol Inflamm 21(2):108–114
65. Velu J, Agarwal S, Gupta V, Sharma K, Sharma A, Gupta A (2013) Hypopyon uveitis – a rare presentation of intraocular tuberculosis. Ocul Immunol Inflamm 21(3):251–253
66. Rathinam SR, Rao NA (2004) Tuberculous intraocular infection presenting with pigmented hypopyon: a clinicopathological case report. Br J Ophthalmol 88(5):721–722
67. Parchand S, Tandon M, Gupta V, Gupta A (2011) Intermediate uveitis in Indian population. J Ophthal Inflamm Infect 1:65–70
68. Gupta A, Gupta V (2005) Tubercular posterior uveitis. Int Ophthalmol Clin 45(2):71–88
69. Gupta V, Shoughy SS, Mahajan S, Khairallah M, Rosenbaum JT, Curi A et al (2015) Clinics of ocular tuberculosis. Ocul Immunol Inflamm 23(1):14–24
70. Gupta A, Sharma A, Bansal R, Sharma K (2015) Classification of intraocular tuberculosis. Ocul Immunol Inflamm 23(1):7–13
71. Morton CA (1892) A group of cases of Tubercles in the choroid presenting some unusual features. Br Med J 1(1640):1190–1191
72. Shiono T, Abe S, Horiuchi T (1990) A case of miliary tuberculosis with disseminated choroidal haemorrhages. Br J Ophthalmol 74(5):317–319
73. Randolph RL, Schmeisser HC (1916) A clinical and pathological study of two cases of miliary tubercles of the choroid. Trans Am Ophthalmol Soc 14(Pt 2):585–592
74. Mehta S, Chauhan V, Hastak S, Jiandani P, Dalal P (2006) Choroidal tubercles in neurotuberculosis: prevalence and significance. Ocul Immunol Inflamm 14(6):341–345
75. Biswas J, Shome D (2002) Choroidal tubercles in disseminated tuberculosis diagnosed by the polymerase chain reaction of aqueous humor. A case report and review of the literature. Ocul Immunol Inflamm 10(4):293–298
76. Bowyer JD, Gormley PD, Seth R, Downes RN, Lowe J (1999) Choroidal tuberculosis diagnosed by polymerase chain reaction. A clinicopathologic case report. Ophthalmology 106(2):290–294
77. Mehta S (2004) Ocular lesions in acute disseminated tuberculosis. Ocul Immunol Inflamm 12(4):311–315
78. Illingworth RS, Wright T (1948) Tubercles of the choroid. Br Med J 2(4572):365–368
79. Mehta S (2006) Fundus fluorescein angiography of choroidal tubercles: case reports and review of literature. Indian J Ophthalmol 54(4):273–275
80. Mehta S (2012) Healing patterns of choroidal tubercles after antitubercular therapy: a photographic and OCT study. J Ophthalmic Inflamm Infect 2(2):95–97
81. Berinstein DM, Gentile RC, McCormick SA, Walsh JB (1997) Primary choroidal tuberculoma. Arch Ophthalmol 115(3):430–431
82. Gupta V, Gupta A, Arora S, Sachdeva N, Bambery P (2005) Simultaneous choroidal tuberculoma and epididymo-orchitis caused by Mycobacterium tuberculosis. Am J Ophthalmol 140(2):310–312
83. Levecq LJ, De Potter P (2005) Solitary choroidal tuberculoma in an immunocompetent patient. Arch Ophthalmol 123(6):864–866
84. Zhang M, Zhang J, Liu Y (2012) Clinical presentations and therapeutic effect of presumed choroidal tuberculosis. Retina 32:805–813
85. Biswas J, Madhavan HN, Gopal L, Badrinath SS (1995) Intraocular tuberculosis: clinicopathologic study of five cases. Retina 15:461–468
86. Gupta V, Gupta A, Sachdeva N, Arora S, Bambery P (2006) Successful management of tubercular subretinal granulomas. Ocul Immunol Inflamm 14(1):35–40

87. Demirci H, Shields CL, Shields JA, Eagle RC (2004) Ocular tuberculosis masquerading as ocular tumors. Surv Ophthalmol 49(1):78–89
88. Saxena S, Singhal V, Akduman L (2013) Three-dimensional spectral domain optical coherence tomography imaging of the retina in choroidal tuberculoma. BMJ Case Rep. Published online doi:10.1136/bcr-2012-008156
89. Bansal R, Gupta A, Gupta V, Dogra MR, Sharma A, Bambery P (2012) Tubercular serpiginous-like choroiditis presenting as multifocal serpiginoid choroiditis. Ophthalmology 119(11):2334–2342
90. Gupta V, Gupta A, SK A et al (2003) Presumed tubercular serpiginous-like choroiditis: clinical presentations and management. Ophthalmology 110:1744–1749
91. Vasconcelos-Santos DV, Rao PK, Davies JB, Sohn EH, Rao NA (2010) Clinical features of tuberculous serpiginouslike choroiditis in contrast to classic serpiginous choroiditis. Arch Ophthalmol 128(7):853–858
92. Cunningham ET Jr, Gupta A, Zierhut M (2014) The creeping choroiditides- serpiginous and multifocal serpiginoid choroiditis. Ocul Immunol Inflamm 22(5):345–348
93. Nayak S, Basu S, Singh MK (2011) Presumed tubercular retinal vasculitis with serpiginous-like choroiditis in the other eye. Ocul Immunol Inflamm 19(5):361–362
94. Bansal R, Gupta A, Gupta V (2012) Imaging in the diagnosis and management of serpiginous choroiditis. Int Ophthal Clinics 52:229–236
95. Wolfensberger TJ, Piguet B, Herbort CP (1999) Indocynanine green angiographic features in tuberculous chorioretinitis. Am J Ophthalmol 127:350–353
96. Gupta A, Bansal R, Gupta V, Sharma A (2012) Fundus autofluorescence in serpiginous-like choroiditis. Retina 32:814–825
97. Bansal R, Kulkarni P, Gupta A, Gupta V, Dogra MR (2011) High-resolution spectral domain optical coherence tomography and fundus autofluorescence correlationin tubercular serpiginouslike choroiditis. J Ophthalmic Inflamm Infect 1:157–163
98. Biswas J, Sharma T, Gopal L, Madhavan HN, Sulochana KN, Ramakrishnan S (2002) Eales disease – an update. Surv Ophthalmol 47(3):197–214
99. Biswas J, Ravi RK, Naryanasamy A, Kulandai LT, Madhavan HN (2013) Eales' disease – current concepts in diagnosis and management. J Ophthalmic Inflamm Infect 3(1):11
100. Singh R, Toor P, Parchand S, Sharma K, Gupta V, Gupta A (2012) Quantitative polymerase chain reaction for Mycobacterium tuberculosis in so-called Eales' disease. Ocul Immunol Inflamm 20(3):153–157
101. Gupta A, Gupta V, Arora S, Dogra MR, Bambery P (2001) PCR-positive tubercular retinal vasculitis: clinical characteristics and management. Retina 21(5):435–444
102. Babu K, Kini R, Mehta R, Philips M, Subbakrishna DK, Murthy KR (2012) Predictors for tubercular uveitis: a comparison between biopsy-proven cases of tubercular and sarcoid uveitis. Retina Phila Pa 32(5):1017–1020
103. Yuksel E, Ozdek S (2013) Unusual presentation of ocular tuberculosis: multiple chorioretinitis, retinal vasculitis and ischaemic central retinal vein occlusion. Clin Exp Optom J Aust Optom Assoc 96(4):428–429
104. Zhao H, Guan J, Zhou L, Zhang Q, Si Y (2012) Frosted branch angiitis in a woman with Mycobacterium tuberculosis infection. Ocul Immunol Inflamm 20(3):227–229
105. Ostheimer TA, Dunn JP, Eberhart CG, Burkholder BM (2015) Intraocular tuberculosis presenting as a large anterior chamber mass. Ocul Immunol Inflamm 23(1):100–101
106. Sheu SJ, Shyu JS, Chen LM, Chen YY, Chirn SC, Wang JS (2001) Ocular manifestations of tuberculosis. Ophthalmology 108(9):1580–1585
107. Chawla R, Garg S, Venkatesh P, Kashyap S, Tewari HK (2004) Case report of tuberculous panophthalmitis. Med Sci Monit Int Med J Exp Clin Res 10(10):CS57–CS59
108. Wadhwani M, Sethi S, Beri S, Jain R, Dsouza P, Nangia A et al (2011) An unusual case of metastatic tubercular panophthalmitis in a 14-year-old boy. J Pediatr Ophthalmol Strabismus 48(5):318–319
109. Mansour AM (1998) Optic disk tubercle. J Neuroophthalmol 18:201–203
110. Stechschulte SU, Kim RY, Cunningham ET Jr (1999) Tuberculous neuroretinitis. J Neuroophthalmol 19:201–204
111. Davis EJ, Rathinam SR, Okada AA, Tow SL, Petrushkin H, Graham EM et al (2012) Clinical spectrum of tuberculous optic neuropathy. J Ophthalmic Inflamm Infect 2(4):183–189
112. Ang M, Htoon HM, Chee SP (2009) Diagnosis of tuberculous uveitis: Clinical application of an Interferon-gamma release assay. Ophthalmology 116:1391–1396
113. Gineys R, Bodaghi B, Carcelain G, Cassoux N, Boutin le TH, Amoura Z et al (2011) QuantiFERON-TB gold cut-off value: Implications for the management of tuberculosis-related ocular inflammation. Am J Ophthalmol 152:433–440
114. Ang M, Wong WL, Li X, Chee SP (2013) Interferon gamma release assay for the diagnosis of uveitis associated with tuberculosis: a Bayesian evaluation in the absence of a gold standard. Br J Ophthalmol 97:1062–1067
115. Babu K, Philips M, Subbakrishna DK (2013) Perspectives of QuantiFERON-TB Gold test among Indian practitioners: a survey. Journal of Ophthal Inflamm Infect 3:9. doi:10.1186/1869-5760-3-9
116. Greenberg SD, Frager D, Suster B et al (1994) Active pulmonary tuberculosis in patients with

AIDS: spectrum of radiographic findings (including a normal appearance). Radiology 193:115
117. Kim HJ, Lee HJ, Kwon SY et al (2006) The prevalence of pulmonary parenchymal tuberculosis in patients with tuberculous pleuritis. Chest 129:1253–1258
118. Wroblewski KJ, Hidayat AA, Neafie RC, Rao NA, Zapor M (2011) Ocular tuberculosis: a clinicopathologic and molecular study. Ophthalmology 118:727–777
119. Doycheva D, Deuter C, Hetzel J et al (2011) The use of positron emission tomography/CT in the diagnosis of tuberculosis-associated uveitis. Br J Ophthalmol 95:1290–1294
120. Mehta S, Jiandani P (2010) Fluorine-18 Fluorodeoxyglucose positron emission tomography in the evaluation of a patient with presumed ocular tuberculosis. Ocul Immunol Inflamm 18:192–193
121. Mehta S (2012) Patterns of systemic uptake of 18-FDG with positron emission tomography/computed tomography (PET/CT) studies in patients with presumed ocular tuberculosis. Ocul Immunol Inflamm 20:434–437
122. Arora S, Gupta V, Gupta A, Bambery P, Kapoor GS, Sehgal S (1999) Diagnostic efficacy of polymerase chain reaction in granulomatous uveitis. Tuber Lung Dis 79:229–233
123. Gupta V, Arora S, Gupta A, Ram J, Bambery P, Sehgal S (1998) Management of presumed intraocular tuberculosis: possible role of polymerase chain reaction. Acta Ophthalmol Scand 76:679–682
124. Madhavan HN, Therese KL, Gunisha P, Jayanthi U, Biswas J (2000) Polymerase chain reaction for detection of Mycobacterium tuberculosis in epiretinal membrane in Eales disease. Invest Ophthalmol Vis Sci 41:822–825
125. Sharma K, Gupta V, Bansal R, Sharma A, Sharma M, Gupta A (2013) Novel multitargeted polymerase chain reaction for diagnosis of presumed tubercular uveitis. J Ophthalmic Inflamm Infect 3:25
126. Sharma P, Bansal R, Gupta V, Gupta A (2011) Diagnosis of tubercular uveitis by quantitative polymerase chain reaction. J Ophthalmic Inflamm Infect 1:23–27
127. Tan SH, Tan BH, Goh GL et al (1999) Detection of Mycobacterium tuberculosis DNA using polymerase chain reaction in cutaneous tuberculosis and tuberculids. Int J Dermatol 38:122–127
128. Sharma K, Bansal R, Sharma A, Gupta A, Fiorella PD (2015) Successful treatment of rifampicin resistant intraocular tuberculosis. Ocul Immunol Inflamm 23(1):93–96
129. Sharma K, Sharma A, Bansal R, Fiorella PD, Gupta A (2014) Drug-resistant tubercular uveitis. J Clin Microbiol 52(11):4113–4114
130. Bansal R, Sharma K, Gupta A, Sharma A, Singh MP, Gupta V, Mulkutkar S, Dogra M, Dogra MR, Kamal S, Sharma SP, Fiorella PD (2015) Detection of Mycobacterium tuberculosis genome in vitreous fluid of eyes with multifocal serpiginoid choroiditis. Ophthalmol. pii: S0161–6420(14)01115–4. doi: 10.1016/j.ophtha.2014.11.021. [Epub ahead of print]
131. World Health Organization (2011) Automated real-time nucleic acid amplification technology for rapid and simultaneous detection of tuberculosis and rifampicin resistance: Xpert MTB/RIF system. Policy statement. World Health Organization, Geneva http://apps.who.int/iris/handle/10665/44586
132. Boehme CC, Nabeta P, Hillemann D et al (2010) Rapid molecular detection of tuberculosis and rifampin resistance. New Engl J Med 363:1005–1015
133. Marlowke EM, Novak Weekley SM, Cumpio J et al (2011) Evaluation of the Cepheid Xpert MTB/RIF assay for the direct detection of Mycobacterium tuberculosis Complex from respiratory specimens. J Clin Microbiol 49:1621–1623
134. Hillemann D, Ruesch-Gerdes S, Boehme C, Richter E (2011) Rapid molecular detection of extrapulmonary tuberculosis by automated GeneXpert® MTB/RIF system. J Clin Microbiol 49:1202–1205
135. Ling D, Zwerling A, Pai M (2008) GenoType MTBDR assays for the diagnosis of multidrug-resistant tuberculosis: a meta-analysis. Eur Respir J 32:1165–1174
136. Albert H, Bwanga F, Mukkada S et al (2010) Rapid screening of MDR-TB using molecular line probe assay is feasible in Uganda. BMC Infect Dis 10:41
137. Agrawal R, Gupta B, Gonzalez-Lopez JJ, Rahman F, Phatak S, Triantafyllopoulou I, Addison PKF, Westcott M, CE P (2015) The role of anti-tubercular therapy in patients with presumed ocular tuberculosis. Ocul Immunol Inflamm 23(1):40–46
138. Ang M, Hedayatfar A, Wong W, Chee SP (2012) Duration of anti-tubercular therapy in uveitis associated with latent tuberculosis: a case-control study. Br J Ophthalmol 96(3):332–336
139. Centers for Disease Control, American Thoracic Society, CDC and Infectious Diseases Society of America (2003) Treatment of tuberculosis. MMWR Morb Mortal Wkly Rep 52:RR11
140. Vascocelos-Santos DV, Zierhut M, Rao NA (2009) Strengths and weaknesses of diagnostic tools for tuberculous uveitis. Ocul Immunol Inflamm 17:351–355
141. Gupta V, Bansal R, Gupta A (2011) Continuous progression of tubercular serpiginous-like choroiditis after initiating antituberculosis treatment. Am J Ophthalmol 152(5):857–863
142. Rathinam SR, Lalitha P (2007) Paradoxical worsening of ocular tuberculosis in HIV patients after antiretroviral therapy. Eye 21(5):667–668
143. Basu S, Das T (2010) Pitfalls in the management of TB-associated uveitis. Eye 24(11):1681–1684
144. Cheung CM, Chee SP (2009) Jarisch–Herxheimer reaction: paradoxical worsening of tuberculosis chorioretinitis following initiation of antituberculous therapy. Eye 23(6):1472–1473
145. Yilmaz T, Selcuk E, Polat N, Mutlu K (2015) Choroidal tuberculoma showing paradoxical worsening in a patient with miliary TB. Ocul Immunol Inflamm 23(1):97–99

8 Leptospirosis

S.R. Rathinam

8.1 Introduction

Leptospirosis is a reemerging zoonotic water-borne illness in tropical countries caused by the spirochete of the genus *Leptospira* [1–4]. Initially it presents as an acute febrile illness which may be followed by an asymptomatic latent period and a late-onset ocular morbidity in the form of uveitis [5]. Eliciting history of exposure to risk factors and the occurrence of prior systemic illness is the critical step needed in the ocular workup. The ocular signs of leptospirosis are more specific than the systemic signs, and they aid in establishing a diagnosis.

8.2 Epidemiology

Leptospires are widespread throughout the world, and their abundance is due to their ability to infect a wide range of animal species, including human, as well as their ability to survive outside the host, if environmental conditions are favorable. Leptospirosis was first recognized as an endemic occupational disease affecting farmers in rice or sugarcane fields, fishermen, sewer workers, forestry workers, laboratory workers, veterinarians, dairy industry workers, and miners [6–12]. However it has an epidemic potential in rainy season, and outbreaks have been reported after recreational water carnivals. Presently it is recognized as an emerging disease as the incidence is documented to be increasing globally [4, 13–16]. Global climate change, travel, and eco-tourism are considered important for this emergence [8, 13, 17]. High prevalence of the disease is also reported among economically marginalized population in urban slum with inadequate sewage disposal and water treatment. High incidence is seen in tropics and subtropics ranging from 10 to 100 human patients per 1,000,000 individuals [13]. WHO Leptospirosis Burden Epidemiology Reference Group (LERG) estimates 873,000 annual cases and 48,000 deaths due to leptospirosis [18]. However there is a definite underestimation of this disease in endemic countries due to the lack of gold standard diagnostic test, poor surveillance, and clinicians' ability to recognize the disease [8, 9, 13].

8.3 Etiopathogenesis

Leptospira, *Borrelia*, and *Treponema* are three important spirochetes, each of which can cause a primary systemic infection and a late ocular complication, uveitis. *Leptospira interrogans* is a gram-negative bacterium that belongs to the family *Spirochaetaceae* [6]. They are thin, spiral-shaped,

S.R. Rathinam, FAMS, PhD
Uveitis Service, Aravind Eye Hospital and PG. Institute of Ophthalmology, 1, Anna Nagar, Madurai, Tamil Nadu 625020, India
e-mail: rathinam@aravind.org

S.-P. Chee, M. Khairallah (eds.), *Emerging Infectious Uveitis*, DOI 10.1007/978-3-319-23416-8_8

and motile and can only be visualized by dark-field microscopy. Antigenically related serovars are grouped as serogroups whose members cross agglutinate with each other, but they do not cross agglutinate with members of other serogroups. There are nearly 270 serovars grouped into 23 serogroups. Of seven pathogenic leptospiral species, *L. interrogans* is more common [6].

The organism infects a variety of animals including rodents, cattle, swine, dogs, horses, sheep, and goats [7]. Animals may be asymptomatic or develop clinical infection and can shed the leptospires in their urine intermittently or continuously throughout life, resulting in environmental contamination. Cattle and field rat particularly contaminate the agricultural field and stagnant water [8–11].

Infected animal urine contaminates the standing or flowing water bodies. The spirochetes enter the human host through the mucous membrane or abraded skin [6]. After the entry, they spread to all organs via the blood stream. Damage to the endothelial lining of the capillaries and subsequent interference with blood flow appear to be responsible for the lesions associated with leptospirosis. With the appearance of antibody, leptospires start disappearing from the blood, but can persist in immunologically privileged sites such as brain, meninges, uterus, and renal tubules or in the anterior chamber of the eye. Persistence of these organisms in these organs causes late-onset immunological disorders. The host immune response to leptospirosis is mainly a humoral response. Agglutinating antibodies against leptospiral lipopolysaccharide (LPS) have a protective role [19]. However this immunity is protective against homologous serovars. In addition, Toll-like receptor (TLR)2 and TLR4 have also been found to be necessary for effective innate immune control [20]. The pathogenic mechanism of leptospiral uveitis is believed to be endotoxin mediated. A study demonstrated the presence of serovar-specific leptospiral lipopolysaccharide in aqueous humor [21]. This serovar-specific LPS was found to be a useful diagnostic marker for serodiagnosis [20].

Risk factors for systemic leptospirosis include travel to endemic countries and exposure to contaminated water sources. Occupational exposure is reported in rice field workers, mining ranchers, abattoir workers, veterinarians, sewer workers, and military personnel. Recreational activities such as fresh water swimming, canoeing, kayaking, and trail biking can cause outbreaks. Household exposure to infected rodents, pet dogs, and livestock can result in sporadic infections [6].

8.4 Clinical Features

8.4.1 Systemic Disease

The spectrum of clinical presentation of human leptospirosis ranges from asymptomatic to fatal [22–24]. Majority of patients present with a mild fever mimicking a flu-like illness and less than 10 % develop a severe disease. The latter form commences abruptly with severe headache, high fever, and multi-organ hemorrhage and progressive impairment of hepatic and renal function. Renal failure is the most common cause of death. This presentation is known as Weil's disease [2, 6]. During this acute phase, patient may present with conjunctival congestion and chemosis. The disease can also affect the lungs, brain, pericardium, or gastrointestinal tract, resulting in pulmonary hemorrhage, aseptic meningitis, cardiovascular collapse, or pancreatitis. The clinical signs depend, to a large extent, on the organs involved and are not sufficiently characteristic. Physicians may easily miss the diagnosis, as symptoms are extremely variable, and can mimic other infectious diseases. Common systemic signs of systemic leptospirosis are given in Table 8.1.

Table 8.1 Common systemic signs of systemic leptospirosis

▪ Acute fever, rigor, and severe fatigue
▪ Scleral icterus with or without conjunctival congestion
▪ Severe headache and meningeal irritation
▪ Delirium/psychosis
▪ Muscle tenderness, myalgia – particularly involving the calves and lumbar area
▪ Anuria or oliguria
▪ Jaundice
▪ Multi-organ hemorrhages
▪ Cardiac arrhythmia or failure
▪ Acute abdomen

8.4.2 Differential Diagnosis of Systemic Leptospirosis

Dengue fever and leptospirosis are important causes of acute febrile illness whose clinical signs overlap. Clinical diagnosis and confirmation remain a challenge mainly because of the lack of affordable and practical diagnostic tests for both [22, 25]. Other common differential diagnosis of systemic leptospirosis includes hemorrhagic yellow fever, influenza, hantavirus infection, viral hepatitis, malaria, typhoid, Rickettsial relapsing fever, meningitis, and encephalitis.

8.4.3 Laboratory Diagnosis

Complete blood count may reveal neutrophilia, elevated erythrocyte sedimentation rate, thrombocytopenia, and anemia. Renal function tests reveal azotemia and hyponatremia. Urine examination may reveal microscopic hematuria, proteinuria, pyuria, and granular casts.

Diagnosis of systemic leptospirosis is confirmed only by isolation of the organisms which is possible during the first week of infection, before the appearance of antibodies. Alive motile leptospires can be seen under dark-field microscopy in the blood, urine, or cerebrospinal fluid. *Leptospira* can be grown in special media such as Ellinghausen-McCullough-Johnson-Harris (EMJH) medium. Beyond 10 days, the microscopic agglutination test (MAT) is commonly used as a diagnostic gold standard. Motile bacteria in liquid medium are added with titrated amounts of patient's serum. When the serum contains antibodies, agglutination is observed under dark-field microscopy. This test relies on detecting an increase in antibody titer between two serum samples obtained at least 2 weeks apart. Seroconversion or a fourfold rise in paired serum samples or a titer above 1:400 dilution in the presence of a compatible clinical illness is considered diagnostic for systemic leptospirosis. In chronic immunological reactions like uveitis where fourfold raise cannot be demonstrated, a titer of 1:100 dilutions is usually considered significant. MAT requires live organisms and considerable expertise, and it is performed only by reference laboratories. It is not available in primary ophthalmic setup [6, 26].

Other serological tests include ELISA, macroscopic agglutination, indirect hemagglutination, LEPTO dipstick, immunofluorescence assay, microcapsule agglutination tests, microsphere immunoassay, and lateral flow assays. Molecular diagnostics include conventional polymerase chain reaction (PCR) and real-time PCR [27, 28]. In one of the studies, commercial serodiagnostic kits showed varying sensitivity and specificities, and they did not correspond with each other [29]. It is mandatory for the practitioner to check the reliability of the locally available diagnostic kits.

Next-generation sequencing is a very recent technology for determining DNA sequence by analyzing multiple DNA fragments in parallel. It allows sequencing of an exponentially greater number of genes than conventional DNA sequencing. Molecular diagnostics will prove its potential use in future [22]. But these advanced procedures are not available in health centers in tropical countries where the disease is more common.

8.4.4 Treatment of Systemic Leptospirosis

Leptospires are sensitive in vitro to most antimicrobial agents, including penicillin, amoxicillin, doxycycline, and ceftriaxone. Treatment details are given in Table 8.2. In addition to antimicrobial agents, supportive therapy is mandatory in severe cases. Depending upon the organ involved, patient may need management of electrolyte imbalance, renal dialysis, mechanical ventilation, airway protection, and cardiac monitoring and administration of vitamin K in patients with hypoprothrombinemia [30].

Table 8.2 Treatment of systemic leptospirosis

Systemic leptospirosis	Drug	Dosage
Severe form with hepatorenal damage	IV Penicillin G	1.5 MU every 6 h for 1 week
Mild to moderate fever	Doxycycline	100 mg BD for 1 week
Chemoprophylaxis	Doxycycline	200 mg/week

8.4.5 Ocular Disease

The spectrum of ocular manifestation leptospirosis can be seen both in septicemic phase and in immune phase. In a febrile patient, conjunctival chemosis and congestion are pathognomonic signs for the diagnosis of systemic leptospirosis, but they are frequently overlooked. In one case series, chemosis and congestion occurred in 55 % of patients with systemic leptospirosis [31].

8.5 Leptospiral Uveitis

Uveitis is an important late complication of leptospirosis [26, 32]. The precise incidence of uveitis in patients with systemic leptospirosis is not known, but it is estimated to be about 10–45 % [33]. Uveitis manifests within 2 months after infection or may be delayed for up to 1 year. The onset and severity of leptospiral uveitis is quite variable, and the severity of ocular inflammation does not correlate with the severity of systemic infection. Leptospiral uveitis more commonly occurs as single episode than recurrent episodes. The primary anatomical location of inflammation tends to be either anterior or panuveitis. Nongranulomatous uveitis is the most common presentation.

Ocular signs of leptospirosis are given in Table 8.3. Anterior uveitis is usually mild in contrast to severe course characteristic of panuveitis. Leptospiral uveitis is one of the most common causes of hypopyon uveitis in leptospiral endemic areas. Early onset, rapid progression, and spontaneous absorption of cataractous lens are unique features in this uveitis; however it is seen only in 10 % of leptospiral uveitis [34] (Fig. 8.1).

Dense vitreous inflammation with the formation of veil-like vitreous membranes is a pathognomonic sign seen in posterior segment. Although these membranes persist for several months, most patients regain good vision. Exudative retinal vasculitis with perivascular sheathing of the vein is frequently seen in leptospiral uveitis; however occlusion and neovascularization are uncommon. Disc hyperemia and edema are seen in 40 % of leptospiral uveitis patients. Retinitis and choroiditis are never seen in leptospiral uveitis. Although leptospiral uveitis is a common entity, it remains underdiagnosed mainly because of the lack of laboratory support in ophthalmic setup (Figs. 8.2 and 8.3).

Differential diagnosis of leptospiral uveitis includes Behcet's disease, HLA-B27-associated anterior uveitis, syphilis, Lyme disease, endogenous endophthalmitis, sarcoidosis, and early stage of acute retinal necrosis.

Table 8.3 Common ocular signs in leptospirosis

Common ocular signs in leptospirosis
Septicemic phase
Conjunctival chemosis and congestion
Scleral icterus as a manifestation of leptospiral jaundice
Immune phase
Interstitial keratitis
Cranial nerve palsies
Uveitis
Leptospiral anterior uveitis
Nongranulomatous anterior uveitis
Hypopyon
Pearly white cataract
Leptospiral panuveitis
Vitreous cells
Membranous vitreous opacities
Papillitis
Retinal vasculitis
Vitreous hemorrhage
Neuroretinitis

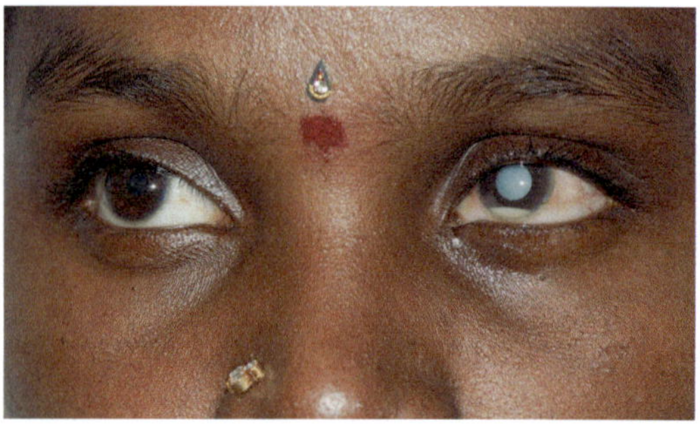

Fig. 8.1 Hypopyon and pearly white cataract in leptospiral uveitis in a young female patient

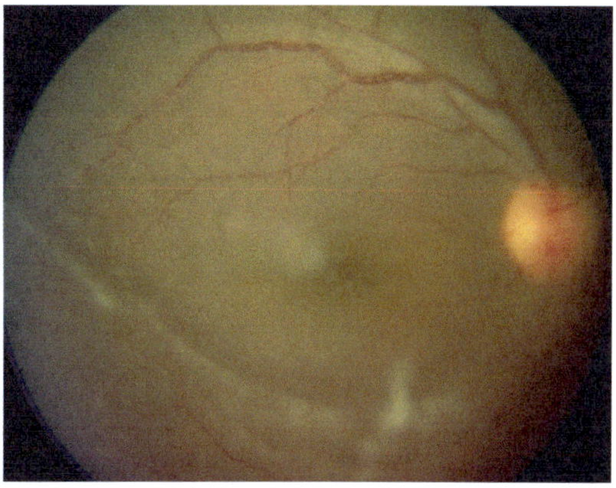

Fig. 8.2 Retinal vasculitis and vitreous membranes in leptospiral uveitis patient

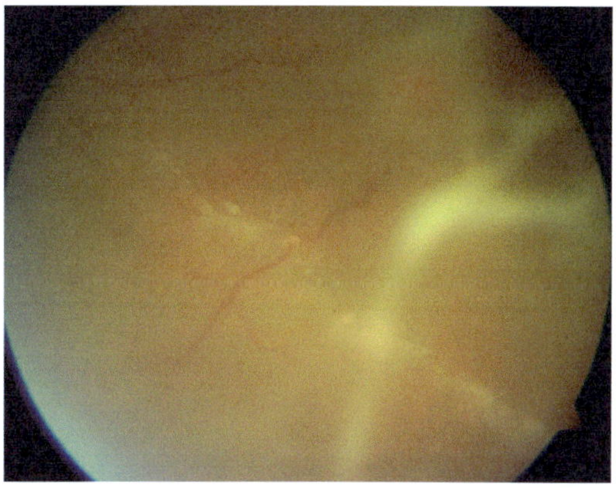

Fig. 8.3 Vitreous inflammatory reaction with freely floating veil-like vitreous membranes and a string of pearls appearance below and hazy view of hyperemic disc in the background

Core Messages

- Leptospirosis, borreliosis, and syphilis are three important spirochetal diseases, which can cause systemic disease and after a latent period, they result in uveitis.
- Unlike syphilis, leptospires can live outside the human body, if environmental conditions are favorable, and can infect a wide range of animal species.
- It is a zoonotic tropical disease of global concern can affect travelers and water sports players.
- Serious and potentially life-threatening complications of systemic leptospirosis can cause multi-organ dysfunction and death in a matter of days. It is critical to suspect and recognize the disease early, in order to initiate early treatment.
- Uveitis is a late complication that presents after an asymptomatic latent period.
- In a patient coming from an endemic area, with uveitis, a past history of exposure to animal urine contaminated environment and a past febrile illness could raise a suspicion of leptospiral etiology.
- Commonly presents as unilateral or bilateral acute, nongranulomatous panuveitis with or without hypopyon, optic disc edema, retinal vasculitis, and membranous vitreous opacities [35].
- Although the systemic morbidity is high, leptospiral uveitis carries good prognosis.

8.5.1 Management of Leptospiral Uveitis

Corticosteroids are the mainstay of treatment for leptospiral uveitis. The preferred mode of delivery depends upon the severity, laterality, and anatomical location of the inflammation [5, 26]. Severe anterior uveitis is treated with hourly topical corticosteroid eye drops, like prednisolone acetate 1 %, together with a cycloplegic/mydriatic eye drops. Patients with unilateral panuveitis will need a posterior sub-tenon depot-corticosteroids injection, such as triamcinolone acetonide, 40 mg, in addition to topical treatment. Bilateral panuveitis is treated with oral corticosteroids (0.5–1 mg/Kg body weight/day). It is not known whether the systemic antibiotic treatment during the systemic phase of illness has any protective role on long-term complications such as uveitis [5, 26].

8.5.2 Prognosis

Leptospiral uveitis carries a good prognosis. The inflammation is transient, and a complete resolution with restoration of vision is the commonly seen. Rapid maturation of cataract with phacolysis can rarely complicate the course. Steroids are useful to control the inflammation in such scenario, and cataract extractions followed by intraocular lens implantation carry an excellent prognosis [5, 26, 34].

Conclusion

Systemic leptospirosis is a globally distributed and highly transmissible zoonotic disease [4]. The typical systemic presentation of the disease is an acute biphasic febrile illness with or without jaundice. Uveitis is a late complication which can be treated with steroids. Leptospiral uveitis carries good visual prognosis.

References

1. Haake DA, Levett PN (2015) Leptospirosis in humans. Curr Top Microbiol Immunol 387:65–97
2. Goris MGA, Kikken V, Straetemans M, Alba S, Goeijenbier M, van Gorp ECM et al (2013) Towards the burden of human leptospirosis: duration of acute illness and occurrence of post-leptospirosis symptoms of patients in the Netherlands. PLoS ONE 8(10):e76549
3. Hartskeerl RA, Collares-Pereira M, Ellis WA (2011) Emergence, control and re-emerging leptospirosis: dynamics of infection in the changing world. Clin Microbiol Infect 17:494–501
4. Durski KN, Jancloes M, Chowdhary T, Bertherat E (2014) A global, multi-disciplinary, multi-sectorial initiative to combat leptospirosis: Global Leptospirosis Environmental Action Network (GLEAN). Int J Environ Res Public Health 11:6000–6008
5. Rathinam SR (2002) Ocular leptospirosis. Curr Opin Ophthalmol 13:381–386
6. Faine S, Adler B, Bolin C, Perolat P (1999) Leptospira and leptospirosis, 2nd edn. MediSci, Melbourne
7. Major A, Schweighauser A, Francey T (2014) Increasing incidence of canine leptospirosis in Switzerland. Int J Environ Res Public Health 11:7242–7260
8. Bandara M, Ananda M, Wickramage K, Berger E, Agampodi S (2014) Globalization of leptospirosis through travel and migration. Global Health 10:61
9. Victoriano AFB, Smythe LD, Gloriani-Barzaga N, Cavinta LL, Kasai T, Limpakarnjanarat K, Ong BL, Gongal G, Hall J, Coulombe CA, Yanagihara Y, Yoshida S, Adler B (2009) Leptospirosis in the Asia Pacific region. BMC Infect Dis 9:147
10. Cosson JF, Picardeau M, Mielcarek M, Tatard C, Chaval Y, Suputtamongkol Y, Buchy P, Jittapalapong S, Herbreteau V, Morand S (2014) Epidemiology of Leptospira transmitted by rodents in southeast Asia. PLoS Negl Trop Dis 8:e2902
11. Costa F, Ribeiro GS, Felzemburgh RDM, Santos N, Reis RB, Santos AC, Fraga DB, Araujo WN, Santana C, Childs JE, Reis MG, Ko AI (2014) Influence of household rat infestation on Leptospira transmission in the urban slum environment. PLoS Negl Trop Dis 8:e3338
12. Richard S, Oppliger A (2015) Zoonotic occupational diseases in forestry workers – Lyme borreliosis, tularemia and leptospirosis in Europe. Ann Agric Environ Med 22:43–50
13. Guerra MA (2013) Leptospirosis: public health perspectives. Biologicals 41:295–297
14. Dupouey J, Faucher B, Edouard S, Richet H, Kodjo A, Drancourt M, Davoust B (2014) Human leptospirosis: an emerging risk in Europe? Comp Immunol Microbiol Infect Dis 37:77–83
15. Desvars A, Michault A, Bourhy P (2013) Leptospirosis in the western Indian Ocean islands: what is known so far? Vet Res 44:80
16. Traxler RM, Callinan LS, Holman RC, Steiner C, Guerra MA (2014) Leptospirosis-associated hospitalizations, United States, 1998–2009. Emerg Infect Dis 20:1273
17. Yaita K, Suzuki T, Yoshimura Y, Tachikawa N (2013) Leptospirosis: a Japanese traveler returned from Laos. Intern Med 52:1439
18. WHO. Leptospirosis Burden Epidemiology Reference Group (LERG) [Internet]. WHO. [cited 2015 Apr 20]. Available from: http://www.who.int/zoonoses/diseases/lerg/en/
19. Priya CG, Bhavani K, Rathinam SR, Muthukkaruppan VR (2003) Identification and evaluation of LPS antigen for serodiagnosis of uveitis associated with leptospirosis. J Med Microbiol 52:667–673
20. Chassin C, Picardeau M, Goujon JM, Bourhy P, Quellard N, Darche S, Badell E, d'Andon MF, Winter N, Lacroix-Lamandé S, Buzoni-Gatel D, Vandewalle A, Werts C (2009) TLR4- and TLR2-mediated B cell responses control the clearance of the bacterial pathogen, leptospirainterrogans. J Immunol 183:2669–2677
21. Priya CG, Rathinam SR, Muthukkaruppan V (2008) Evidence for endotoxin as a causative factor for leptospiral uveitis in humans. Invest Ophthalmol Vis Sci 49:5419–5424
22. Wilson MR, Naccache SN, Samayoa E, Biagtan M, Bashir H, Yu G, Salamat SM, Somasekar S, Federman S, Miller S, Sokolic R, Garabedian E, Candotti F, Buckley RH, Reed KD, Meyer TL, Seroogy CM, Galloway R, Henderson SL, Gern JE, DeRisi JL, Chiu CY (2014) Actionable diagnosis of neuroleptospirosis by next-generation sequencing. N Engl J Med 370:2408–2417

23. Pushpakumara J, Prasath T, Samarajiwa G, Priyadarshani S, Perera N, Indrakumar J (2015) Myocarditis causing severe heart failure – an unusual early manifestation of leptospirosis: a case report. BMC Res Notes 8:80
24. Alian S, Taghipour M, Sharifian R, Fereydouni MA (2014) Cavernous sinus thrombosis syndrome and brainstem involvement in patient with leptospirosis: two rare complications of leptospirosis. J Res Med Sci 19:907–910
25. Conroy AL, Gélvez M, Hawkes M, Rajwans N, Liles WC, Villar-Centeno LA, Kain KC (2014) Host biomarkers distinguish dengue from leptospirosis in Colombia: a case-control study. BMC Infect Dis 14:35
26. Rathinam SR, Rathnam S, Selvaraj S, Dean D, Nozik RA, Namperumalsamy P (1997) Uveitis associated with an epidemic outbreak of leptospirosis. Am J Ophthalmol 124:71–79
27. Picardeau M, Bertherat E, Jancloes M, Skouloudis AN, Durski K, Hartskeerl RA (2014) Rapid tests for diagnosis of leptospirosis: current tools and emerging technologies. Diagn Microbiol Infect Dis 78:1–8
28. Wynwood SJ, Burns MA, Graham GC, Weier SL, McKay DB, Craig SB (2015) Validation of a microsphere immunoassay for serological leptospirosis diagnosis in human serum by comparison to the current gold standard. PLoS Negl Trop Dis 9:e0003636
29. Kannan A, Priya CG, Prajna L, Rathinam SR (2012) Efficiency of two commercial kits in serodiagnosis of leptospiral uveitis. Indian J Med Microbiol 30:418–422
30. Ressner RA, Griffith ME, Beckius ML, Pimentel G, Miller RS, Mende K, Fraser SL, Galloway RL, Hospenthal DR, Murray CK (2008) Antimicrobial susceptibilities of geographically diverse clinical human isolates of Leptospira. Antimicrob Agents Chemother 52:2750–2754
31. Vanasco NB, Schmeling MF, Lottersberger J, Costa F, Ko AI, Tarabla HD (2008) Clinical characteristics and risk factors of human leptospirosis in Argentina (1999–2005). Acta Trop 107:255–258
32. Verma A, Stevenson B (2012) Leptospiral uveitis – there is more to it than meets the eye! Zoonoses Public Health 59:132–141
33. Duke-Elder S, Perkins ES (1966) System of ophthalmology: diseases of the uveal tract, vol IX. Hendry Kimpton, London, pp. 322–325
34. Rathinam SR, Namperumalsamy P, Cunningham ET (2000) Spontaneous cataract absorption in patients with leptospiral uveitis. Br J Ophthalmol 84:1135–1141
35. Rathinam SR, Vijayakumar B, Priya CG (2016) Visali Jeyaseelan Leptospiral uveitis: Usefulness of clinical signs as diagnostic predictors. Ocul Immunol Inflamm 6:1–8. [Epub ahead of print] PMID: 27598430 DOI: 10.1080/09273948.2016.1217341

9 Other Bacterial Infections: Vancomycin-Resistant *Enterococcus* (VRE), Methicillin-Resistant *Staphylococcus aureus* (MRSA)

Sarakshi Mahajan and Vishali Gupta

9.1 Introduction

Gram-positive bacteria are the most common causative organisms both for exogenous and endogenous endophthalmitis. In the Endophthalmitis Vitrectomy Study, 100 % of Gram-positive organisms were susceptible to vancomycin [1]. Thus, vancomycin is the most widely used glycopeptide antibiotic used for empiric coverage of Gram-positive organisms in endophthalmitis. Multidrug-resistant bacteria especially vancomycin-resistant *Enterococcus* (VRE) and methicillin-resistant *Staphylococcus aureus* (MRSA) are emerging as an increasing threat in ophthalmology with increasing reports of these organisms causing endophthalmitis [2–7]. Further, there are also reports of prophylactic use of vancomycin either in the irrigating solution or intracamerally during the cataract surgery that would possibly increase the chances of developing drug resistance [8–10]. The diagnosis and management of these rarer infections poses a major challenge as these infections closely resemble the infections caused by *Staphylococcus aureus* but do not respond to the standard treatment for endophthalmitis. One has to have a high index of suspicion for these infections that may present with endogenous or exogenous endophthalmitis associated with severe intraocular inflammation.

9.2 Epidemiology

The exogenous endophthalmitis due to VRE and MRSA is quite rare, and there are only isolated published case reports and few case series. The Gram-positive bacteria reported in Endophthalmitis Vitrectomy Study were all susceptible to vancomycin [1]. The reported incidence of MRSA-induced exogenous endophthalmitis has been reported to vary between 1.56% and 41% in different reported series (Table 9.1). A recent series reported a statistically significant increase in the trend toward microbial resistance against a variety of antibiotics including methicillin [6].

There is no series reporting the incidence of MRSA-related endogenous endophthalmitis. HoV et al. [13] have recently reported the largest series on eight patients with endogenous methicillin-resistant *S. aureus* who had a virulent disease course.

9.3 Pathophysiology

MRSA: These organisms may be present on the ocular surface, thus increasing the chances of acquiring infection. The culture swabs taken from the ocular surface of patients scheduled for

S. Mahajan, MBBS (✉) • V. Gupta, MD
Advanced Eye Centre, Post Graduate Institute of Medical Education and Research, Chandigarh, India

S.-P. Chee, M. Khairallah (eds.), *Emerging Infectious Uveitis*, DOI 10.1007/978-3-319-23416-8_9

Table 9.1 Incidence of MRSA-induced endophthalmitis

Study/country	Period of the study	Number of eyes	MRSA positivity
Das et al. [10] India	1991–1998	31	10/31 (32.3 %)
Chen and Adelman [3] Northeast United States	1988–2008	143	Nil
Major et al. [11] United States	1995–2008	32	13 (41 %)
Khera et al. [12] India	2005–2010	448	7/448 (1.56 %)

cataract surgery in Uganda showed 31.9 % (29/91) methicillin-resistant coagulase-negative *Staphylococcus* (MRS) and 27.6 % (8/29) methicillin-resistant *S. aureus* (MRSA), respectively. All Gram-positive bacterial isolates were sensitive to vancomycin [14].

Infections caused by methicillin-resistant *S. aureus* (MRSA) strains, in general, have been reported to be seen in health care (hospital-acquired MRSA [HA-MRSA]) as well as in the community-based setting (community-acquired MRSA [CA-MRSA]). The intraocular infections are mostly HA-MRSA. *S. aureus* has a tendency to develop resistance to methicillin due to the presence of penicillin-binding protein coded for by a mobile genetic element called methicillin-resistant gene. In the last few years, this gene has continued to evolve so that many MRSA strains are becoming resistant to several antibiotics including oxacillin, penicillin, and amoxicillin. Many antibiotic-resistant genes and toxins are bundled and get transferred together to be passed on to other bacteria that enhance the development of resistant strains of MRSA [14, 15].

VRS: Vancomycin is a very commonly used antibiotic against most Gram-positive bacteria including *Staphylococcus*, *Streptococcus*, as well as *Bacillus* species. In addition, it is also effective against methicillin-resistant coagulase-negative *Staphylococcus* and methicillin-resistant *Staphylococcus aureus* (MRSA) infections. Vancomycin is a glycoprotein that binds irreversibly to D-alanyl-D-alanine moieties of the N-acetylmuramic acid (NAM) and N-acetylglucosamine (NAG) peptides that inhibit the synthesis and cross-linking of the NAM/NAG polymers. These polymers form the backbone of the cell wall. The mechanism of acquiring vancomycin resistance includes conversion of D-Ala-D-Ala to the depsipeptide D-Ala-D-Lac or to D-Ala-D-Ser, which in turn results in altered cross-linkages in the peptidoglycans of the cell wall contributing to the development of resistance to vancomycin [16].

9.4 Clinical Symptoms

9.4.1 Ocular

1. Acute onset: The onset is acute with majority of patients presenting within 1 week of the onset of infection.
2. Virulent course: The presenting visual acuity is reported to be poor with majority of patients presenting with LP vision alone [12] (Figs. 9.1, 9.2 and 9.3).
3. Predisposing risk factors: The patients may give history of trauma or surgery in case of exogenous and history of hospitalization, parental therapy, indwelling catheter, intravenous drug abuse, and some focus of infection in case of endogenous endophthalmitis.

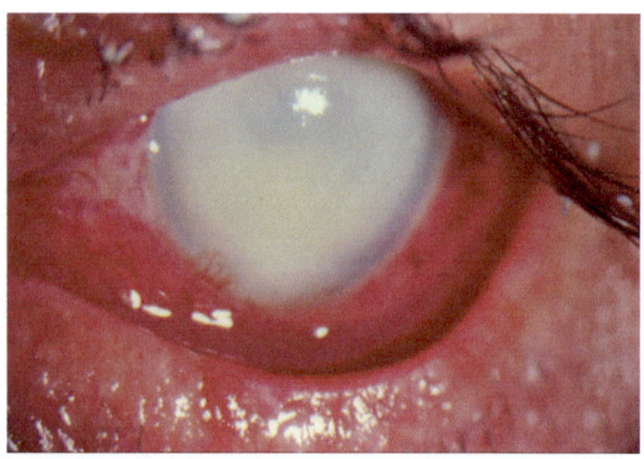

Fig. 9.1 (Patient #1): Anterior segment photograph of the right eye of a patient following extracapsular cataract extraction 4 days ago. The patient developed fulminant endophthalmitis in the early postoperative period with corneal involvement, and culture showed MRSA

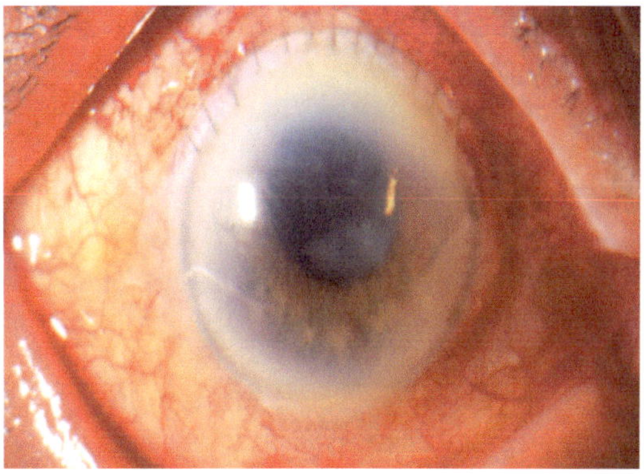

Fig. 9.2 (Patient #2): Fundus photograph of the right eye of a patient following complicated cataract surgery with IOL implant. The patient developed endophthalmitis with corneal infiltration at the section noticed 2 weeks after cataract surgery

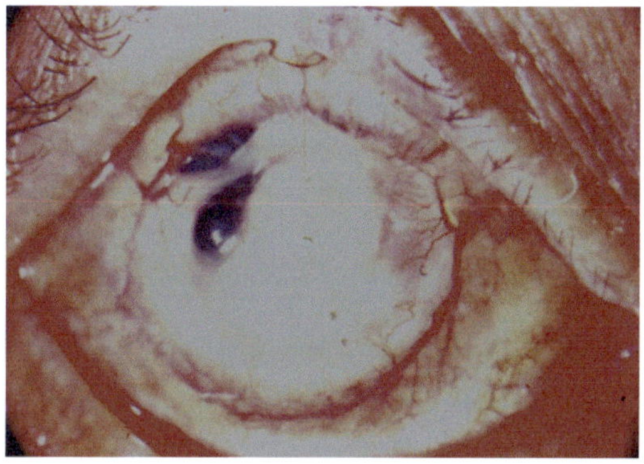

Fig. 9.3 (Patient # 2): Anterior segment photograph of the same patient as in Fig. 9.2, 6 weeks later showing no response to treatment received with total corneal infiltration. The cultures showed MRSA

In a short series by Ness and Schneider [9], all the three patients had predisposing factors including B cell lymphoma, steroid therapy, diabetes mellitus, or gastrointestinal symptoms.

4. Signs: The features that may help in differentiating endogenous endophthalmitis of infective variety like MRSA from noninfectious uveitis include the presence of lid edema, swelling, corneal infiltrates in some cases, exudates in the anterior chamber or vitreous cavity, and loss of red reflex in the infective variety.
5. Endogenous variety: Sometimes, patients with endogenous endophthalmitis may present with mild to moderate anterior segment inflammation, vitreous haze, and retinitis [17].
6. Systemic: The systemic features of these infections are variable; however, formation of the pus is common, e.g., boils, abscesses, impetigo, etc.

9.5 Diagnosis

The most common factor causing the diagnostic delay is the lack of suspicion for these organisms and not testing for them because of the rarity of the infection. What makes the infection suspicious, as being caused by one of these organisms, is when there is worsening of infection despite adequate treatment.

For diagnosing MRSA, *S. aureus* is isolated and identified by standard microbiological techniques, and then these bacteria are cultured in the presence of methicillin; if *S. aureus* grows in the presence of methicillin, the bacteria are termed as MRSA.

Similarly, the definitive diagnosis of VRE is made when the enterococci grow in the culture media in the presence of vancomycin.

9.6 Differential Diagnosis

1. Severe panuveitis: The endogenous variety of endophthalmitis may be mistaken for severe panuveitis especially when the appropriate history is not available. The patients affected with infections from one of these organisms tend to have poorer vision, lid edema, yellow reflex from the fundus, more fulminant course, and poor or no response to therapy.
2. Endogenous fungal endophthalmitis: Endogenous endophthalmitis due to fungus has more chronic, smoldering course, and fungal hyphae can be detected by smear examination of the smear from intraocular fluids.

9.7 Management

1. History of risk factors: These patients need a detailed history including demography, history of trauma, surgery, duration of symptoms, or any risk factor in case of endogenous infections like history of admission to the hospital, intravenous fluid administration, indwelling catheter, immunosuppression, intravenous drug abuse, etc.
2. Ocular examination: The examination should include visual acuity, presence of hypopyon, vitreous haze, and media clarity. In case the media haze, the ultrasonography should be done to look for the presence of vitreous membranes and to rule out retinal detachment.
3. Surgical management: These patients generally have a severe infection and poor visual acuity at presentation and would need pars plana vitrectomy. The undiluted vitreous sample should be sent for smears, PCR, and cultures along with antibiotic sensitivity testing. The diagnosis can be established by doing culture sensitivity test.
4. Medical management: Once the diagnosis is established, the next step is to choose an antibiotic that the organism would be sensitive to. Various antibiotics including linezolid, daptomycin, quinupristin-dalfopristin, and tigecycline have been used to treat systemic infections caused by vancomycin-resistant bacteria, but there are no recommendations for the systemic use of these antibiotics in endophthalmitis patients. However, a recent study has shown that the intravenous administration of daptomycin could achieve therapeutic intravitreal concentration greater than minimum inhibitory concentration for MRSA [16]. Daptomycin is a lipopeptide that binds to the bacterial cytoplasmic membrane resulting in the release of intracellular ions with concentration-dependent depolarization of cytoplasmic membrane and cell death and is effective against vancomycin-resistant strains of bacteria accounting for endophthalmitis, including *S. epidermidis*, *S. aureus*, *S. pneumoniae*, *E. faecalis*, and *E. faecium* [18]. In an animal study, daptomycin was found to safe by intravitreal injection given in the dose of 200 μg in adult belted rabbits and was reported to kill 99.9 % of the Gram-positive bacteria within a duration of 6–8 hours [19]. Buzzacco and Carroll [20] have reported the successful use of single injection of intravitreal daptomycin (200 ug/0.1 mL) in a patient with bilateral endogenous endophthalmitis. Their patient also received intravenous daptomycin for her endocarditis. The bactericidal activity of daptomycin with good intravitreal concentration following systemic administration and safe intravitreal administration makes it a drug of choice to be tried in patients infected with resistant organisms. In addition, early pars plana vitrectomy would be advisable.

9.8 Prognosis

The prognosis of exogenous endophthalmitis is poor mainly because of the lack of suspicion causing delay in the diagnosis, and the disease keeps progressing in the meantime, as the usual antibiotics have no effect on these organisms. In the series published by Khera et al. [12] reporting seven patients with vancomycin-resistant endophthalmitis, the favorable outcome could be achieved only in one patient (14.3 %). Five eyes went into phthisis, while one patient achieved counting fingers at 1 m.

Major et al. [11] reported significantly worse prognosis with MRSA compared to methicillin-sensitive *S. aureus* (MSSA) with a final visual acuity of 20/400 or better seen in 59 % of MSSA compared to 36 % of MRSA patients at the end of 3 months.

In the largest series reported by Ho et al. [13] on the endogenous MRSA infections in seven patients (eight eyes), five of the eight eyes showed improvement in visual acuity from presentation and only one eye required enucleation. The risk of retinal detachment was high with six of eight eyes showing development of retinal detachment.

Conclusions

Methicillin and vancomycin resistance among Gram-positive isolates, though rare, is an emerging problem. One has to keep these resistant strains in mind especially when the patients are not responding to the usual treatment. There is a need for ongoing surveillance and periodic reporting from the laboratories so that the magnitude of antibiotic resistance can be accessed.

Core Message

Methicillin and vancomycin resistance among Gram-positive isolates, though rare, is an emerging problem and should be considered in patients not responding to usual antibiotics.

References

1. Han DP, Wisniewski SR, Wilson LA, Barza M, Vine AK, Doft BH, Kelsey SF (1996) Spectrum and susceptibilities of microbiologic isolates in the Endophthalmitis Vitrectomy Study. Am J Ophthalmol 122:1–17
2. Bains HS, Weinberg DV, Feder RS, Noskin GA (2007) Postoperative vancomycin-resistant Enterococcus faecium endophthalmitis. Arch Ophthalmol 125: 1292–1293
3. Chen X, Adelman RA (2012) Microbial spectrum and resistance patterns in endophthalmitis: a 21-year (1988–2008) review in northeast United States. J Ocul Pharmacol Ther 28(4):329–334. doi:10.1089/jop.2011.0204 Epub 2012 Apr 16
4. Ness T (2010) Multiresistant bacteria in ophthalmology. Ophthalmologe 107(4):318–322. doi:10.1007/s00347-009-2076-0
5. Sharma S, Desai RU, Pass AB, Saffra NA (2010) Vancomycin-resistant enterococcal endophthalmitis. Arch Ophthalmol 128(6):794–795. doi:10.1001/archophthalmol.2010.77
6. Gentile RC, Shukla S, Shah M, Ritterband DC, Engelbert M, Davis A, Hu DN (2014) Microbiological spectrum and antibiotic sensitivity in endophthalmitis: a 25-year review. Ophthalmology 121(8):1634–1642. doi:10.1016/j.ophtha.2014.02.001 Epub 2014 Apr 2
7. Ness T, Schneider C (2009) Endogenous endophthalmitis caused by methicillin-resistant Staphylococcus aureus (MRSA). Retina 29(6):831–834. doi:10.1097/IAE.0b013e3181a3b7a1
8. Anijeet DR, Palimar P, Peckar CO (2010) Intracameral vancomycin following cataract surgery: an eleven-year study. Clin Ophthalmol 26:321–326
9. Sobaci G, Tuncer K, Taş A, Ozyurt M, Bayer A, Kutlu U (2003) The effect of intraoperative antibiotics in irrigating solutions on aqueous humor contamination and endophthalmitis after phacoemulsification surgery. Eur J Ophthalmol 13:773–778
10. Das T, Choudhury K, Sharma S, Jalali S, Nuthethi R (2001) Clinical profile and outcome in Bacillus endophthalmitis. Ophthalmology 108:1819–1825
11. Major JC Jr, Engelbert M, Flynn HW Jr et al (2010) Staphylococcus aureus endophthalmitis: antibiotic susceptibilities, methicillin resistance and clinical outcomes. Am J Ophthalmol 149:278–283
12. Khera M, Pathengay A, Jindal A et al (2013) Vancomycin-resistant Gram-positive bacterial endophthalmitis: epidemiology, treatment options and outcomes. J Ophthalmic Inflamm Infect 3:46. doi:10.1186/1869-5760-3-46
13. Ho V, Ho LY, Ranchord TM et al (2011) Endogenous methicillin-resistant Staphylococcus aureus endophthalmitis. Retina 32(3):596–601
14. Mshangila B, Kajumbula H, Paddy M et al (2013) External ocular surface bacterial isolates and their antimicrobial susceptibility patterns among preoperative cataract patients at Mulago National Hospital in Kampala, Uganda. BMC Ophthalmol 13:71
15. Gordon RJ, Lowy FD (2008) Pathogenesis of Methicillin-resistant Staphylococcus aureus infection. Clin Infect Dis 46:S350–S359
16. Bisicchia P, Bui NK, Aldridge C, Vollmer W, Devine KM (2011) Acquisition of VanB-type vancomycin resistance by Bacillus subtilis: the impact on gene expression, cell wall composition and morphology. Mol Microbiol 81:157–178
17. Rybak MJ, Hershberger E, Moldovan T, Grucz RG (2000) In vitro activities of daptomycin, vancomycin, linezolid, and quinupristin-dalfopristin against staphylococci and enterococci, including vancomycin-intermediate and resistant strains. Antimicrob Agents Chemother 44:1062–1066
18. Sheridan KR, Potoski BA, Shields RK, Nau GJ (2010) Presence of adequate intravitreal concentrations of daptomycin after systemic intravenous administration in a patient with endogenous endophthalmitis. Pharmacother 30(12):1247–1251
19. Comer GM, Miller JB, Schneider EW et al (2011) Intravitreal daptomycin: a safety and efficacy study. Retina 31(6):1199–1206
20. Buzzacco DM, Carroll P (2012) Intravitreal daptomycin in a case of bilateral endogenous endophthalmitis. Arch Ophthalmol 130:940

Part II

Emerging Viral Infections

10 Cytomegalovirus Anterior Uveitis

Soon-Phaik Chee and Aliza Jap

10.1 Introduction

Cytomegalovirus (CMV) infection is extremely common but often passes unnoticed in healthy individuals. However, it is a significant cause of morbidity in the immunocompromised and in neonates of infected mothers. As with most viruses, there is no vaccine against CMV, and as asymptomatic infected persons may continue to shed the virus in their secretions for prolonged periods, prevention of its spread is difficult, especially where there is social crowding.

S.-P. Chee (✉)
Singapore National Eye Centre,
11 Third Hospital Avenue, 168751 Singapore,
Singapore

Department of Ophthalmology, Yong Loo Lin School of Medicine, National University of Singapore,
1E Kent Ridge Road, Singapore 119228, Singapore

Duke-NUS Graduate Medical School,
8 College Road, Singapore 169857, Singapore

Singapore Eye Research Institute,
11 Third Hospital Avenue, Singapore 168751,
Singapore
e-mail: chee.soon.phaik@snec.com.sg

A. Jap
Singapore National Eye Centre,
11 Third Hospital Avenue, 168751 Singapore,
Singapore

Division of Ophthalmology, Changi General Hospital, 2 Simei Street 3,
Singapore 529889, Singapore

In congenital CMV and in immunocompromised individuals such as those with acquired immunodeficiency syndrome (AIDS) or solid organ transplant recipients, ocular CMV manifests primarily in the posterior segment as a retinitis and/or optic atrophy, with rare reports of concomitant anterior segment involvement [1–14], whereas in immunocompetent individuals, CMV affects mainly the anterior segment structures. This chapter will focus on CMV anterior uveitis in immunocompetent hosts.

10.2 Epidemiology

Humans are the only host for the human cytomegalovirus which is transmitted via various secretions including saliva, respiratory tract secretions, urine, semen, tears, and breast milk as well as through blood transfusions and transplacentally. It has been shown that CMV secreted in saliva can survive for up to 6 hours on wet highly absorbent surfaces [15]. Hence, it is easily transmitted via close contact especially among young children in day care centers, their carers, and their parents [16–21].

The overall prevalence of CMV in adults varies from 40 to 100 % with the highest prevalence in developing countries. In addition to place of birth, socioeconomic factors, ethnicity, and gender, its seroprevalence is also influenced by age [22–31]. The incidence of CMV disease in organ transplant patients is determined by a number of

S.-P. Chee, M. Khairallah (eds.), *Emerging Infectious Uveitis*, DOI 10.1007/978-3-319-23416-8_10

factors including the use of preventive measures such as prophylatic or preemptive ganciclovir or valganciclovir, donor and recipient serostatus, and nature of the organ transplant. In relation to solid organ transplants, the highest risk of infection and disease occurs in seropositive donor and seronegative recipient pairs where the immunosuppressed recipient is most vulnerable to the latent virus transmitted in the graft. On the contrary, in the case of hematopoietic stem cell transplants, a seropositive recipient has a greater likelihood of morbidity especially if the graft is obtained from a HLA-mismatched or non-related donor, and a seropositive donor may possibly confer a certain amount of immunity to the recipient. Among solid organ transplants, lung transplants have the highest incidence of CMV disease of 15 %, while in hematopoietic stem cell transplants, it is about 5 % [9, 32–40]. Among human immunodeficiency virus (HIV)-positive individuals, the prevalence of CMV ranges from 5 to 85 % and is negatively correlated with CD4 cell counts and highly active antiretroviral therapy (HAART), with about one third developing CMV retinitis [4, 41–50]. The prevalence of congenital CMV is estimated to be between 0.04 % and 6 %, with primary maternal infection being a more common source of transmission than recurrent maternal infection [51–56]. Nonetheless non-primary maternal infection is responsible for a larger proportion of cases of congenital CMV especially in countries with a high seroprevalence.

The prevalence of CMV anterior uveitis varies considerably from 0 to 80 %, depending on the criteria for aqueous analysis, the diagnostic tests used, as well as the population studied [57–87]. Of the 239 reported cases (235 patients) of CMV anterior uveitis, the majority was from Asian countries where there is higher prevalence of CMV, with only 46 (19.0 %) coming from non-Asian populations. There are very few systematic surveys of its prevalence in the eyes with anterior uveitis [57, 58, 60, 62, 63, 65, 71–87]. The data suggest that there is higher prevalence of CMV anterior uveitis in populations with a high seroprevalence and that CMV is a common cause of acute recurrent hypertensive uveitis (44–77 %), regardless of population [58, 60, 62–64]. On the other hand, while CMV is a fairly common cause of hypertensive chronic anterior uveitis in most Asian populations with a prevalence of 40–80 % in Singapore and Korea, with South Indians having an exceptionally low rate of 2 % [57, 61, 64], it is on the whole rare (0.0–3.4 %) in Western populations [66–69]. However, the prevalence of CMV anterior uveitis may be further underestimated as most authors performed either polymerase chain reaction (PCR) for viral nucleic acid or ELISA for serum and intraocular antibody production and not both. The sensitivities and specificities of these tests will be discussed below.

10.3 Pathophysiology

Human CMV is also known as human herpes virus 5 and is a DNA virus belonging to the family *Herpesviridae*. In common with the other members of the herpes family, following a primary infection, it remains latent in various sites, the most important of which are the myeloid progenitor cells in the bone marrow. Recent studies show that instead of lying truly dormant, CMV maintains a state of apparent latency in immunocompetent individuals by active expression of gene products to evade the host's immune response among which CMV-specific CD4+ and CD8+ T cells are the most critical components. An imbalance between the viral load and the immune response such as occurs in HIV-infected individuals whose CD4/CD8 cell counts become depleted, hence, has the potential to result in clinically apparent reactivation. The manifestations are also more likely to be severe in the immunocompromised as CMV replicates fairly rapidly in these persons particularly in primary infections [88–93].

Similarly the occurrence of congenital CMV and its severity is a result of the interaction of multiple factors such as direct viral infection of the fetus and placenta and maternal immune response [94]. CMV has also been implicated in atherosclerotic-related diseases, possibly from a subclinical infection, where it may either have a direct effect on endothelial cell function or an indirect effect by inhibiting the tumor suppressor protein, p53, and hence permitting the proliferation of smooth muscle cells, as well as by activating inflammatory pathways which further contribute to formation of atherosclerotic plaques [95–103]. There are also studies which suggest that subclinical CMV infection plays a role in the pathogenesis of certain tumors. [104–106] As with atherosclerosis, whether it exerts an oncogenic effect directly by the expression of oncogenes or indirectly via a chronic inflammatory mechanism remains to be determined [107–109].

CMV retinitis is one of the most common opportunistic infections in patients with AIDS, and CMV anterior uveitis has increasingly been reported in immunocompetent individuals. Ocular CMV may be a result of viral invasion via the retinal vessels during viremia in immunosuppressed patients [110–112] or represent a reactivation from an ocular reservoir such as the retinal pigment epithelium or the uveal tract especially in immunocompetent individuals who are typically negative for CMV antigen and CMV IgM although they may be positive for CMV IgG [62, 71, 76, 80, 113].

As with systemic CMV, the spectrum of manifestations of ocular CMV in immunocompetent persons reflects an imbalance between viral load and host immune response as retinitis or endotheliitis tends to occur in patients who have received periocular or intravitreal corticosteroids and/or are diabetic, whereas the milder acute recurrent anterior uveitis tends to occur in younger healthy individuals [64, 114–123]. However, the ocular sites of CMV persistence remain to be definitely established [124–129].

10.4 Clinical Features

1. Systemic disease

(A) In immunocompetent individuals

Although primary CMV infection is extremely common in many parts of the world, it often passes unnoticed or causes at most a self-limiting mononucleosis-like syndrome of fever, lethargy, pharyngitis, lymphadenopathy, rash, and lymphocytosis [130]. Severe organ-specific disease is characteristically seen in immunocompromised individuals but has also been described following primary infection in the immunocompetent. The most common presentation is colitis, followed by neurological manifestations, hematological abnormalities, pneumonia, and myocarditis [131].

(B) In immunocompromised individuals

In severely immunocompromised individuals such as those with HIV infections or transplant recipients, reactivation or infection from a seropositive host usually results in multiple organ disease including the gastrointestinal tract and central nervous and respiratory systems and was an important cause of mortality in HIV-infected patients prior to the availability of HAART [132].

(C) Congenital CMV

As with primary infection in adults, congenital CMV is common, but symptomatic disease is relatively uncommon occurring in only 10 to 15 %. The most devastating complications of congenital CMV include intrauterine growth retardation, neurological deficits such as mental retardation, microcephaly, sensorineural hearing loss, and optic atrophy. Other manifestations of congenital CMV include hepatosplenomegaly and hematological abnormalities.

Even among infants who were asymptomatic, about 10 % eventually develop hearing loss later in life [1].

2. Ocular disease

(A) In immunocompromised individuals and congenital CMV

A comprehensive description of the manifestations of CMV retinitis which is the principal sign of ocular CMV in the immunocompromised and in congenital disease is beyond the scope of this chapter, but in brief, there are three main morphological variants of which one is a fulminant necrotizing retinitis with areas of retinal whitening which progressively enlarge along the retinal vessels to become confluent, with accompanying exudates and intraretinal hemorrhages. As the borders advance, the central areas may clear with atrophic changes giving rise to the characteristic brushfire appearance. A second variant consists of a more indolent granular retinitis, and lastly there is an extensive diffuse vasculitis or frosted branch angiitis. Optic atrophy has also been described possibly as a result of a vasculitis or neuritis. Rarely endothelial deposits and anterior chamber inflammation have also been reported [1–3, 5, 6, 10–14].

(B) In immunocompetent individuals

10.4.1 Anterior Uveitis

An anterior uveitis is the hallmark of CMV infection in immunocompetent individuals. It is usually unilateral and may manifest as an acute recurrent hypertensive uveitis or as a chronic uveitis associated with ocular hypertension [57, 58, 60–63, 65, 71–76, 78–85, 87].

(a) Acute recurrent uveitis

These patients tend to be younger (mean age of 37 years) than those with chronic anterior uveitis (mean age of 65 years) [64]. They present characteristically with episodic complaints of mild headache, blurring of vision, and seeing haloes. There is minimal conjunctival injection with corneal epithelial edema and elevated intraocular pressure (IOP). There are only few keratic precipitates (KPs) located inferiorly or paracentrally which may range from fine to large (Fig. 10.1a, b). Nodular endothelial lesions consisting of white nodular deposits with brown pigments and surrounding translucent halo may be seen in about a quarter of the eyes (Fig. 10.2) [64]. The anterior chamber activity is mild with less than 2+ cells. Diffuse or patchy iris atrophy may be seen but posterior synechiae is not a feature. These attacks are usually short-lived, and although the IOP is often in the 50s, it responds well to glaucoma medications. However, with repeated episodes, about 20 % may develop glaucomatous optic neuropathy (GON) [64].

(b) Chronic anterior uveitis

Similarly, there is only minimal injection and AC activity. The KPs may be pigmented and are more numerous and diffusely distributed ranging in size from fine stellate to mutton fat (Fig. 10.3). Nodular endothelial lesions may be present in about 60% of the eyes. The AC activity in these eyes is again mild, but diffuse iris atrophy is more common. The IOP is often elevated, but the mean of the highest IOP (33 to 39 mmHg) is

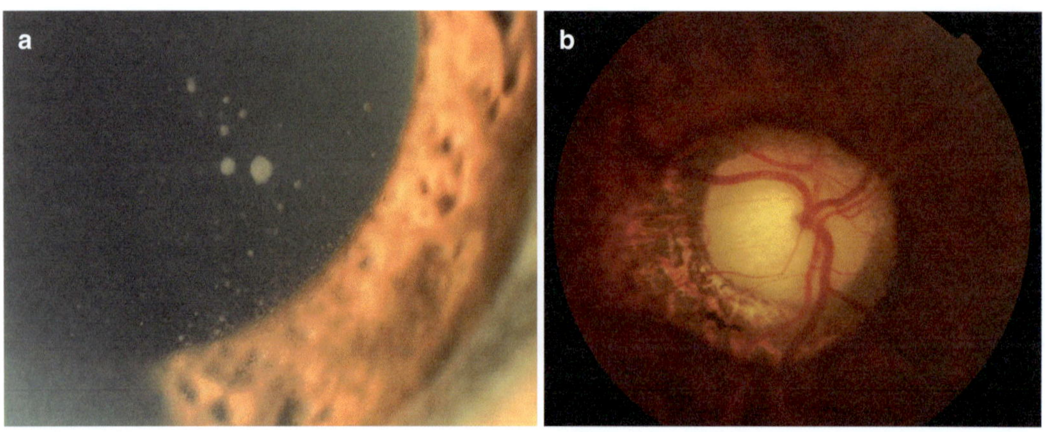

Fig. 10.1 (**a**) Slit lamp photograph of an eye with acute recurrent *Cytomegalovirus* anterior uveitis showing a few fine to large keratic precipitates with diffuse iris atrophy. (**b**) Fundal photograph of the same eye showing advanced cupping form repeated episodes of recurrences

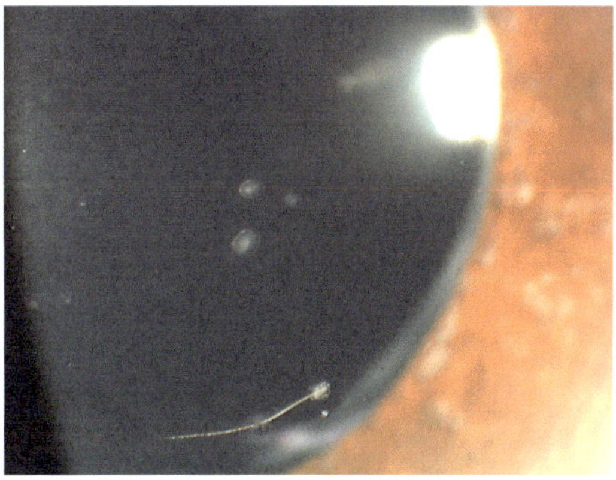

Fig. 10.2 Slit lamp photograph of another eye with acute recurrent *Cytomegalovirus* anterior uveitis showing nodular endothelial lesions

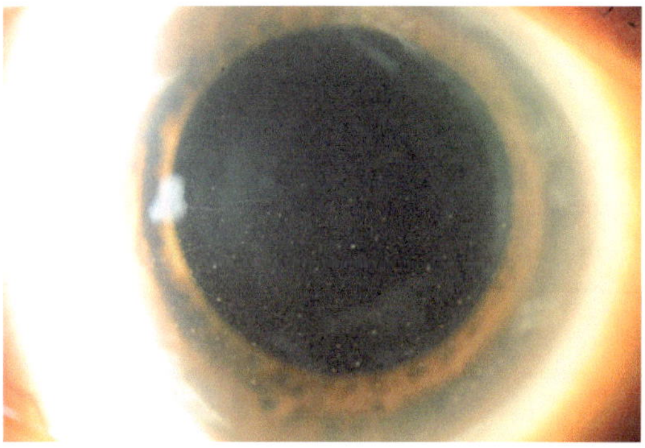

Fig. 10.3 Slit lamp photograph of an eye with chronic persistent *Cytomegalovirus* anterior uveitis showing diffuse fine- to medium-sized keratic precipitates

generally lower than in the acute form. Nonetheless 36 % of the eyes eventually developed GON [61, 64].

10.4.2 Complications of CMV Anterior Uveitis

The main causes of visual loss are GON, cataract, and corneal endothelial damage. However, there are few systematic analyses of their prevalence, and the wide variations in the definition of outcomes and patients may have had previous glaucoma or cataract surgery. Hence, it is difficult to derive their true prevalence.

Glaucoma as defined by the presence of GON or need for glaucoma surgery is estimated to vary from 12 to 60 % [62, 71–73, 78–82, 87, 133] and the prevalence of cataract at 14 to 60 % [71, 78–80].

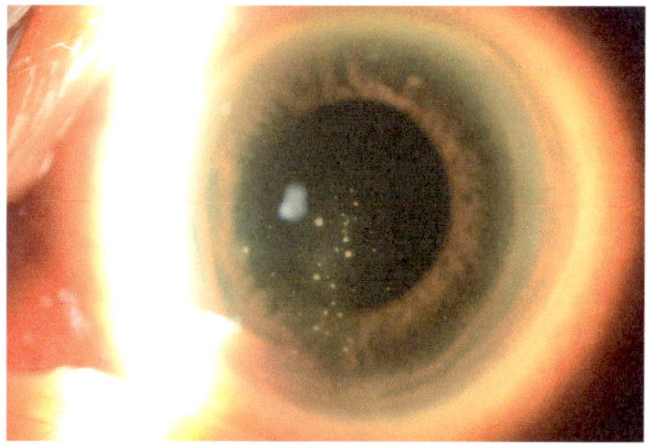

Fig. 10.4 Slit lamp photograph of an eye with chronic *Cytomegalovirus* anterior uveitis showing fine to large keratic precipitates with a small area of mild stromal edema

Some patients with CMV anterior segment infection present as a corneal endotheliitis with areas of stromal edema ranging from small localized lesions to diffuse edema (Fig. 10.4). Some of these patients were diagnosed during investigation for graft failure post-corneal transplant surgery, but some also had a history of previous hypertensive anterior uveitis. While small focal lesions may resolve with therapy, up to 63 % of eyes developed persistent diffuse edema causing visual loss despite medical therapy [75, 79, 87, 134–142]. Endothelial cell loss has been shown to occur in eyes with CMV anterior uveitis and is correlated with the viral load [81, 133]. Hence, the endothelial damage may be a consequence of repeated episodes of inflammation or related to the use of corticosteroids in some of these eyes [122, 123].

10.4.3 Posterior Uveitis

Although CMV predominantly affects the anterior segment in immunocompetent patients, there have been isolated case reports of retinitis. Although these patients were not HIV-positive nor transplant recipients, a significant number had received corticosteroids including periocular or intravitreal injections or corticosteroid implants or had associated systemic conditions which may impair the immune response such as diabetes mellitus. In contrast to HIV-infected patients with CMV retinitis, anterior chamber inflammation, vitritis, and vascular occlusion were common associated findings in the immunocompetent patients [114, 118–121].

Even more of an enigma was the development of an autoimmune retinopathy in a patient with recurrent CMV anterior uveitis. This otherwise healthy man had multiple relapses with oral valganciclovir and eventually required intravitreal ganciclovir implants for control. Although the anterior segment was quiet, he developed progressive retinal atrophy in the affected eye with constriction of visual fields and ablation of electroretinogram responses. Since the fellow eye was entirely normal, despite the presence of antiretinal autoantibodies in his serum, a retinal dystrophy or paraneoplastic retinopathy was felt to be unlikely cause of the changes [143].

A small case series suggest that posterior segment changes in eyes with CMV anterior uveitis may be more common than what was previously thought. Although none of the 11 patients in this series had retinitis, nine (82 %) had some form of retinal abnormalities including prolonged arm retinal time (mean of 25 seconds) on fundus fluorescein angiography (FFA) in all nine (100 %), disc swelling in three patients of which two were only evident on FFA, and macula edema in four eyes. Only one of the 11 patients, who had macula edema, had atherosclerotic risk factors including diabetes mellitus, hypertension, and hyperlipidemia. Therefore, these changes may be secondary to a subclinical CMV vasculitis [144].

10.5 Diagnosis

There are no clinical features that are pathognomic of CMV anterior uveitis, and the only diagnostic test available today that can distinguish it from an idiopathic hypertensive uveitis or that caused by other viruses is aqueous analysis using polymerase chain reaction (PCR) techniques for viral nucleic acid and/or intraocular antibody production as these patients are usually negative for sera CMV antigen and CMV IgM. Conventional stains or cytologic techniques require much larger volumes of fluid than what can be obtained via an aqueous tap, and the sensitivity of viral cultures is highly vulnerable to the condition of the specimen and contamination. Unfortunately even with PCR or intraocular antibody production techniques, a significant proportion of cases may be missed due to various reasons. Firstly, even with PCR, which enables the amplification of miniscule amounts of viral nucleic acid, the viral load in the limited volume of aqueous available may be below the detection limits of the test. Secondly, due to short-lived nature of the inflammation in eyes with acute recurrent disease, the detection of actively replicating virus may be subject to the timing of the tap. In addition, there is also data showing that there are differences in the load of viral antigen and viral antibody production between immunocompetent and immunocompromised patients [145–148]. Hence, these two tests complement each other and both should be done if available. In the series by Kongyai et al., the combination of antigen detection by PCR with the detection of a rise in the ratio of intraocular IgG to serum IgG of more than three (Goldmann-Witmer coefficient) resulted in a higher sensitivity than if only either had been done alone. Only 60 % of the cases would have detected using PCR alone, and using GWC alone would have detected only 70 % of the cases [65].

Although an aqueous tap is a relatively safe procedure with only rare reports of introduction of air into the anterior chamber, transient hyphema, wound leak, and localized lens damage, these tests are costly and not readily accessible [59, 149, 150]. Therefore, other diagnostic techniques such as confocal microscopy have been assessed as for their potential in aiding diagnosis as it has been able to demonstrate the presence of an "owl's eye sign," which represents CMV inclusion bodies, in eyes with corneal endotheliitis [151]. It has not been proven though to be sufficiently sensitive nor specific in its ability to differentiate between infectious and noninfectious cases of anterior uveitis [152–156].

10.6 Differential Diagnosis

10.6.1 Systemic Disease

The infectious mononucleosis-like syndrome characteristically results from infection by the Epstein-Barr virus where a lymphadenopathy is more common and the heterophile antibody is usually positive. However, a number of other viruses such as the human herpes virus 6, HIV, hepatitis virus, and rubella as well as other microbes including *Toxoplasma gondii* have also been implicated as causative organisms [157].

10.6.2 Ocular Disease

Hypertensive anterior uveitis may be idiopathic in origin as in the Posner-Schlossman syndrome and Fuchs' uveitis syndrome or be caused by other viruses including herpes simplex virus (HSV), varicella zoster virus (VZV), and rubella. Unless there are accompanying dermatological or corneal manifestations of HSV/VZV such as a vesicular rash or a disciform stromal keratitis or dendritic epitheliopathy, it remains difficult to distinguish between the various viruses as well as an idiopathic cause based on clinical features alone as there is considerable overlap of features with none that is pathognomic [64, 73, 158] (Table 10.1). For example, sector iris atrophy that was initially attributed solely to VZV was subsequently seen also in CMV and HSV infections [76, 113, 159]. Moreover skin lesions are absent in zoster sine herpete [160], and there is also a possibility of concomitant infection by two viruses [161].

Table 10.1 Comparison of clinical features of viral anterior uveitis

Clinical features	Rubella	HSV	VZV	CMV
Mean age at presentation (SD/range) years	35 (12)	43 (15) to 50 (range 15–83)	53 (23) to 61 (32–80	Acute – 37 (12) Chronic – 54 (17–79) to 65 (9)
Clinical course	Chronic 52/54 (96 %)	Acute 23/38 (61 %)	Acute 6/10 (60 %)	Acute recurrent 35/50 (70 %)
Keratic precipitates				Nodular endothelial lesions Acute recurrent – 9/35 (26 %) Chronic – 9/15 (60 %)
>2+ AC cells	8/56 (14 %)	21/39 (54 %)	2/10 (20 %)	
Fibrin formation	–	1/8 (13 %)	1/20 (5 %)	Nil
Iris changes				
Segmental/focal atrophy	3/54 (5.5 %)	1/8 (13 %) to 18/37 (48.6 %)	1/10 (10 %) to 8/20 (40 %)	Nil
Diffuse	8/54 (14.8 %)	3/37 (8.1 %) to 1/8 (13 %)	0 to 1/20 (5 %)	Acute 15/35(43 %) Chronic 6/18 (33 %) to 9/15 (60 %)
Iridoplegia			4/20 (20 %)	
Vitritis	45/55 (88 %)	10/23 (43 %)	5/6 (83 %)	Nil
Posterior synechiae	4/55 (7.3 %)	2/8 (25 %) to 14/37 (38 %)	6/20 (30 %) to 4/10 (40 %)	None to 1/18 (5 %)
Mean of maximum IOP (range)	–	30 (18–42)	35 (17–60)	Acute recurrent, 50 (28–80) Chronic, 35 (18–64) to 41(14–70)
IOP > 30 mmHg	13/53 (25 %)	18/39 (46 %)	5/10 (50 %)	Acute 34/35 (97 %) Chronic 8/14 (57 %)
Corneal changes				
Keratitis	2/56 (3.6 %)	Nil to 12/36 (33 %)	1/20 (5 %) to 2/10 (25 %)	Nil
Coin-shaped lesions				Chronic 2/18 (11 %)
Endotheliitis		2/8 (25 %)	4/20 (20 %)	1/18 (6 %)

Data from references [64, 73, 158]

10.7 Management

10.7.1 Antiviral Therapy

Ganciclovir, a guanosine analogue, was the main antiviral drug used in the management of systemic as well as CMV anterior uveitis. It is administered as an initial induction dose of 5 mg/kg/body weight twice daily for 2–3 weeks followed by oral ganciclovir maintenance. It may be given prophylactically or preemptively in transplant patients (Table 10.2). Valganciclovir, its prodrug, does not require an intravenous induction dose due to its significantly better bioavailability that has largely replaced systemic ganciclovir. It is given orally commencing with an induction dose of 900 mg twice daily for 2–4 weeks followed by maintenance dose 450 mg twice daily for 6 or more weeks according to the immune status of the patient and may be discontinued when this normalizes. In addition, in HIV-infected patients with CMV retinitis, it may also be administered as intravitreal injections of 2 mg/0.1 ml weekly or as an intravitreal implant containing 4.5 mg of the drug released over 5 to 8 months. Other antiviral options in the management of systemic CMV as well as CMV retinitis are foscarnet and cidofovir.

Table 10.2 Ganciclovir/valganciclovir regimes for treatment of viral anterior uveitis

Antiviral agents	CMV
Initial	*Ganciclovir* Intravenous 5 mg/kg/body weight twice daily for 2–3 weeks Intravitreal injections 2 mg/0.1 ml weekly for 12 weeks Intravitreal implant 4.5 mg slow release over 5 to 8 months (Vitrasert™ – not available) *Topical ganciclovir gel* 4 to 5 times daily for 12 weeks *Valganciclovir oral* 900 mg twice daily for 2–3 weeks
Maintenance	*Topical ganciclovir gel* 4–5 times daily tapered after 12 weeks to 3 times daily if quiescent *Valganciclovir* *Oral* 450 mg twice daily for 6 weeks

Systemic and intravitreal ganciclovir and oral valganciclovir have been used in a similar fashion to treat CMV anterior uveitis. Ganciclovir is also commercially available as a topical 0.15 % ophthalmic gel. However, the optimal therapeutic regime is uncertain as there are considerable variations in the baseline characteristics of patients, treatment duration, as well as endpoints of treatment. Generally, 75 % of treated patients respond to therapy with resolution of the inflammation within a month, but the relapse rate is also as high. Hence, most studies advocate long-term treatment. This however poses issues of costs as well as potential for severe adverse effects such as hematological abnormalities (neutropenia, thrombocytopenia, anemia), neurological (confusion, hallucinations), and gastrointestinal symptoms (abdominal pain, vomiting, diarrhea), among others. Topical ganciclovir gel, while it had a lower response rate of 67 %, has minimal adverse effects, is fairly well tolerated, and is less costly. A 2 % solution may be prepared from lyophilized ganciclovir and all treated eyes responded, with resolution of the AC inflammation and control of the IOP, and were negative for CMV on repeat taps. Relapse however similarly occurred upon stopping treatment [71, 72, 76–87, 133, 162].

10.7.2 Anti-inflammatory Agents

Most authors advocate adjunctive anti-inflammatory agents such as topical corticosteroids and/or nonsteroidal anti-inflammatory drugs in reducing the inflammation in eyes with anterior uveitis. However, corticosteroids should be used judiciously as there is concern that they may possibly potentiate the infection resulting in permanent endothelial damage as discussed above.

10.7.3 Glaucoma Management

Glaucomatous optic neuropathy is a major cause of visual loss in CMV anterior uveitis. Hence, IOP management is a vital component in their management. While there have been sporadic reports suggesting that the prostaglandin analogues may induce or potentiate a viral anterior uveitis, they are effective options if the IOP remains uncontrolled, with careful monitoring for any exacerbation of the inflammation. Pilocarpine on the other hand is contraindicated as it increases the blood-ocular permeability. Glaucoma surgery may be required in refractory cases or where there is progressive optic nerve damage.

10.8 Prognosis

The visual outcome of CMV anterior uveitis is not well studied as most authors examine mainly recurrences with few reports of visual acuity. The prevalence of the main causes of visual loss is also not well documented with considerable variations in the definition of glaucoma as well as the population analyzed. However, the inflammation in acute recurrent anterior uveitis is short-lived, and the attacks may be few and far between. Although the IOP is more refractory in chronic uveitis, it is less elevated than in the acute form, and hence central vision may be preserved in these eyes. In most studies, at least 80 % of eyes have 20/40 or better vision at the last visit. In a series by Hwang et al., 13 of 20 eyes had a final vision worse than 20/40, four of which were possibly due to GON [71, 76, 78, 79, 82, 87, 133, 162].

Conclusion

CMV anterior uveitis presents predominantly as a hypertensive uveitis and may be acute recurrent or chronic in its course. There are considerable similarities with other viral as well as idiopathic causes, and it can only be diagnosed by aqueous analysis for viral nucleic acid by PCR and/or intraocular antibody synthesis. While it responds to all formulations of ganciclovir/valganciclovir, the relapse rate is also high and long-term treatment may be required. Most patients achieve a good visual outcome unless they develop severe GON or corneal endothelial damage.

Core Message

Ocular CMV classically presents as a retinitis in immunocompromised individuals with rare instances of anterior segment involvement. On the other hand, in immunocompetent persons, CMV anterior uveitis is increasingly recognized as a cause of hypertensive uveitis especially in Asia. Hence, it is important to avoid the use of corticosteroids alone unless aqueous analysis can be performed to exclude a viral etiology.

References

1. Boppana SB, Ross SA, Fowler KB (2013) Congenital cytomegalovirus infection: clinical outcome. Clin Infect Dis 57(Suppl 4):S178–S181
2. Coats DK, Demmler GJ, Paysse EA, Du LT, Libby C (2000) Ophthalmologic findings in children with congenital cytomegalovirus infection. J AAPOS 4(2):110–116
3. Anderson KS, Amos CS, Boppana S, Pass R (1996) Ocular abnormalities in congenital cytomegalovirus infection. J Am Optom Assoc 67(5):273–278
4. Jabs DA (2011) Cytomegalovirus retinitis and the acquired immunodeficiency syndrome – bench to bedside: LXVII Edward Jackson Memorial Lecture. Am J Ophthalmol 151(2):198–216
5. Vendrell CP, Ramírez-Ronda CH (1994) Cytomegalovirus retinitis in AIDS patients: a clinical review. Bol Asoc Med P R 86(7–9):62–67
6. Drew WL (1992) Nonpulmonary manifestations of cytomegalovirus infection in immunocompromised patients. Clin Microbiol Rev 5(2):204–210 Review
7. Gupta PK, Patel NV, Patel SD, Patel KJ (2014) Cytomegalovirus retinitis in acquired immunodeficiency syndrome patients: a problem worth giving attention to. Indian J Sex Transm Dis 35(1):21–24
8. Sungkanuparph S, Chakriyanuyok T, Butthum B (2008) Antiretroviral therapy in AIDS patients with CMV disease: impact on the survival and long-term treatment outcome. J Infect 56(1):40–43
9. Jeon S, Lee WK, Lee Y, Lee DG, Lee JW (2012) Risk factors for cytomegalovirus retinitis in patients with cytomegalovirus viremia after hematopoietic stem cell transplantation. Ophthalmology 119(9):1892–1898
10. Cheng L, Rao NA, Keefe KS, Avila CP Jr, Macdonald JC, Freeman WR (1998) Cytomegalovirus iritis. Ophthalmic Surg Lasers 29(11):930–932
11. Daicker B (1988) Cytomegalovirus panuveitis with infection of corneo-trabecular endothelium in AIDS. Ophthalmologica 197(4):169–175

12. Walter KA, Coulter VL, Palay DA, Taravella MJ, Grossniklaus HE, Edelhauser HF (1996) Corneal endothelial deposits in patients with cytomegalovirus retinitis. Am J Ophthalmol 121(4):391–396
13. Mitchell SM, Barton K, Lightman S (1994) Corneal endothelial changes in cytomegalovirus retinitis. Eye (Lond) 8(Pt 1):41–43
14. Althaus C, Best J, Hintzmann A, Schimkat M, Hudde T, Cepin A, Sundmacher R (1996) Endothelial precipitates and laser flare photometry in patients with acquired immunodeficiency syndrome: a screening test for cytomegalovirus retinitis? Ger J Ophthalmol 5(6):443–448
15. Stowell JD, Forlin-Passoni D, Din E, Radford K, Brown D, White A, Bate SL, Dollard SC, Bialek SR, Cannon MJ, Schmid DS (2012) Cytomegalovirus survival on common environmental surfaces: opportunities for viral transmission. J Infect Dis 205(2):211–214
16. Pass RF, Hutto C, Lyon MD, Cloud G (1990) Increased rate of cytomegalovirus infection among day care center workers. Pediatr Infect Dis J 9(7):465–470
17. Pass RF, Hutto C, Ricks R, Cloud GA (1986) Increased rate of cytomegalovirus infection among parents of children attending day-care centers. N Engl J Med 314(22):1414–1418
18. Pass RF, Hutto SC, Reynolds DW, Polhill RB (1984) Increased frequency of cytomegalovirus infection in children in group day care. Pediatrics 74(1):121–126
19. Adler SP (1989) Cytomegalovirus and child day care. Evidence for an increased infection rate among day-care workers. N Engl J Med 321(19):1290–1296
20. Adler SP (1988) Molecular epidemiology of cytomegalovirus: viral transmission among children attending a day care center, their parents, and caretakers. J Pediatr 112(3):366–372
21. Taber LH, Frank AL, Yow MD, Bagley A (1985) Acquisition of cytomegaloviral infections in families with young children: a serological study. J Infect Dis 151(5):948–952
22. Cannon MJ, Schmid DS, Hyde TB (2010) Review of cytomegalovirus seroprevalence and demographic characteristics associated with infection. Rev Med Virol 20(4):202–213
23. Korndewal MJ, Mollema L, Tcherniaeva I, van der Klis F, Kroes AC, Oudesluys-Murphy AM, Vossen AC, de Melker HE (2015) Cytomegalovirus infection in the Netherlands: Seroprevalence, risk factors, and implications. J Clin Virol 63:53–58
24. Bate SL, Dollard SC, Cannon MJ (2010) Cytomegalovirus seroprevalence in the United States: the national health and nutrition examination surveys, 1988–2004. Clin Infect Dis 50(11):1439–1447
25. Tookey PA, Ades AE, Peckham CS (1992) Cytomegalovirus prevalence in pregnant women: the influence of parity. Arch Dis Child 67(7 Spec No):779–783.
26. Gratacap-Cavallier B, Bosson JL, Morand P, Dutertre N, Chanzy B, Jouk PS, Vandekerckhove C, Cart-Lamy P, Seigneurin JM (1998) Cytomegalovirus seroprevalence in French pregnant women: parity and place of birth as major predictive factors. Eur J Epidemiol 14(2):147–152
27. Varga M, Görög D, Kári D, Környei E, Kis É, Túryné HJ, Jankovics I, Péter A, Toronyi É, Sárváry E, Fazakas J, Reusz G (2011) Cytomegalovirus seroprevalence among solid organ donors in Hungary: correlations with age, gender, and blood group. Transplant Proc 43(4):1233–1235
28. Preiksaitis JK, Larke RP, Froese GJ (1988) Comparative seroepidemiology of cytomegalovirus infection in the Canadian Arctic and an urban center. J Med Virol 24(3):299–307
29. Wong A, Tan KH, Tee CS, Yeo GS (2000) Seroprevalence of cytomegalovirus, toxoplasma and parvovirus in pregnancy. Singapore Med J 41(4):151–155
30. Seale H, MacIntyre CR, Gidding HF, Backhouse JL, Dwyer DE, Gilbert L (2006) National serosurvey of cytomegalovirus in Australia. Clin Vaccine Immunol 13(11):1181–1184
31. Enders G, Daiminger A, Lindemann L, Knotek F, Bäder U, Exler S, Enders M (2012) Cytomegalovirus (CMV) seroprevalence in pregnant women, bone marrow donors and adolescents in Germany, 1996–2010. Med Microbiol Immunol 201(3):303–309
32. Ramanan P, Razonable RR (2013) Cytomegalovirus infections in solid organ transplantation: a review. Infect Chemother 45(3):260–271
33. George B, Pati N, Gilroy N, Ratnamohan M, Huang G, Kerridge I, Hertzberg M, Gottlieb D, Bradstock K (2010) Pre-transplant cytomegalovirus (CMV) serostatus remains the most important determinant of CMV reactivation after allogeneic hematopoietic stem cell transplantation in the era of surveillance and preemptive therapy. Transpl Infect Dis 12(4):322–329
34. Liu YC, Lu PL, Hsiao HH, Chang CS, Liu TC, Yang WC, Lin SF (2012) Cytomegalovirus infection and disease after allogeneic hematopoietic stem cell transplantation: experience in a center with a high seroprevalence of both CMV and hepatitis B virus. Ann Hematol 91(4):587–595
35. Razonable RR (2005) Epidemiology of cytomegalovirus disease in solid organ and hematopoietic stem cell transplant recipients. Am J Health Syst Pharm 62(8 Suppl 1):S7–13
36. Razonable RR (2005) Epidemiology of cytomegalovirus disease in solid organ and hematopoietic stem cell transplant recipients. Am J Health Syst Pharm 62(8 Suppl 1):S7–13
37. Schmidt-Hieber M, Labopin M, Beelen D, Volin L, Ehninger G, Finke J, Socié G, Schwerdtfeger R, Kröger N, Ganser A, Niederwieser D, Polge E, Blau

IW, Mohty M (2013) CMV serostatus still has an important prognostic impact in de novo acute leukemia patients after allogeneic stem cell transplantation: a report from the Acute Leukemia Working Party of EBMT. Blood 122(19):3359–3364
38. Ugarte-Torres A, Hoegh-Petersen M, Liu Y, Zhou F, Williamson TS, Quinlan D, Sy S, Roa L, Khan F, Fonseca K, Russell JA, Storek J (2011) Donor serostatus has an impact on cytomegalovirus-specific immunity, cytomegaloviral disease incidence, and survival in seropositive hematopoietic cell transplant recipients. Biol Blood Marrow Transplant 17(4):574–585
39. Boeckh M, Nichols WG (2004) The impact of cytomegalovirus serostatus of donor and recipient before hematopoietic stem cell transplantation in the era of antiviral prophylaxis and preemptive therapy. Blood 103(6):2003–2008
40. Ljungman P (2014) The role of cytomegalovirus serostatus on outcome of hematopoietic stem cell transplantation. Curr Opin Hematol 21(6):466–469
41. Fielding K, Koba A, Grant AD, Charalambous S, Day J, Spak C, Wald A, Huang ML, Corey L, Churchyard GJ (2011) Cytomegalovirus viremia as a risk factor for mortality prior to antiretroviral therapy among HIV-infected gold miners in South Africa. PLoS One 6(10):e25571
42. Deayton JR, Prof Sabin CA, Johnson MA, Emery VC, Wilson P, Griffiths PD (2004) Importance of cytomegalovirus viraemia in risk of disease progression and death in HIV-infected patients receiving highly active antiretroviral therapy. Lancet 363(9427):2116–2121
43. Weinberg A, Tierney C, Kendall MA, Bosch RJ, Patterson-Bartlett J, Erice A, Hirsch MS, Polsky B, AIDS Clinical Trials Group 360 Team (2006) Cytomegalovirus-specific immunity and protection against viremia and disease in HIV-infected patients in the era of highly active antiretroviral therapy. J Infect Dis 193(4):488–493
44. Micol R, Buchy P, Guerrier G, Duong V, Ferradini L, Dousset JP, Guerin PJ, Balkan S, Galimand J, Chanroeun H, Lortholary O, Rouzioux C, Fontanet A, Leruez-Ville M (2009) Prevalence, risk factors, and impact on outcome of cytomegalovirus replication in serum of Cambodian HIV-infected patients (2004–2007). J Acquir Immune Defic Syndr 51(4):486–491
45. Wohl DA, Kendall MA, Andersen J, Crumpacker C, Spector SA, Feinberg J, Alston-Smith B, Owens S, Chafey S, Marco M, Maxwell S, Lurain N, Jabs D, Benson C, Keiser P, Jacobson MA, A5030 Study Team (2009) Low rate of CMV end-organ disease in HIV-infected patients despite low CD4+ cell counts and CMV viremia: results of ACTG protocol A5030. HIV Clin Trials 10(3):143–152
46. Durier N, Ananworanich J, Apornpong T, Ubolyam S, Kerr SJ, Mahanontharit A, Ferradini L, Ruxrungtham K, Avihingsanon A (2013) Cytomegalovirus viremia in Thai HIV-infected patients on antiretroviral therapy: prevalence and associated mortality. Clin Infect Dis 57(1):147–155
47. Deayton JR, Wilson P, Sabin CA, Davey CC, Johnson MA, Emery VC, Griffiths PD (2000) Changes in the natural history of cytomegalovirus retinitis following the introduction of highly active antiretroviral therapy. AIDS 14(9):1163–1170
48. Lin DY, Warren JF, Lazzeroni LC, Wolitz RA, Mansour SE (2002) Cytomegalovirus retinitis after initiation of highly active antiretroviral therapy in HIV infected patients: natural history and clinical predictors. Retina 22(3):268–277
49. Sugar EA, Jabs DA, Ahuja A, Thorne JE, Danis RP, Meinert CL, Studies of the Ocular Complications of AIDS Research Group (2012) Incidence of cytomegalovirus retinitis in the era of highly active antiretroviral therapy. Am J Ophthalmol 153(6):1016–1024
50. Ford N, Shubber Z, Saranchuk P, Pathai S, Durier N, O'Brien DP, Mills EJ, Pascual F, Hoen E', Holland GN, Heiden D (2013) Burden of HIV-related cytomegalovirus retinitis in resource-limited settings: a systematic review. Clin Infect Dis 57(9):1351–1361
51. Ruffini E, Compagnoni L, Tubaldi L, Infriccioli G, Vianelli P, Genga R, Bonifazi V, Dieni A, Guerrini D, Basili G, Salvatori P, DeColli R, Leone L, Gesuita R (2014) Congenital and perinatal infections in the Marche region (Italy): an epidemiological study and differences between ethnic groups. Infez Med 22(3):213–221
52. Satilmiş A, Güra A, Ongun H, Mendilcioğlu I, Colak D, Oygür N (2007) CMV seroconversion in pregnants and the incidence of congenital CMV infection. Turk J Pediatr 49(1):30–36
53. Kenneson A, Cannon MJ (2007) Review and meta-analysis of the epidemiology of congenital cytomegalovirus (CMV) infection. Rev Med Virol 17(4): 253–276
54. Lanzieri TM, Dollard SC, Bialek SR, Grosse SD (2014) Systematic review of the birth prevalence of congenital cytomegalovirus infection in developing countries. Int J Infect Dis 22:44–48 Jul-Aug;17(4):253–276
55. Basha J, Iwasenko JM, Robertson P, Craig ME, Rawlinson WD (2014) Congenital cytomegalovirus infection is associated with high maternal socio-economic status and corresponding low maternal cytomegalovirus seropositivity. J Paediatr Child Health 50(5):368–372
56. de Vries JJ, van Zwet EW, Dekker FW, Kroes AC, Verkerk PH, Vossen AC (2013) The apparent paradox of maternal seropositivity as a risk factor for congenital cytomegalovirus infection: a population-based prediction model. Rev Med Virol 23(4):241–249
57. Babu K, Kini R, Philips M, Subbakrishna DK (2014) Clinical profile of isolated viral anterior uveitis in a South Indian patient population. Ocul Immunol Inflamm 22(5):356–359

58. Rodier-Bonifas C, Cornut PL, Billaud G, Lina B, Burillon C, Denis P (2011) Cytomegalovirus research using polymerase chain reaction in Posner-Schlossman syndrome. J Fr Ophtalmol 34(1):24–29
59. Anwar Z, Galor A, Albini TA, Miller D, Perez V, Davis JL (2013) The diagnostic utility of anterior chamber paracentesis with polymerase chain reaction in anterior uveitis. Am J Ophthalmol 155(5):781–786
60. Bloch-Michel E, Dussaix E, Cerqueti P, Patarin D (1987) Possible role of cytomegalovirus infection in the etiology of the Posner-Schlossman syndrome. Int Ophthalmol 11(2):95–96
61. Park SW, Yu HG (2013) Association of cytomegalovirus with idiopathic chronic anterior uveitis with ocular hypertension in Korean patients. Ocul Immunol Inflamm 21(3):192–196
62. Hedayatfar A, Chee SP (2014) Posner-Schlossman syndrome associated with cytomegalovirus infection: a case series from a non-endemic area. Int Ophthalmol 34(5):1123–1129
63. Kandori M, Miyazaki D, Yakura K, Komatsu N, Touge C, Ishikura R, Inoue Y (2013) Relationship between the number of cytomegalovirus in anterior chamber and severity of anterior segment inflammation. Jpn J Ophthalmol 57(6):497–502
64. Chee SP, Jap A (2008) Presumed Fuchs heterochromic iridocyclitis and Posner-Schlossman syndrome: comparison of cytomegalovirus-positive and negative eyes. Am J Ophthalmol 146(6):883–889
65. Kongyai N, Sirirungsi W, Pathanapitoon K, Tananuvat N, Kunavisarut P, Leechanachai P, de Groot-Mijnes JD, Rothova A (2012) Viral causes of unexplained anterior uveitis in Thailand. Eye (Lond) 26(4):529–534
66. Mitchell SM, Phylactou L, Fox JD, Kilpatrick MW, Murray PI (1996) The detection of herpesviral DNA in aqueous fluid samples from patients with Fuchs' heterochromic cyclitis. Ocul Immunol Inflamm 4(1):33–38
67. Cimino L, Aldigeri R, Parmeggiani M, Belloni L, Zotti CA, Fontana L, Invernizzi A, Salvarani C, Cappuccini L (2013) Searching for viral antibodies and genome in intraocular fluids of patients with Fuchs uveitis and non-infectious uveitis. Graefes Arch Clin Exp Ophthalmol 251(6):1607–1612
68. Stunf S, Petrovec M, Žigon N, Hawlina M, Kraut A, de Groot-Mijnes JD, Valentinčič NV (2012) High concordance of intraocular antibody synthesis against the rubella virus and Fuchs heterochromic uveitis syndrome in Slovenia. Mol Vis 18:2909–2914
69. Ruokonen PC, Metzner S, Ucer A, Torun N, Hofmann J, Pleyer U (2010) Intraocular antibody synthesis against rubella virus and other microorganisms in Fuchs' heterochromic cyclitis. Graefes Arch Clin Exp Ophthalmol 248(4):565–571
70. Babu K, Adiga M, Govekar SR, Kumar BR, Murthy KR (2013) Associations of Fuchs heterochromic iridocyclitis in a South Indian patient population. J Ophthalmic Inflamm Infect 3(1):14
71. Accorinti M, Gilardi M, Pirraglia MP, Amorelli GM, Nardella C, Abicca I, Pesci FR (2014) Cytomegalovirus anterior uveitis: long-term follow-up of immunocompetent patients. Graefes Arch Clin Exp Ophthalmol 252(11):1817–1824
72. Sobolewska B, Deuter C, Doycheva D, Zierhut M (2014) Long-term oral therapy with valganciclovir in patients with Posner-Schlossman syndrome. Graefes Arch Clin Exp Ophthalmol 252(1):117–124
73. Takase H, Kubono R, Terada Y, Imai A, Fukuda S, Tomita M, Miyanaga M, Kamoi K, Sugita S, Miyata K, Mochizuki M (2014) Comparison of the ocular characteristics of anterior uveitis caused by herpes simplex virus, varicella-zoster virus, and cytomegalovirus. Jpn J Ophthalmol 58(6):473–482
74. Woo JH, Lim WK, Ho SL, Teoh SC (2014) Characteristics of cytomegalovirus uveitis in immunocompetent patients. Ocul Immunol Inflamm 10:1–6
75. Yamauchi Y, Suzuki J, Sakai J, Sakamoto S, Iwasaki T, Usui M (2007) A case of hypertensive keratouveitis with endotheliitis associated with cytomegalovirus. Ocul Immunol Inflamm 15(5):399–401
76. Markomichelakis NN, Canakis C, Zafirakis P, Marakis T, Mallias I, Theodossiadis G (2002) Cytomegalovirus as a cause of anterior uveitis with sectoral iris atrophy. Ophthalmology 109(5): 879–882
77. Kawaguchi T, Sugita S, Shimizu N, Mochizuki M (2007) Kinetics of aqueous flare, intraocular pressure and virus-DNA copies in a patient with cytomegalovirus iridocyclitis without retinitis. Int Ophthalmol 27(6):383–386
78. Chee SP, Jap A (2010) Cytomegalovirus anterior uveitis: outcome of treatment. Br J Ophthalmol 94(12):1648–1652
79. Hwang YS, Shen CR, Chang SH, Lai CC, Liu CL, Chen KJ, Lin KK, Chen TL, Hsiao CH (2011) The validity of clinical feature profiles for cytomegaloviral anterior segment infection. Graefes Arch Clin Exp Ophthalmol 249(1):103–110
80. van Boxtel LA, van der Lelij A, van der Meer J, Los LI (2007) Cytomegalovirus as a cause of anterior uveitis in immunocompetent patients. Ophthalmology 114(7):1358–1362
81. Miyanaga M, Sugita S, Shimizu N, Morio T, Miyata K, Maruyama K, Kinoshita S, Mochizuki M (2010) A significant association of viral loads with corneal endothelial cell damage in cytomegalovirus anterior uveitis. Br J Ophthalmol 94(3):336–340
82. de Schryver I, Rozenberg F, Cassoux N, Michelson S, Kestelyn P, Lehoang P, Davis JL, Bodaghi B (2006) Diagnosis and treatment of cytomegalovirus iridocyclitis without retinal necrosis. Br J Ophthalmol 90(7):852–855
83. Sira M, Murray PI (2007) Treatment of cytomegalovirus anterior uveitis with oral valaciclovir. Ocul Immunol Inflamm 15(1):31–32

84. Chung RS, Chua CN (2006) Intravitreal ganciclovir injections in aqueous cytomegalovirus DNA positive hypertensive iritis. Eye (Lond) 20(9):1080
85. Mietz H, Aisenbrey S, Ulrich Bartz-Schmidt K, Bamborschke S, Krieglstein GK (2000) Ganciclovir for the treatment of anterior uveitis. Graefes Arch Clin Exp Ophthalmol 238(11):905–909
86. Hart WM Jr, Reed CA, Freedman HL, Burde RM (1978) Cytomegalovirus in juvenile iridocyclitis. Am J Ophthalmol 86(3):329–331
87. Wong VW, Chan CK, Leung DY, Lai TY (2012) Long-term results of oral valganciclovir for treatment of anterior segment inflammation secondary to cytomegalovirus infection. Clin Ophthalmol 6:595–600
88. Mendelson M, Monard S, Sissons P, Sinclair J (1996) Detection of endogenous human cytomegalovirus in CD34+ bone marrow progenitors. J Gen Virol 77(Pt 12):3099–3102
89. Sindre H, Tjøonnfjord GE, Rollag H, Ranneberg-Nilsen T, Veiby OP, Beck S, Degré M, Hestdal K (1996) Human cytomegalovirus suppression of and latency in early hematopoietic progenitor cells. Blood 88(12):4526–4533
90. Noriega V, Redmann V, Gardner T, Tortorella D (2012) Diverse immune evasion strategies by human cytomegalovirus. Immunol Res 54(1–3):140–151
91. Sinclair JH, Reeves MB (2013) Human cytomegalovirus manipulation of latently infected cells. Viruses 5(11):2803–2824
92. Griffiths P, Baraniak I, Reeves M (2015) The pathogenesis of human cytomegalovirus. J Pathol 235(2):288–297
93. Emery VC, Hassan-Walker AF, Burroughs AK, Griffiths PD (2002) Human cytomegalovirus (HCMV) replication dynamics in HCMV-naive and -experienced immunocompromised hosts. J Infect Dis 185(12):1723–1728
94. Schleiss MR (2011) Congenital cytomegalovirus infection: molecular mechanisms mediating viral pathogenesis. Infect Disord Drug Targets 11(5):449–465
95. Ji YN, An L, Zhan P, Chen XH (2012) Cytomegalovirus infection and coronary heart disease risk: a meta-analysis. Mol Biol Rep 39(6):6537–6546
96. Speir E, Modali R, Huang ES, Leon MB, Shawl F, Finkel T, Epstein SE (1994) Potential role of human cytomegalovirus and p53 interaction in coronary restenosis. Science 265(5170):391–394
97. Dengler TJ, Raftery MJ, Werle M, Zimmermann R, Schönrich G (2000) Cytomegalovirus infection of vascular cells induces expression of pro-inflammatory adhesion molecules by paracrine action of secreted interleukin-1beta. Transplantation 69(6):1160–1168
98. Rahbar A, Söderberg-Nauclér C (2005) Human cytomegalovirus infection of endothelial cells triggers platelet adhesion and aggregation. J Virol 79(4):2211–2220
99. Potena L, Valantine HA (2007) Cytomegalovirus-associated allograft rejection in heart transplant patients. Curr Opin Infect Dis 20:425–431
100. Melnick JL, Petrie BL, Dreesman GR, Burek J, McCollum CH, DeBakey ME (1983) Cytomegalovirus antigen within human arterial smooth muscle cells. Lancet 2:644–647
101. Adam E, Melnick JL, Probtsfield JL, Petrie BL, Burek J, Bailey KR, McCollum CH, DeBakey ME (1987) High levels of cytomegalovirus antibody in patients requiring vascular surgery for atherosclerosis. Lancet 2:291–293
102. Hendrix MG, Salimans MM, van Boven CP, Bruggeman CA (1990) High prevalence of latently present cytomegalovirus in arterial walls of patients suffering from grade III atherosclerosis. Am J Pathol 136:23–28
103. Burns LJ, Pooley JC, Walsh DJ, Vercellotti GM, Weber ML, Kovacs A (1999) Intercellular adhesion molecule-1 expression in endothelial cells is activated by cytomegalovirus immediate early proteins. Transplantation 67:137–144
104. Chen HP, Chan YJ (2014) The oncomodulatory role of human cytomegalovirus in colorectal cancer: implications for clinical trials. Front Oncol 4:314
105. Herbein G, Kumar A (2014) The oncogenic potential of human cytomegalovirus and breast cancer. Front Oncol 4:230
106. Jin J, Hu C, Wang P, Chen J, Wu T, Chen W, Ye L, Zhu G, Zhang L, Xue X, Shen X (2014) Latent infection of human cytomegalovirus is associated with the development of gastric cancer. Oncol Lett 8(2):898–904
107. Melnick M, Sedghizadeh PP, Allen CM, Jaskoll T (2012) Human cytomegalovirus and mucoepidermoid carcinoma of salivary glands: cell-specific localization of active viral and oncogenic signaling proteins is confirmatory of a causal relationship. Exp Mol Pathol 92(1):118–125
108. Barami K (2010) Oncomodulatory mechanisms of human cytomegalovirus in gliomas. J Clin Neurosci 17(7):819–823
109. Ranganathan P, Clark PA, Kuo JS, Salamat MS, Kalejta RF (2012) Significant association of multiple human cytomegalovirus genomic loci with glioblastoma multiforme samples. J Virol 86(2):854–864
110. Rao NA, Zhang J, Ishimoto S (1998) Role of retinal vascular endothelial cells in development of CMV retinitis. Trans Am Ophthalmol Soc 96:111–123
111. Zhang M, Xin H, Atherton SS (2005) Murine cytomegalovirus (MCMV) spreads to and replicates in the retina after endotoxin-induced disruption of the blood-retinal barrier of immunosuppressed BALB/c mice. J Neurovirol 11(4):365–375
112. Duan Y, Hernandez R, Pang L, Atherton SS (1996) Spread of murine cytomegalovirus to inner ocular structures following disruption of the blood-retina barrier in immunosuppressed BALB/c mice. Invest Ophthalmol Vis Sci 37(5):935–940

113. Chee SP, Bacsal K, Jap A, Se-Thoe SY, Cheng CL, Tan BH (2008) Clinical features of cytomegalovirus anterior uveitis in immunocompetent patients. Am J Ophthalmol 145(5):834–834
114. Takakura A, Tessler HH, Goldstein DA, Guex-Crosier Y, Chan CC, Brown DM, Thorne JE, Wang R, Cunningham ET Jr (2014) Viral retinitis following intraocular or periocular corticosteroid administration: a case series and comprehensive review of the literature. Ocul Immunol Inflamm 22(3):175–182
115. Zghal I, Malek I, Amel C, Soumaya O, Bouguila H, Nacef L (2013) Viral retinitis following intravitreal triamcinolone injection. J Fr Ophtalmol 36(7):e129–e132
116. Cho WB, Kim HC, Moon JW (2012) Spontaneous resolution of intravitreal steroid-induced bilateral cytomegalovirus retinitis. Korean J Ophthalmol 26(2):151–155
117. Van Damme E, Sauviller S, Lau B, Kesteleyn B, Griffiths P, Burroughs A, Emery V, Sinclair J, Van Loock M (2015) Glucocorticosteroids trigger reactivation of human cytomegalovirus from latently infected myeloid cells and increase the risk for HCMV infection in D+R+ liver transplant patients. J Gen Virol 96(Pt 1):131–143
118. Or C, Press N, Forooghian F (2013) Acute retinal necrosis secondary to cytomegalovirus following successful treatment of cytomegalovirus anterior uveitis in an immunocompetent adult. Can J Ophthalmol 48(2):e18–e20
119. Radwan A, Metzinger JL, Hinkle DM, Foster CS (2013) Cytomegalovirus retinitis in immunocompetent patients: case reports and literature review. Ocul Immunol Inflamm 21(4):324–328
120. Davis JL, Haft P, Hartley K (2013) Retinal arteriolar occlusions due to cytomegalovirus retinitis in elderly patients without HIV. J Ophthalmic Inflamm Infect 3(1):17
121. Gupta S, Vemulakonda GA, Suhler EB, Yeh S, Albini TA, Mandelcorn E, Flaxel CJ (2013) Cytomegalovirus retinitis in the absence of AIDS. Can J Ophthalmol 48(2):126–129
122. Sims JL, Chee SP (2010) Cytomegalovirus endotheliitis following fluocinolone acetonide (retisert) implant. Eye (Lond) 24(1):197–198
123. Park UC, Kim SJ, Yu HG (2011) Cytomegalovirus endotheliitis after fluocinolone acetonide (retisert) implant in a patient with Behçet uveitis. Ocul Immunol Inflamm 19(4):282–283
124. Zhang M, Xin H, Duan Y, Atherton SS (2005) Ocular reactivation of MCMV after immunosuppression of latently infected BALB/c mice. Invest Ophthalmol Vis Sci 46(1):252–258
125. Rabinovitch T, Oh JO, Minasi P (1990) In vivo reactivation of latent murine cytomegalovirus in the eye by immunosuppressive treatment. Invest Ophthalmol Vis Sci 31(4):657–663
126. Hayashi K, Kurihara I, Uchida Y (1985) Studies of ocular murine cytomegalovirus infection. Invest Ophthalmol Vis Sci 26(4):486–493
127. Bale JF Jr, O'Neil ME, Lyon B, Perlman S (1990) The pathogenesis of murine cytomegalovirus ocular infection. Anterior chamber inoculation. Invest Ophthalmol Vis Sci 31(8):1575–1581
128. Scholz M, Doerr HW, Cinatl J (2003) Human cytomegalovirus retinitis: pathogenicity, immune evasion and persistence. Trends Microbiol 11(4):171–178
129. Vogel JU, Fleckenstein C, Wagner M, Gümbel HO, Theegarten D, Cinatl J Jr, Doerr HW (2005) The human eye (retina): a site of persistent HCMV infection? Graefes Arch Clin Exp Ophthalmol 243(7):671–676
130. Cohen JI, Corey GR (1985) Cytomegalovirus infection in the normal host. Medicine (Baltimore) 64(2):100–114
131. Rafailidis PI, Mourtzoukou EG, Varbobitis IC, Falagas ME (2008) Severe cytomegalovirus infection in apparently immunocompetent patients: a systematic review. Virol J 5:47
132. Yust I, Fox Z, Burke M, Johnson A, Turner D, Mocroft A, Katlama C, Ledergerber B, Reiss P, Kirk O, EuroSIDA (2004) Retinal and extraocular cytomegalovirus end-organ disease in HIV-infected patients in Europe: a EuroSIDA study, 1994–2001. Eur J Clin Microbiol Infect Dis 23(7):550–559
133. Su CC, Hu FR, Wang TH, Huang JY, Yeh PT, Lin CP, Wang IJ (2014) Clinical outcomes in cytomegalovirus-positive Posner-Schlossman syndrome patients treated with topical ganciclovir therapy. Am J Ophthalmol 158(5):1024–1031
134. Zamir E, Stawell R, Jhanji V, Vajpayee RB (2011) Corneal endotheliitis triggered by cataract surgery in a Chinese patient with cytomegalovirus anterior uveitis. Clin Experiment Ophthalmol 39(9):913–915
135. Koizumi N, Inatomi T, Suzuki T, Shiraishi A, Ohashi Y, Kandori M, Miyazaki D, Inoue Y, Soma T, Nishida K, Takase H, Sugita S, Mochizuki M, Kinoshita S, Japan Corneal Endotheliitis Study Group (2015) Clinical features and management of cytomegalovirus corneal endotheliitis: analysis of 106 cases from the Japan corneal endotheliitis study. Br J Ophthalmol 99(1):54–58
136. Chee SP, Bacsal K, Jap A, Se-Thoe SY, Cheng CL, Tan BH (2007) Corneal endotheliitis associated with evidence of cytomegalovirus infection. Ophthalmology 114(4):798–803
137. Kandori M, Inoue T, Takamatsu F, Kojima Y, Hori Y, Maeda N, Tano Y (2010) Prevalence and features of keratitis with quantitative polymerase chain reaction positive for cytomegalovirus. Ophthalmology 117(2):216–222
138. Sonoyama H, Araki-Sasaki K, Osakabe Y et al (2010) Detection of cytomegalovirus DNA from cytomegalovirus corneal endotheliitis after penetrating keratoplasty. Cornea 29(6):683–685
139. Chu HY, Sun CC, Chuang WY, Liou SW, Ma DH, Lai CC, Hwang YS, Hsiao CH (2012) Cytomegalovirus associated corneal endotheliitis after penetrating keratoplasty in a patient with Fuchs corneal endothelial dystrophy. Br J Ophthalmol 96(2):300–301

140. Chu HY, Sun CC, Chuang WY, Liou SW, Ma DH, Lai CC, Hwang YS, Hsiao CH (2012) Cytomegalovirus associated corneal endotheliitis after penetrating keratoplasty in a patient with Fuchs corneal endothelial dystrophy. Br J Ophthalmol. 96(2): 300–301.
141. Chee SP, Jap A (2012) Treatment outcome and risk factors for visual loss in Cytomegalovirus endotheliitis. Graefes Arch Clin Exp Ophthalmol 250(3):383–389
142. Anshu A, Chee SP, Mehta JS, Tan DT (2009) Cytomegalovirus endotheliitis in Descemet's stripping endothelial keratoplasty. Ophthalmology 116(4):624–630
143. Cheung CM, Chee SP (2010) Anti-retinal autoantibodies-positive autoimmune retinopathy in cytomegalovirus-positive anterior uveitis. Br J Ophthalmol 94(3):380–381
144. Wong MH, Cheung GC, Chee SP (2014) Posterior segment findings of ocular cytomegalovirus infection in immunocompetent patients. Graefes Arch Clin Exp Ophthalmol 252(11):1811–1816
145. De Groot-Mijnes JD, Rothova A, Van Loon AM, Schuller M, Ten Dam-Van Loon NH, De Boer JH, Schuurman R, Weersink AJ (2006) Polymerase chain reaction and Goldmann-Witmer coefficient analysis are complimentary for the diagnosis of infectious uveitis. Am J Ophthalmol 141(2):313–318
146. Doornenbal P, Seerp Baarsma G, Quint WG, Kijlstra A, Rothbarth PH, Niesters HG (1996) Diagnostic assays in cytomegalovirus retinitis: detection of herpes virus by simultaneous application of the polymerase chain reaction and local antibody analysis on ocular fluid. Br J Ophthalmol 80(3):235–240
147. de Boer JH, Verhagen C, Bruinenberg M, Rothova A, de Jong PT, Baarsma GS, Van der Lelij A, Ooyman FM, Bollemeijer JG, Derhaag PJ, Kijlstra A (1996) Serologic and polymerase chain reaction analysis of intraocular fluids in the diagnosis of infectious uveitis. Am J Ophthalmol 121(6):650–658
148. Fardeau C, Romand S, Rao NA, Cassoux N, Bettembourg O, Thulliez P, Lehoang P (2002) Diagnosis of toxoplasmic retinochoroiditis with atypical clinical features. Am J Ophthalmol 134(2):196–203
149. Van der Lelij A, Rothova A (1997) Diagnostic anterior chamber paracentesis in uveitis: a safe procedure? Br J Ophthalmol 81(11):976–979
150. Cheung CM, Durrani OM, Murray PI (2004) The safety of anterior chamber paracentesis in patients with uveitis. Br J Ophthalmol 88(4):582–583
151. Shiraishi A, Hara Y, Takahashi M, Oka N, Yamaguchi M, Suzuki T, Uno T, Ohashi Y (2007) Demonstration of "owl's eye" morphology by confocal microscopy in a patient with presumed cytomegalovirus corneal endotheliitis. Am J Ophthalmol 143(4):715–717
152. Mahendradas P, Shetty R, Narayana KM, Shetty BK (2010) In vivo confocal microscopy of keratic precipitates in infectious versus noninfectious uveitis. Ophthalmology 117(2):373–380
153. Kanavi MR, Soheilian M, Yazdani S, Peyman GA (2010) Confocal scan features of keratic precipitates in Fuchs heterochromic iridocyclitis. Cornea 29(1):39–42
154. Kanavi MR, Soheilian M, Naghshgar N (2010) Confocal scan of keratic precipitates in uveitic eyes of various etiologies. Cornea 29(6):650–654
155. Fd O, Oliveira Motta AC, Muccioli C (2009) Corneal specular microscopy in infectious and noninfectious uveitis. Arq Bras Oftalmol 72(4):457–461
156. Mocan MC, Kadayifcilar S, Irkeç M (2012) In vivo confocal microscopic evaluation of keratic precipitates and endothelial morphology in Fuchs' uveitis syndrome. Eye(Lond) 26(1):119–125
157. Klemola E, Von Essen R, Henle G, Henle W (1970) Infectious-mononucleosis-like disease with negative heterophil agglutination test. Clinical features in relation to Epstein-Barr virus and cytomegalovirus antibodies. J Infect Dis 121(6):608–614
158. Wensing B, Relvas LM, Caspers LE, Valentincic NV, Stunf S, de Groot-Mijnes JD, Rothova A (2011) Comparison of rubella virus- and herpes virus-associated anterior uveitis: clinical manifestations and visual prognosis. Ophthalmology 118(10): 1905–1910
159. Van der Lelij A, Ooijman FM, Kijlstra A, Rothova A (2000) Anterior uveitis with sectoral iris atrophy in the absence of keratitis: a distinct clinical entity among herpetic eye diseases. Ophthalmology 107(6):1164–1170
160. Chen MJ, Chen KH, Chung YM, Li AF, Chou CK, Hsu WM (2006) Detection of varicella-zoster virus DNA in the iris of a zoster sine herpete patient. Int J Biomed Sci 2(3):302–304
161. Kasetsuwan N, Tangmonkongvoragul C (2013) Concomitant herpes simplex virus and cytomegalovirus endotheliitis in immunocompetent patient. BMJ Case Rep 9:2013
162. Hwang YS, Lin KK, Lee JS, Chang SH, Chen KJ, Lai CC, Huang JC, Kuo YH, Hsiao CH (2010) Intravitreal loading injection of ganciclovir with or without adjunctive oral valganciclovir for cytomegalovirus anterior uveitis. Graefes Arch Clin Exp Ophthalmol 248(2):263–269

11 West Nile Virus Infection

Nesrine Abroug, Bechir Jelliti, Salim Ben Yahia, and Moncef Khairallah

11.1 Introduction

The West Nile virus (WNV) is a single-stranded RNA arbovirus of the family *Flaviviridae* [1, 2]. It is the most widespread member of the Japanese encephalitis serocomplex [2]. The virus is transmitted among birds by mosquitoes (primarily the *Culex* species) which may pass the virus to humans and other vertebrates. Less common routes of transmission include blood transfusion [3], organ transplantation [4], transplacental transmission [5], laboratory transmission, and breastfeeding [6, 7]. WNV infection is often subclinical, but systemic disease may vary from mild febrile illness to severe neurologic disease [6]. Ocular involvement, typically self-limited multifocal chorioretinitis, is common in patients with WNV infection associated with neurologic disease. Diagnosis of WNV infection is usually based on clinical features and is confirmed by positive serologic testing. Prevention remains the mainstay of WNV infection control.

Financial disclosure: No financial interest for all authors.

N. Abroug • B. Jelliti • S. Ben Yahia
• M. Khairallah, MD (✉)
Department of Ophthalmology, Fattouma Bourguiba University Hospital, Faculty of Medicine, University of Monastir, 5019 Monastir, Tunisia
e-mail: moncef.khairallah@rns.tn; moncef.khairallah@yahoo.fr

11.2 Epidemiology

WNV, first identified in 1937 in the West Nile District of Uganda [1], was recognized as the etiologic agent of severe meningoencephalitis in 1957 in Israel [8]. Subsequently multiple sporadic cases and outbreaks occurred worldwide, throughout the 1950s–1980s [9, 10]. Since the mid-1990s, an apparent change in the WNV epidemiology was observed. Increasing frequency of severe WNV-related neuroinvasive disease in both humans and equines was reported with outbreaks in the Northern Africa, the Middle East, and Europe [9, 11–17]. After the initial North American outbreak in 1999 [18], WNV has spread rapidly throughout the Western Hemisphere, including the United States, Canada, Mexico, and the Caribbean, and into parts of Central and South America [10, 19]. In each of these outbreaks, mortality among patients with meningitis and encephalitis was approximately 10 % and occurred more often in elderly patients [6].

During 2014, 2122 cases of human WNV illness have been reported to the Centers for Disease Control and Prevention (CDC) in the United States and the District of Columbia. Of these, 1283 (60 %) were classified as neuroinvasive disease (such as meningitis or encephalitis), and 839 (40 %) were classified as non-neuroinvasive disease [20]. Most cases of WNV infection were caused by lineage 1 of the virus, whereas lineage 2 was involved in African enzootic strains [6].

S.-P. Chee, M. Khairallah (eds.), *Emerging Infectious Uveitis*, DOI 10.1007/978-3-319-23416-8_11

A recent new epidemiological scenario is the spread of lineage 2 strains across European and Mediterranean countries in regions where lineage 1 strain is still circulating creating favorable conditions for genetic reassortment and emergence of new strains [21].

11.3 Pathophysiology

The pathogenesis of WNV infection is complex and involves viral and host factors as well as antiviral immunity in the periphery and the CNS [7]. Following peripheral inoculation, initial WNV replication is thought to occur in skin Langerhans dendritic cells. These cells migrate to regional lymph nodes, where virus replication produces a primary viremia that seeds various peripheral organs and tissues, such as the spleen, liver, and kidneys. By the end of first week, WNV is largely cleared from the serum and peripheral organs, and infection of the CNS is observed in a subset of immunocompetent animals. WNV may enter the brain through a combination of mechanisms that facilitates viral neuroinvasion, such as direct infection with or without a breakdown of the blood-brain barrier, transport by infected immune cells that traffic to the CNS, and/or retrograde virus transport along peripheral nerve axons. The host's response to infection mediated by humoral and cellular immunity may also contribute to WNV pathogenesis, as demonstrated in animal models and extreme susceptibility to severe infection in persons with certain immunocompromising conditions [22].

The exact pathogenesis of WNV-associated chorioretinitis remains speculative. It is likely a combination of direct cell damage by WNV and secondary effects associated with inflammatory response to the virus. The route by which WNV reaches the eye also remains unknown. It may result from viral hematogenous dissemination to the choroidal circulation [6] or from a contiguous spread from CNS via the optic nerve fibers to the retina, retinal pigment epithelial, and choroid, as suggested by the typical linear clustering of chorioretinal lesions in parallel with the path of retinal nerve fibers [23]. Retinal vasculitis likely results from immune-mediated mechanisms associated with WNV infection.

11.4 Clinical Features

11.4.1 Systemic Disease

The peak onset of the disease occurs in late summer, but onset can occur anytime between July and December [6]. Following the incubation period which ranges from 3 to 14 days, systemic disease has three possible presentations: asymptomatic disease, West Nile fever, and meningoencephalitis. About 80 % of human infections are apparently asymptomatic. Only approximately 20 % of infected persons develop symptoms, with a self-limiting flu-like syndrome in most cases [2, 6]. Severe, potentially lethal, neurologic involvement can occur in less than 1 % of infected individuals [7]. It mainly includes aseptic meningitis and/or encephalitis characterized by rapid onset of headache, photophobia, back pain, confusion, and continued fever [22]. A poliomyelitis-like syndrome with asymmetric paralysis of acute onset and absent reflexes without pain and movement disorders such as tremor, myoclonus, and parkinsonism have been also reported [2, 6, 20, 24].

11.4.2 Ocular Disease

Since the first descriptions of ocular involvement secondary to WNV infection in 2002 and 2003, several ophthalmologic findings have been recognized, including chorioretinitis, retinitis, anterior uveitis, retinal vasculitis, optic neuropathy, and congenital chorioretinal scarring [6, 13, 25–48].

11.4.2.1 Chorioretinitis

A bilateral or rarely unilateral multifocal chorioretinitis, with typical clinical and fluorescein angiographic features, is the most common finding, occurring in almost 80 % of patients with acute WNV infection associated with neurologic illness [30]. Most patients are above 50 years in age, suffer from diabetes mellitus, and have no ocular symptoms or present with mildly reduced vision. An associated mild to moderate vitreous inflammation is frequently observed. The chorioretinal lesions commonly develop early in the course of the disease, appearing to be active (35 %) or already inactive (65 %) at presentation [30]. Active chorioretinal lesions appear as circular, deep, creamy lesions on ophthalmoscopy, with early hypofluorescence and late staining on fluorescein angiography [30] (Fig. 11.1a–c). Inactive chorioretinal lesions are typically partially atrophic and partially pigmented with a "target-like appearance": central hypofluorescence by blockage from pigment and peripheral hyperfluorescence on fluorescein angiography [30] (Fig. 11.2a, b). Some atrophic lesions are not pigmented. Chorioretinal lesions vary in number (from less than 20 to more than 50 per eye) and size (200–1500 μm), being distributed throughout the mid zone and/or periphery in almost all eyes. The posterior pole is involved in nearly 2/3 of eyes. Linear clustering of chorioretinal lesions is a

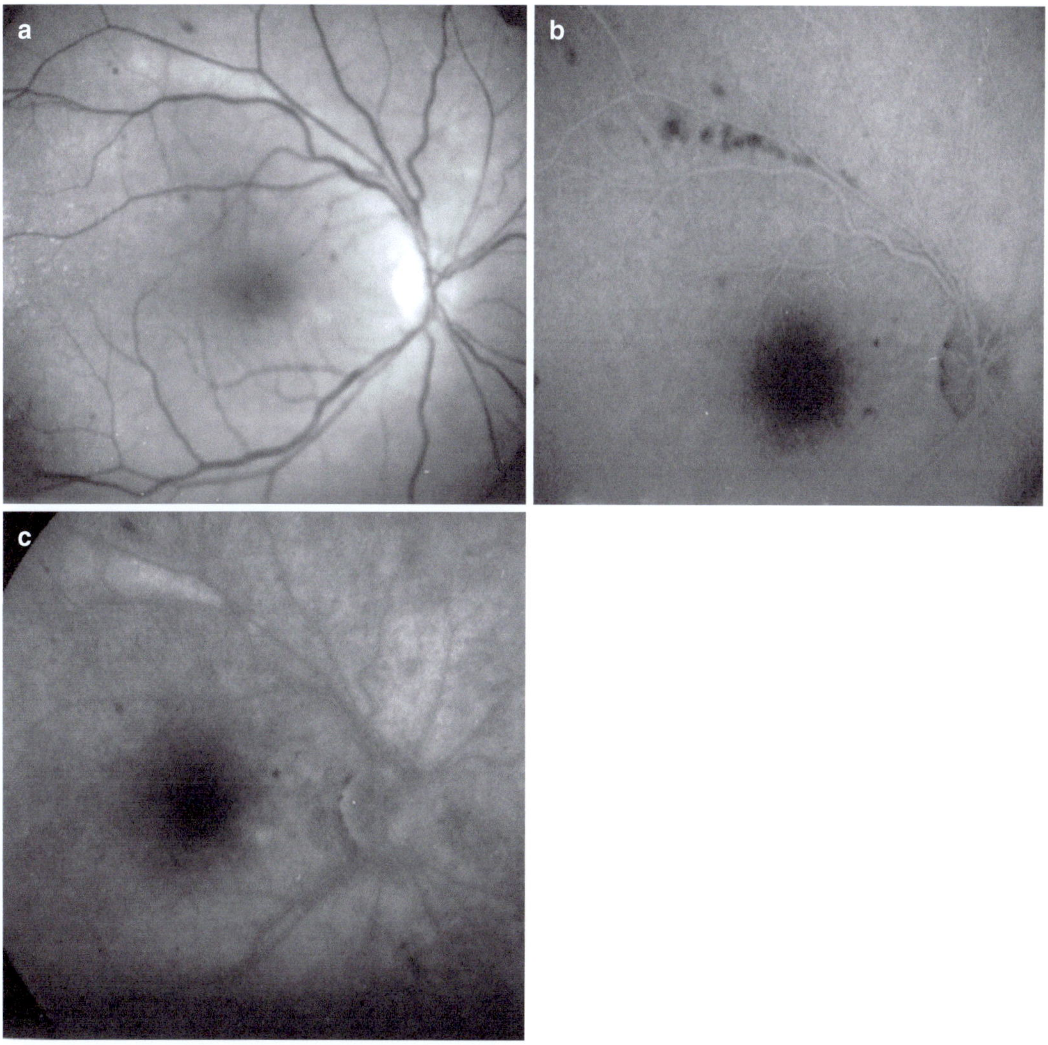

Fig. 11.1 (**a**) Red-free fundus photograph of the right eye of a diabetic 57-year-old woman with a recent history of WNV infection shows superotemporal linear clusterings of deep, chorioretinal lesions and associated faint intraretinal hemorrhages. Fluorescein angiography shows (**b**) early hypofluorescence and (**c**) late staining of the chorioretinal lesions

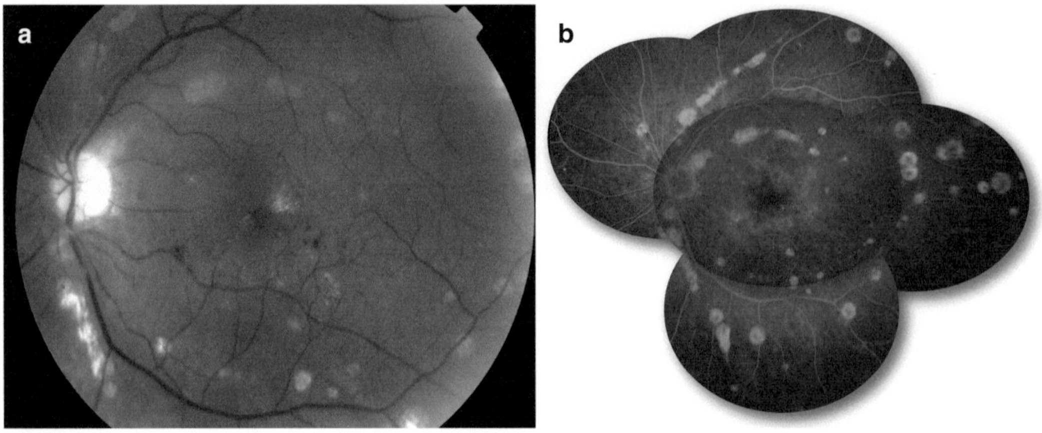

Fig. 11.2 (**a**) Red-free photograph of the left eye of a 64-year-old diabetic patient with serologically confirmed WNV infection shows multiple deep chorioretinal lesions, marked diffuse arterial sheathing, and diabetic macular edema. (**b**) Mid-phase fluorescein angiogram shows chorioretinal lesions with central hypofluorescence and peripheral hyperfluorescence and capillary leakage resulting from diabetic maculopathy. Several chorioretinal lesions extend superiorly and inferiorly in a linear pattern from the optic disc

prominent feature, occurring in more than 80 % of eyes with chorioretinitis. The streaks vary in number, from one to more than three per eye, and in length approximately from 2 to 15 mm [30]. They are typically oriented radially in the nasal and peripheral fundus or arranged in a curvilinear pattern in the temporal posterior fundus [30]. Indocyanine green angiography shows well-delineated hypofluorescent choroidal lesions, which are more numerous than those appreciated by fluorescein angiography or clinically [43].

Typical multifocal chorioretinitis, commonly associated with advanced age and/or diabetes, was found to be a specific marker of WNV infection, particularly in patients who present with meningoencephalitis [44, 49].

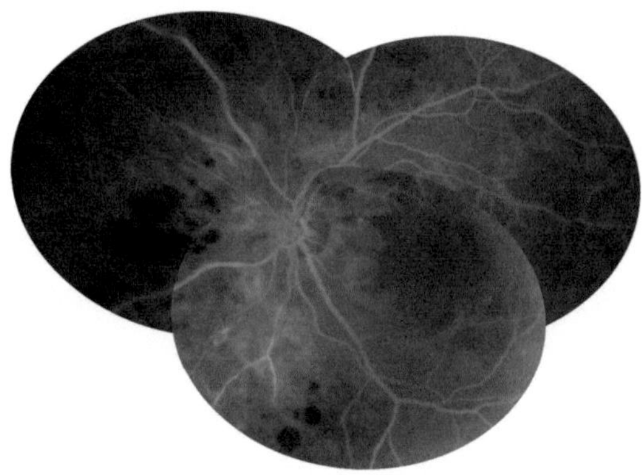

Fig. 11.3 Fluorescein angiogram of the left eye of a 62-year-old patient with serologically confirmed WNV infection shows retinal hemorrhages with extensive areas of retinal capillary non-perfusion suggestive of occlusive vasculitis

11.4.2.2 Other Ophthalmic Manifestations

Other ocular findings have been reported in association with WNV infection including iridocyclitis in the absence of chorioretinitis, retinitis, retinal hemorrhages, focal or diffuse vascular sheathing, vascular leakage, macular edema, occlusive vasculitis (Fig. 11.3), severe ischemic maculopathy, and segmental wedge-shaped zones of atrophy and mottling of the retinal pigment epithelium [29, 34, 37, 38, 48, 49]. WNV-associated optic nerve involvement may occur, including optic disc swelling, optic neuritis, neuroretinitis, papilledema (personal unpublished data), and optic disc staining on fluorescein angiography [29]. Other reported neuro-ophthalmic manifestations include ocular nerve palsy and nystagmus [29]. Congenital chorioretinal scarring secondary to intrauterine transmission of WNV infection has been reported [25].

11.5 Diagnosis

Diagnosis of WNV infection requires a high index of suspicion and specific laboratory testing. WNV should be strongly considered in patients who present with unexplained febrile illness, meningoencephalitis, or flaccid paralysis during mosquito season, particularly in endemic areas. The presence of mosquito bites on the skin will assist in diagnosis. The most common efficient diagnostic method is detection of WNV-specific IgM antibody in serum, cerebrospinal fluid, or both using the antibody-capture enzyme-linked immunosorbent assay (MAC-ELISA). This test is most accurate when performed within 8 to 21 days after the appearance of clinical symptoms [2, 24]. Since IgM antibody does not cross the blood-brain barrier, its presence in the cerebrospinal fluid strongly suggests infection of the central nervous system. Based on CDC guidelines (www.cdc.gov/ncidod/dvbid/westnile/resources/ wnvguidelines-aug-2003.pdf), the diagnosis of WNV meningoencephalitis is confirmed if the IgM from cerebrospinal fluid is positive for WNV. A fourfold or greater increase serum antibody titer in serum samples collected 2–3 weeks apart can also be used to make a diagnosis of WNV infection. Serum IgM antibody to WNV can persist for six months or longer after onset of illness. Flaviviruses may exhibit antigenic cross-reactivity; therefore persons, who have recently been vaccinated with yellow fever or Japanese encephalitis vaccines or have infections with related flaviviruses, may generate a false-positive result in the serum. The plaque-reduction neutralization test can help distinguish false-positive results of MAC-ELISA or other assays as well as to help to distinguish serologic cross-reactions among the flaviviruses [2, 20].

Recently, PCR-based detection systems for the rapid detection of WNV infection in clinical specimens that are negative for virus isolation have been reported, suggesting that nucleic acid-based assays hold great promise for the detection of WNV infection [42]. In addition, other PCR-based methods, including real-time PCR (RT-PCR), reverse transcription loop-mediated isothermal gene amplification (RT-LAMP) assay, and qRT-PCR, have been developed for the detection of WNV RNA [42, 50, 51].

Cerebrospinal fluid generally shows normal glucose, elevated protein, and pleocytosis (>5 leukocytes/μL) [20]. The unique pattern of multifocal chorioretinitis can help establish an early diagnosis of the disease while serologic testing is pending [49].

11.6 Differential Diagnosis

The differential diagnosis of WNV systemic disease include other arthropod-borne viral encephalitides, enteroviral aseptic meningitis, herpesvirus encephalitis, encephalopathy from systemic illnesses (Legionnaires' disease, rickettsiosis, Epstein-Barr virus infectious mononucleosis, and systemic lupus erythematosus), epidural abscess, hypertensive encephalopathy, and drug-induced meningitis. Many infectious and inflammatory conditions may present with chorioretinitis. The differential diagnosis includes syphilis, tuberculosis, histoplasmosis, sarcoidosis, and idiopathic multifocal chorioretinitis [6, 30]. WNV-associated chorioretinitis can be distinguished from these entities on the basis of history, systemic signs and symptoms, and particularly the unique pattern of chorioretinitis [30].

11.7 Management

There is, at present, no proven treatment for WNV infection. In cases of severe systemic disease, intensive supportive therapy is indicated, often involving hospitalization, intravenous fluids, respiratory support, prevention of secondary infections, and good nursing care [24].

Clinical trials of antiviral agents such as ribavirin interferon α -2b, interferon b, high-titer intravenous immunoglobulin, and pluripotent immunomodulator AS101 will allow new and more effective therapeutic approaches to emerge in future [52–54].

Passively transferring anti-WNV immunoglobulin has been shown to be effective in animal models and may be helpful in patients [7].

Specific ophthalmic treatment may be required: topical steroids for anterior uveitis, peripheral retinal photocoagulation for neovascularization due to occlusive vasculitis, pars plana vitrectomy for non-clearing vitreous hemorrhage or tractional retinal detachment, and intravitreal injection of anti-vasoendothelial growth factor (anti-VEGF) agent for choroidal neovascularization or macular edema [35, 55].

Prevention is the mainstay of WNV infection control: measures to reduce the number of mosquitoes (draining standing water, larvicides) and personal protection (repellents, window screen, protective clothing). Vaccination, a possible long-term solution, is still in the research phase [56, 57]. Although the cost-effectiveness of WNV vaccination is uncertain, vaccination of populations at risk of developing severe WNV infection may reduce the number of fatalities due to WNV.

11.8 Prognosis

Prognosis of WNV systemic disease is good in most patients. Full recovery is the norm for patients with uncomplicated West Nile fever or meningitis; however, initial symptoms, particularly extreme fatigue, may be prolonged [20]. However, severe cases may result in neurologic sequelae or death, especially in patients who are elderly or debilitated [7, 20]. Advanced age is the most important risk factor for death, ranging from 0.8 % among those aged less than 40 years to 17 % among those aged at least 70 years [20]. Encephalitis with severe muscle weakness, changes in the level of consciousness, diabetes, cardiovascular disease, hepatitis C virus infection, and immunosuppression are possible risk factors for death [20].

Ocular involvement usually has a self-limited course. Active chorioretinal lesions at presentation evolved to the typical inactive stage [6, 30]. Some inactive lesions become more prominent on both ophthalmoscopy and fluorescein angiography. Visual acuity returns to baseline in most patients [30]. However, persistent visual impairment may occur due to a foveal chorioretinal scar, choroidal neovascularization, complicated occlusive retinal vasculitis (vitreous hemorrhage secondary to retinal neovascularization, severe ischemic maculopathy), optic atrophy, or retrogeniculate damage [35, 37, 38]. Recently, one case of reactivation of WNV infection-related chorioretinitis has been reported [45].

Conclusion

WNV infection is among the most important emergent and resurgent infections that are tending to expand worldwide, mainly due to climate changes and globalization. Most frequently, systemic disease is subclinical or manifest as a mild febrile illness, but a severe, potentially lethal systemic involvement with neurologic disease also can occur. Chorioretinal involvement, frequently asymptomatic and self-limited, is the most common finding in patients with WNV infection associated with neurologic disease. The unique pattern of multifocal chorioretinitis can help establish an early diagnosis of the disease while serologic testing is pending. Therefore, an ocular examination, including ophthalmoscopy and fluorescein angiography in selected cases, should be part of the routine evaluation of patients with clinically suspected WNV infection.

Core Messages

- Systemic WNV disease: often subclinical, but may vary from mild febrile illness to very severe neurologic involvement
- Ocular disease: typical bilateral multifocal chorioretinitis with linear clustering of chorioretinal lesions, retinal vasculitis, anterior uveitis, optic neuropathy
- Fundus examination: useful diagnostic tool while serologic testing is pending in patients with suspected WNV neurologic disease
- Laboratory diagnosis: serology (WNV-specific IgM), real-time polymerase chain reaction (PCR)
- Management: mostly supportive

- Prognosis:
  - Systemic disease: usually good, but potentially lethal in patients who are elderly or debilitated
  - Ocular disease: usually self-limiting, rarely persistent visual loss
- Prevention: personal protection against tick bites, improvement of sanitary conditions

References

1. Smithburn KC, Hughes TP, Burke AW, Paul JH (1940) A neurotropic virus isolated from the blood of a native of Uganda. Am J Trop Med 20:471–492
2. Petersen LR, Marfin AA (2002) West Nile virus: a primer for the clinician. Ann Intern Med 137:173–179
3. Pealer LN, Marfin AA, Petersen LR, Lanciotti RS, Page PL, Stramer SL, Stobierski MG, Signs K, Newman B, Kapoor H, Goodman JL, Chamberland ME, West Nile Virus Transmission Investigation Team (2003) Transmission of West Nile virus through blood transfusion in the United States in 2002. N Engl J Med 349:1236–1245
4. Iwamoto M, Jernigan DB, Guasch A, Trepka MJ, Blackmore CG, Hellinger WC, Pham SM, Zaki S, Lanciotti RS, Lance-Parker SE, DiazGranados CA, Winquist AG, Perlino CA, Wiersma S, Hillyer KL, Goodman JL, Marfin AA, Chamberland ME, Petersen LR, West Nile Virus in Transplant Recipients Investigation Team (2003) Transmission of West Nile virus from an organ donor to four transplant recipients. N Engl J Med 348:2196–2203
5. Alpert SG, Fergerson J, Noël LP (2003) Intrauterine West Nile virus: ocular and systemic findings. Am J Ophthalmol 136:733–735
6. Garg S, Jampol LM (2005) Systemic and intraocular manifestations of West Nile virus infection. Surv Ophthalmol 50:3–13
7. Gyure KA (2009) West Nile virus infections. J Neuropathol Exp Neurol 68:1053–1060
8. Spigland I, Jasinska-Klingberg W, Hofsbi E, Goldblum N (1958) Clinical and laboratory observations in an outbreak of West Nile fever in Israel in 1957. Harefuah 54:275–281
9. Murgue B, Murri S, Triki H, Deubel V, Zeller HG (2001) West Nile in the Mediterranean basin: 1950–2000. Ann N Y AcadSci 951:117–126
10. Mann BR, McMullen AR, Swetnam DM, Barrett AD (2013) Molecular epidemiology and evolution of West Nile virus in North America. Int J Environ Res Public Health 10:5111–5129
11. Schuffenecker I, Peyrefitte CN, el Harrak M, Murri S, Leblond A, Zeller HG (2005) West Nile virus in Morocco, 2003. Emerg Infect Dis 11:306–309
12. Tsai TF, Popovici F, Cernescu C, Campbell GL, Nedelcu NI (1998) West Nile encephalitis epidemic in southeastern Romania. Lancet 352:767–771
13. Bargaoui R, Lecollinet S, Lancelot R (2013) Mapping the serological prevalence rate of West Nile fever in equids, Tunisia. Transbound Emerg Dis. doi:10.1111/tbed.12077
14. Platonov AE, Shipulin GA, Shipulina OY, Tyutyunnik EN, Frolochkina TI, Lanciotti RS, Yazyshina S, Platonova OV, Obukhov IL, Zhukov AN, Vengerov YY, Pokrovskii VI (2001) Outbreak of West Nile virus infection, Volgograd region, Russia, 1999. Emerg Infect Dis 7:128–132
15. Banet-Noach C, Malkinson M, Brill A, Samina I, Yadin H, Weisman Y, Pokamunski S, King R, Deubel V, Stram Y (2003) Phylogenetic relationships of West Nile viruses isolated from birds and horses in Israel from 1997 to 2001. Virus Genes 26:135–141
16. Vittecoq M, Lecollinet S, Jourdain E, Thomas F, Blanchon T, Arnal A, Lowenski S, Gauthier-Clerc M (2013) Recent circulation of West Nile virus and potentially other closely related flaviviruses in southern France. Vector Borne Zoonotic Dis 13:610–613
17. Vrioni G, Mavrouli M, Kapsimali V, Stavropoulou A, Detsis M, Danis K, Tsakris A (2014) Laboratory and clinical characteristics of human West Nile virus infections during 2011 outbreak in southern Greece. Vector Borne Zoonotic Dis 14:52–58
18. Nash D, Mostashari F, Fine A, Miller J, O'Leary D, Murray K, Huang A, Rosenberg A, Greenberg A, Sherman M, Wong S, Layton M, 1999 West Nile Outbreak Response Working Group (2001) The outbreak of West Nile virus infection in the New York City area in 1999. N Engl J Med 344:1807–1814
19. Roehrig JT (2013) West Nile virus in the United States – a historical perspective. Viruses 5:3088–3108
20. The Centers for Disease Control and Prevention (CDC). West Nile virus: statistics and maps. Preliminary maps and data for 2014. Available at: http://www.cdc.gov/westnile/statsmaps/preliminarymapsdata/index.html
21. Di Sabatino D, Bruno R, Sauro F, Danzetta ML, Cito F, Iannetti S, Narcisi V, De Massis F, Calistri P (2014) Epidemiology of West Nile disease in Europe and in the Mediterranean Basin from 2009 to 2013. Biomed Res Int 2014:907852
22. Rossi SL, Ross TM, Evans JD (2010) West Nile virus. Clin Lab Med 30:47–65
23. Khairallah M, Ben Yahia S, Attia S, Zaouali S, Ladjimi A, Messaoud R (2007) Linear pattern of West Nile virus-associated chorioretinitis is related to retinal nerve fibres organization. Eye (Lond) 21:952–955
24. Sejvar JJ (2014) Clinical manifestations and outcomes of West Nile virus infection. Viruses 6:606–623
25. Anninger WV, Lomeo MD, Dingle J, Epstein AD, Lubow M (2003) West Nile virus-associated optic neuritis and chorioretinitis. Am J Ophthalmol 136:1183–1185
26. Bains HS, Jampol LM, Caughron MC, Parnell JR (2003) Vitritis and chorioretinitis in a patient with West Nile virus infection. Arch Ophthalmol 121:205–207

27. Vandenbelt S, Shaikh S, Capone A Jr, Williams GA (2003) Multifocal choroiditis associated with West Nile virus encephalitis. Retina 23:97–99
28. Adelman RA, Membreno JH, Afshari NA, Stoessel KM (2003) West Nile virus chorioretinitis. Retina 23:100–101
29. Hershberger VS, Augsburger JJ, Hutchins RK, Miller SA, Horwitz JA, Bergmann M (2003) Chorioretinal lesions in nonfatal cases of West Nile virus infection. Ophthalmol 110:1732–1736
30. Khairallah M, Ben Yahia S, Ladjimi A, Zeghidi H, Ben Romdhane F, Besbes L, Zaouali S, Messaoud R (2004) Chorioretinal involvement in patients with West Nile virus infection. Ophthalmol 111:2065–2070
31. Shaikh S, Trese MT (2004) West Nile virus chorioretinitis. Br J Ophthalmol 88:1599–1600
32. Eidsness RB, Stockl F, Colleaux KM (2005) West Nile chorioretinitis. Can J Ophthalmol 40:721–724
33. Myers JP, Leveque TK, Johnson MW (2005) Extensive chorioretinitis and severe vision loss associated with West Nile virus meningoencephalitis. Arch Ophthalmol 123:1754–1756
34. Chan CK, Limstrom SA, Tarasewicz DG, Lin SG (2006) Ocular features of West Nile virus infection in North America: a study of 14 eyes. Ophthalmol 113:1539–1546
35. Seth RK, Stoessel KM, Adelman RA (2007) Choroidal néovascularisation associated with West Nile virus chorioretinitis. Semin Ophthalmol 22:81–84
36. Kuchtey RW, Kosmorsky GS, Martin D, Lee MS (2003) Uveitis associated with West Nile virus infection. Arch Ophthalmol 121:648–649
37. Kaiser PK, Lee MS, Martin DA (2003) Occlusive vasculitis in a patient with concomitant West Nile virus infection. Am J Ophthalmol 136:928–930
38. Khairallah M, Ben Yahia S, Attia S, Jelliti B, Zaouali S, Ladjimi A (2006) Severe ischemic maculopathy in a patient with West Nile virus infection. Ophthalmic Surg Lasers Imaging 37:240–242
39. Khairallah M, Jelliti B, Jenzeri S (2009) Emergent infectious uveitis. Middle East Afr J Ophthalmol 16:225–238
40. Khairallah M, Chee SP, Rathinam SR, Attia S, Nadella V (2010) Novel infectious agents causing uveitis. Int Ophthalmol 30:465–483
41. Khairallah M, Ben Yahia S, Attia S (2010) Arthropod vector-borne uveitis in the developing world. Int Ophthalmol Clin 50:125–144
42. Shukla J, Saxena D, Rathinam S, Lalitha P, Joseph CR, Sharma S, Soni M, Rao PV, Parida M (2012) Molecular detection and characterization of West Nile virus associated with multifocal retinitis in patients from southern India. Int J Infect Dis 16:e53–e59
43. Khairallah M, Ben Yahia S, Attia S, Zaouali S, Jelliti B, Jenzeri S, Ladjimi A, Messaoud R (2006) Indocyanine green angiographic features in multifocal chorioretinitis associated with West Nile virus infection. Retina 26:358–359
44. Khairallah M, Ben Yahia S, Letaief M, Attia S, Kahloun R, Jelliti B, Zaouali S, Messaoud R (2007) A prospective evaluation of factors associated with chorioretinitis in patients with West Nile virus infection. Ocul Immunol Inflamm 15:435–439
45. Beardsley R, McCannel C (2012) Reactivation West Nile virus infection related chorioretinitis. Semin Ophthalmol 27:43–45
46. Khairallah M, Kahloun R (2013) Ocular manifestations of emerging infectious diseases. Curr Opin Ophthalmol 24:574–580
47. Khairallah M, Kahloun R, Ben Yahia S, Jelliti B, Messaoud R (2013) New infectious etiologies for posterior uveitis. Ophthalmic Res 49:66–72
48. Sivakumar RR, Prajna L, Arya LK, Muraly P, Shukla J, Saxena D, Parida M (2013) Molecular diagnosis and ocular imaging of West Nile virus retinitis and neuroretinitis. Ophthalmol 120:1820–1826
49. Abroug F, Ouanes-Besbes L, Letaief M, Ben Romdhane F, Khairallah M, Triki H, Bouzouiaia N (2006) A cluster study of predictors of severe West Nile virus infection. Mayo Clin Proc 81:12–16
50. Worwa G, Andrade CC, Thiemann TC, Park B, Maharaj PD, Anishchenko M, Brault AC, Reisen WK (2014) Allele-specific qRT-PCR demonstrates superior detection of single nucleotide polymorphisms as genetic markers for West Nile virus compared to Luminex® and quantitative sequencing. J Virol Methods 195:76–85
51. Lim SM, Koraka P, Osterhaus AD, Martina BE (2013) Development of a strand-specific real-time qRT-PCR for the accurate detection and quantitation of West Nile virus RNA. J Virol Methods 194: 146–153
52. Ben ND, Gershoni YO, Samina I, Khinich Y, Nur I, Laub O, Gottreich A, Simanov M, Porgador A, Rager-Zisman B, Orr N (2009) Using high titer West Nile intravenous immunoglobulin from selected Israeli donors for treatment of West Nile virus infection. BMC Infect Dis 9:18
53. Lazear HM, Pinto AK, Vogt MR, Gale M Jr, Diamond MS (2011) Beta interferon controls West Nile virus infection and pathogenesis in mice. J Virol 85:7186–7194
54. Indenbaum V, Bin H, Makarovsky D, Weil M, Shulman LM, Albeck M, Sredni B, Mendelson E (2012) In vitro and in vivo activity of AS101 against West Nile virus (WNV). Virus Res 166:68–76
55. Afshar AR, Hariprasad SM, Jampol LM, Sheth VS (2012) Use of intravitreous bevacizumab to treat macular edema in West Nile virus chorioretinitis. Arch Ophthalmol 130:396–398
56. Brandler S, Tangy F (2013) Vaccines in development against West Nile virus. Viruses 5:2384–2409
57. Magnusson SE, Karlsson KH, Reimer JM, Corbach-Söhle S, Patel S, Richner JM, Nowotny N, Barzon L, Bengtsson KL, Ulbert S, Diamond MS, Stertman L (2014) Matrix-M™ adjuvanted envelope protein vaccine protects against lethal lineage 1 and 2 West Nile virus infection in mice. Vaccine 32:800–808

12 Chikungunya

Padmamalini Mahendradas

12.1 Introduction

Chikungunya virus is a single-stranded RNA virus of the genus *Alphavirus* in the family *Togaviridae*. It is transmitted to humans by the bite of infected mosquitoes, *Aedes aegypti* and *Aedes albopictus* [1]. It causes chikungunya fever first described by Robinson [2] and Lumsden [3] in 1955. Its name is derived from the Makonade word meaning "that which bends up," in reference to the stooped posture developed due to the arthritis manifestations of the disease.

12.2 Epidemiology

Following the report from Tanganyika in 1952 [2, 3], chikungunya epidemics have been reported from several parts of the world including Asia, Africa, and elsewhere. In Southeast Asia, India, Pakistan, Sri Lanka, Myanmar, the Philippines, Cambodia, Thailand, Indonesia, Vietnam, Hong Kong, and Malaysia have documented the epidemics [4, 5]. Since 2003, there have been outbreaks in the islands of the Pacific Ocean, including Madagascar, Mayotte the Seychelles, Comoros, Mauritius, and the Reunion Island (Indian Ocean). Chikungunya fever has also been documented in Italy, France, Australia, and the USA where international travelers have facilitated the introduction of the virus from endemic areas [6–9].

12.3 Pathophysiology

Following the bite of an infected mosquito, chikungunya virus (CHIKV) is injected into blood capillaries and dermis. During this intradermal stage, CHIKV infects human epithelial cells and dermal fibroblasts. Blood monocytes and macrophages then become infected with CHIKV and viral replication happens (>10^8 copies/ml). Monocytes are then responsible for viral dissemination and systemic infection. The principal secondary infection sites are joints and muscles, endothelial cells of the liver and the brain, and macrophages and stroma cells of the spleen and lymph nodes [10, 11]. In humans, chikungunya infection causes high levels of IFN-α, suggesting strong innate immunity, along with the production of IFN-γ, IL-4, and IL-10, suggesting the engagement of the adaptive immunity [12]. Circulating T lymphocytes showed a CD8+ T lymphocyte response in the early stages of the disease and a CD4+ T lymphocyte-mediated response in the later stages [13]. Interferon gamma and IL-12 levels have been observed to rise dramatically during the acute phase of

P. Mahendradas
Uveitis and Ocular Immunology, Narayana Nethralaya, Bangalore, India
e-mail: m.padmamalini@gmail.com

S.-P. Chee, M. Khairallah (eds.), *Emerging Infectious Uveitis*, DOI 10.1007/978-3-319-23416-8_12

chikungunya fever. The level of IL-12 returns to normalcy in patients who recover. In contrast, patients who develop chronic arthritis show persistently high IL-12 levels.

The systemic manifestations of the fever are related to viremia, while joint involvement is believed to be an immune-mediated reaction to the viral antigen [14]. The exact mechanism of ocular involvement following chikungunya infection is not yet studied in detail. Simultaneous occurrence of systemic and ocular disease suggests the possibility of direct viral involvement such as conjunctivitis, anterior uveitis, optic neuritis, and viral retinitis. Chikungunya virus antigens were detected in keratocytes of the corneal stroma and sclera, in fibroblasts of the iris stroma, and in ciliary bodies suggesting direct ocular involvement [15]. Late involvement of ocular tissue suggests a delayed immune response in cases of episcleritis, viral retinitis, panuveitis, and optic neuritis [16, 17].

12.4 Clinical Features

Chikungunya virus is known to cause a self-limiting illness characterized by sudden onset of fever with chills, headache, vomiting, myalgia, malaise, arthritis or arthralgia, skin rash, and low back pain. Incubation period is about 2–7 days [18, 19]. Although chikungunya fever typically lasts for about a week and recovery is usually the outcome, yet certain patients experience persistent joint symptoms for months or, occasionally, years after the initial onset of illness [17]. The risk of developing polyarthritis has been found to be higher if the initial acute phase lasted longer than 3 weeks [20]. Neurological complications such as meningoencephalitis have been reported during the recent French Reunion island outbreak as well as the first Indian outbreak [21]. Mother-to-child transmission of chikungunya virus was a new observation recorded during the outbreak in the French Reunion island where many complications including death have been reported [21]. The increased virulence has been attributed to absence of the herd immunity and the possible emergence of a new strain [21, 22].

12.5 Ocular Disease

Ocular symptoms include blurred vision, floaters, irritation, pain, watering, redness, photophobia, and diplopia. They can present at the time of fever or after the resolution of the fever. Conjunctivitis, which mimics other viral conjunctivitis and resolves within a week, can be present at the time of acute infection [23]. Numerous ocular features have been described, including episcleritis [24], scleritis, keratitis, anterior uveitis (Fig. 12.1) [24–27], retinitis [25, 28, 29], choroiditis [30], neuroretinitis [25], optic neuritis [25, 31, 32], central retinal artery occlusion [25], exudative retinal detachment [25], panuveitis [25], secondary glaucoma [24] [25], cranial nerve palsies [25], and lagophthalmos [25]. Anterior uveitis can have a granulomatous or nongranulomatous presentation which can be associated with increased intraocular pressure [24]. Fuchs' heterochromic iridocyclitis in association with chikungunya infection has also been reported [33, 34].

Chikungunya retinitis occurs several weeks after the primary illness, which is characterized by minimal vitritis, retinitis, and retinal hemorrhages with retinal edema (Figures), whereas in acute retinal necrosis, multifocal retinitis lesions with severe vitritis are seen primarily in the retinal periphery [24, 28]. Although chikungunya retinitis may morphologically mimic the herpetic viral retinitis, the history of fever, skin rash, and joint pains prior to the onset of the visual symptoms is helpful in the clinical diagnosis, particularly in endemic regions [24, 35]. Optic neuritis can present with sudden decrease in vision secondary to chikungunya virus infection and prompt visual recovery after immediate administration of systemic steroid therapy [25, 32] (Fig. 12.2).

12.6 Diagnosis

Laboratory investigations such as virus isolation, serological tests, and molecular techniques are used to diagnose chikungunya infection [34]. Real-time polymerase chain reaction (RT-PCR) and virus isolation are useful during the initial

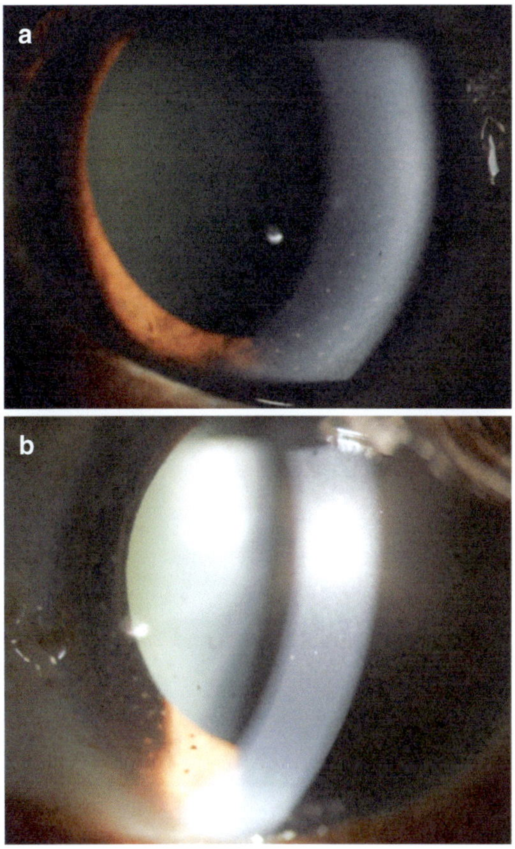

Fig. 12.1 Slit lamp anterior segment photographs of both eyes. From a 45-year-old woman who presented with complaints of discomfort and photophobia 6 weeks following the resolution of chikungunya fever. The photograph shows pigmented keratic precipitates in the inferior cornea of the right eye (**a**) and pigmented and stellate keratic precipitates in the left eye (**b**), with 1+ cells and 2+ flare in the anterior chamber of both eyes (Mahendradas et al. [33])

viremic phase of illness, whereas antibody demonstration from the serum is of use in the later phases of the disease [34]. RT-PCR assay that quantifies viral load in clinical samples can be used as an indicator of active infection [36]. More recently, RT-PCR with real-time loop-mediated isothermal amplification (RT-LAMP) has been developed for rapid diagnosis of chikungunya infection [37].

Enzyme-linked immunosorbent assay (ELISA), indirect immunofluorescent method, and immunochromatographic test (ICT) may be used to detect chikungunya IgM and IgG antibodies in the serum [28].

12.7 Differential Diagnosis

Chikungunya clinically resembles dengue and can be differentiated by the absence of dengue IgM and IgG antibodies in the serum and also by normal platelet count [12]. The differential diagnosis also includes rickettsiosis, herpes, cytomegalovirus, human immunodeficiency virus, syphilis, West Nile virus, tuberculosis, and sarcoidosis.

Chikungunya virus infection can be distinguished from these entities on the basis of history, systemic signs and symptoms, and ocular manifestations with laboratory confirmation of chikungunya infection [4, 12, 20, 21].

12.8 Treatment

There is no specific antiviral drug available for the treatment of chikungunya virus infection [12, 20]. There is no commercial vaccine against chikungunya virus infection even though a lot of research is happening to prepare the vaccine. Symptomatic treatment of the acute stage of the disease is with antipyretics and analgesics such as nonsteroidal anti-inflammatory drugs (NSAIDs) [38]. Chronic arthritis due to chikungunya infection has been treated with corticosteroids, with chloroquine phosphate [39], disease-modifying antirheumatic drugs (DMARDS), and even tumor necrosis factor blockers [40].

Anterior uveitis has been treated with topical steroids and cycloplegic agents [24]. The associated ocular hypertension has been managed with topical beta-blockers and oral or topical carbonic anhydrase inhibitors. Systemic steroids have been required to control the inflammation in posterior uveitis, panuveitis, and optic neuritis [24–26, 30–32]. Preventive measures against mosquito bite continue to be the mainstay for control of chikungunya disease [28].

12.9 Prognosis

Prognosis of chikungunya infection is good in most patients. However, severe cases may result in persistent arthralgia, especially in patients who are elderly or debilitated.

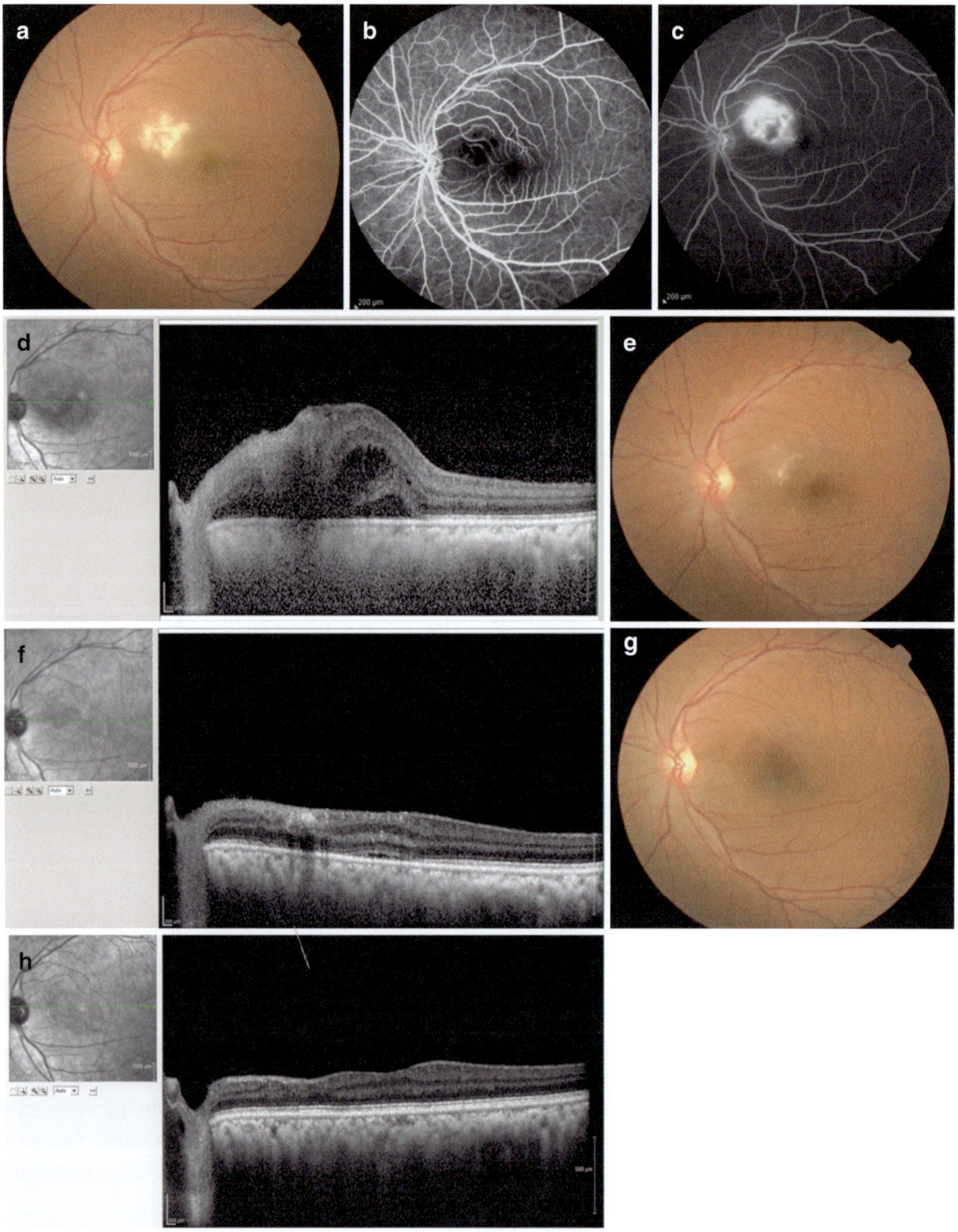

Fig. 12.2 Ocular involvements in chikungunya infection. (**a**) Fundus photograph of the left eye showing confluent area of retinal whitening suggestive of retinitis. Fundus fluorescence in angiography reveals (**b**) early hypofluorescence in the posterior pole and (**c**) late hyperfluorescence in the posterior pole. (**d**) Spectral domain optical coherence tomography (SD OCT) revealed increased reflectivity in the nerve fiber layer zone corresponding to the areas of retinitis with after shadowing and fluid-filled spaces in the outer retina with serous retinal detachment. (**e**) Fundus photograph showing resolving retinitis lesion 2 weeks after initiation of systemic steroid therapy. (**f**) SD OCT showing decreased area of hyper-reflectivity in the inner retina with resolving retinal detachment. (**g**) Fundus photograph after 4 months, showing complete resolution of retinitis. (**h**) SD OCT showing resolution of retinitis with thinning of the inner retinal layers nasal to the fovea (Mahendradas et al. [28])

Ocular involvement usually has a good prognosis except in some cases of optic neuritis, and retinitis occur due to foveal ischemia and optic atrophy [17, 31, 32].

Conclusion

Ocular manifestations of chikungunya infection can be present at the time of fever or may manifest after few weeks. Anterior uveitis, retinitis, and optic neuritis are the commonest manifestations. In the absence of a specific antiviral regimen, the treatment of ocular disease is supportive. The development of specific antiviral therapy and vaccination against chikungunya are the fields under research [28].

Core Messages

- Chikungunya should be considered in the differential diagnosis of viral anterior uveitis, optic neuritis, or multifocal retinitis in patients living in or returning from specific endemic regions.
- Chikungunya infection is diagnosed by RT-PCR from the ocular fluids and serum or by the demonstration of IgM antibodies in the serum.
- In the absence of special antiviral regimen, the treatment of ocular disease is symptomatic and supportive with topical and systemic steroid therapy.

References

1. Calisher CH, Shope RE, Brandt W et al (1980) Proposed antigenic classification of registered arboviruses I (Togaviridae, Alphavirus). Intervirology 14:229–232
2. Robinson MC (1955) An epidemic of virus disease in Southern Province, Tanganyika Territory, in 1952–53. I. Clinical features. Trans R Soc Trop Med Hyg 49:28–32
3. Lumsden WH (1955) An epidemic of virus disease in Southern Province, Tanganyika Territory, in 1952–53; II. General description and epidemiology. Trans Royal Society Trop Med Hyg 49:33–57
4. Pialoux G, Gaüzère BA, Jauréguiberry S, Strobel M (2007) Chikungunya, an epidemic arbovirosis. Lancet Infect Dis 7:319–327
5. World Health Organization (2009) Guidelines for prevention and control of chikungunya fever. World Health Organization, Regional Office for South-East Asia, New Delhi
6. Centers for Disease Control and Prevention (2005–2006) Chikungunya fever diagnosed among international travelers – United States. MMWR Morb Mortal Wkly Rep 55:1040–1042
7. Rezza G, Nicoletti L, Angelini R, Romi R, Finarelli AC, Panning M et al (2007) Infection with chikungunya virus in Italy: an outbreak in a temperate region. Lancet 370:1840–1846
8. Pistone T, Ezzedine K, Schuffenecker I, Receveur MC, Malvy D (2009) An imported case of chikungunya fever from Madagascar: use of the sentinel traveller for detecting emerging arboviral infections in tropical and European countries. Travel Med Infect Dis 7:52–54
9. Rougeron V, Sam IC, Caron M, Nkoghe D, Leroy E, Roques P (2014) Chikungunya, a paradigm of neglected tropical disease that emerged to be a new health global risk. J Clin Virol. Oct 22. pii: S1386–6532(14)00371–0
10. Her Z, Malleret B, Chan M, Ong EK, Wong SC, Kwek DJ et al (2010) Active infection of human blood monocytes by Chikungunya virus triggers an innate immune response. J Immunol 184:5903–5913
11. Das T, Jaffar-Bandjee MC, Hoarau JJ, Krejbich Trotot P, Denizot M, Lee-Pat-Yuen G et al (2010) Chikungunya fever: CNS infection and pathologies of a re-emerging arbovirus. Prog Neurobiol 91:121–129
12. Tang BL (2012) The cell biology of chikungunya virus infection. Cell Microbiol Sep 14(9):1354–1363
13. Wauquier N, Becquart P, Nkoghe D, Padilla C, Ndjoyi-Mbiguino A, Leroy EM (2011) The acute phase of chikungunya virus infection in humans is associated with strong innate immunity and T CD8 cell activation. J Infect Dis 204(1):115–123
14. Jaffar-Bandjee MC, Gasque P (2012) Physiopathology of chronic arthritis following chikungunya infection in man. Med Trop (Mars) 72(Spec No):86–87
15. Couderc T, Gangneux N, Chrétien F, Caro V, Le Luong T, Ducloux B, Tolou H, Lecuit M, Grandadam M (2012) Chikungunya virus infection of corneal grafts. J Infect Dis 206(6):851–859 15
16. Powers AM, Logue CH (2007) Changing patterns of chikungunya virus: reemergence of a zoonotic arbovirus. J Gen Virol 88:2363–2377
17. Mahendradas P (2009) Chikungunya in uveitis: text & imaging, 1st edn. Jaypee Brothers, New Delhi, pp. 706–712
18. Simon F, Savini H, Parola P (2008) Chikungunya: a paradigm of emergence and globalization of vector-borne diseases. Med Clin North Am 92:1323–1343
19. Powers AM, Logue CH (2007) Changing patterns of chikungunya virus: re-emergence of a zoonotic arbovirus. J Gen Virol 88:2363–2377
20. Ribéra A, Degasne I, Jaffar Bandjee MC, Gasque P (2012) Chronic rheumatic manifestations following chikungunya virus infection: clinical description and therapeutic considerations. Med Trop (Mars) 72(Spec No):83–5.

21. Schuffenecker I, Iteman I, Michault A, Murri S, Frangeul L, Vaney MC et al (2006) Genome microevolution of chikungunya viruses causing the Indian Ocean outbreak. PLoS Med 3:e263
22. Mourya DT, Mishra AC (2006) Chikungunya fever. Lancet 368:186–187
23. Parola P, de Lamballerie X, Jourdan J et al (2006) Novel chikungunya virus variant in travelers returning from Indian Ocean islands. Emerg Infect Dis 12:1493–1499
24. Mahendradas P, Ranganna SK, Shetty R, Balu R, Narayana KM, Babu RB, Shetty BK (2008) Ocular manifestations associated with chikungunya. Ophthalmology 115(2):287–291
25. Lalitha P, Rathinam S, Banushree K, Maheshkumar S, Vijayakumar R, Sathe P (2007) Ocular involvement associated with an epidemic outbreak of chikungunya virus infection. Am J Ophthalmol 144(4):552–556
26. Mittal A, Mittal S, Bharathi JM, Ramakrishnan R, Sathe PS (2007) Uveitis during outbreak of chikungunya fever. Ophthalmology 114(9):1798
27. Babu K, Kini R, Philips M, Subbakrishna DK (2014) Clinical profile of isolated viral anterior uveitis in a South Indian patient population. Ocul Immunol Inflamm 22(5):356–359
28. Mahendradas P, Avadhani K, Shetty R (2013) Chikungunya and the eye: a review. J Ophthalmic Inflamm Infect 3:35. doi:10.1186/1869-5760-3-35
29. Vishwanath S, Badami K, Sriprakash KS, Sujatha BL, Shashidhar SD, Shilpa YD (2014) Post-fever retinitis: a single center experience from south India. Int Ophthalmol 34(4):851–857
30. Chanana B, Azad RV, Nair S (2007) Bilateral macular choroiditis following chikungunya virus infection. Eye 21(7):1020–1021
31. Mittal A, Mittal S, Bharati MJ, Ramakrishnan R, Saravanan S, Sathe PS (2007) Optic neuritis associated with chikungunya virus infection in South India. Arch Ophthalmol 125(10):1381–1386
32. Rose N, Anoop TM, John AP, Jabbar PK, George KC (2011) Acute optic neuritis following infection with chikungunya virus in southern rural India. Int J Infect Dis 15(2):e147–e150
33. Mahendradas P, Shetty R, Malathi J, Madhavan HN (2010) Chikungunya virus iridocyclitis in Fuchs' heterochromic iridocyclitis. Indian J Ophthalmol 58(6):545–547
34. Babu K, Murthy GJ (2012) Chikungunya virus iridocyclitis in Fuchs' heterochromic iridocyclitis. Indian J Ophthalmol 60(1):73–74
35. Mahendradas P, Avadhani K (2013) Chikungunya retinitis: spectral-domain optical coherence tomography imaging of the eye. Elsevier, a division of Reed Elsevier India Private Limited, New Delhi, pp. 415–417
36. Pastorino B, Bessaud M, Grandadam M, Murri S, Tolou HJ, Peyrefitte CN (2005) Development of a TaqMan RT-PCR assay without RNA extraction step for the detection and quantification of African chikungunya viruses. J Virol Methods 124:65–71
37. Lakshmi V, Neeraja M, Subbalaxmi MV, Parida MM, Dash PK, Santhosh SR et al (2005) Clinical features and molecular diagnosis of chikungunya fever from South India. Clin Infect Dis 46:1436–1442
38. Couderc T, Khandoudi N, Grandadam M et al (2008) Prophylaxis and therapy for chikungunya virus infection. J Infect Dis 200:516–523
39. Brighton SW (1984) Chloroquine phosphate treatment of chronic chikungunya arthritis. An open pilot study. S Afr Med J 66:217–218
40. Bouquillard E, Combe B (2009) A report of 21 cases of rheumatoid arthritis following chikungunya fever. A mean follow-up of 2 years. Joint Bone Spine 76:654–657

13 Dengue-Related Ocular Disease

Soon-Phaik Chee and Aliza Jap

13.1 Introduction

Despite intense public health efforts, dengue remains an important cause of morbidity and mortality particularly in Asia and Latin America. It has proven difficult to eradicate due to a few factors, one of which is its transmission via the *Aedes aegypti* mosquito. Other major factors that render dengue difficult to eradicate is the non-specific nature of the initial symptoms leading to delays in identifying an outbreak, as well as the existence of several serotypes which is further compounded by the lack of cross immunity. This in turn has hampered efforts to produce an effective and easily deliverable vaccine.

S.-P. Chee (✉)
Singapore National Eye Centre,
11 Third Hospital Avenue, 168751 Singapore, Singapore

Department of Ophthalmology, Yong Loo Lin School of Medicine, National University of Singapore,
1E Kent Ridge Road, Singapore 119228, Singapore

Duke-NUS Graduate Medical School,
8 College Road, Singapore 169857, Singapore

Singapore Eye Research Institute,
11 Third Hospital Avenue, Singapore 168751, Singapore
e-mail: chee.soon.phaik@snec.com.sg

A. Jap
Singapore National Eye Centre,
11 Third Hospital Avenue, 168751 Singapore, Singapore

Division of Ophthalmology, Changi General Hospital, 2 Simei Street 3,
Singapore 529889, Singapore

13.2 Epidemiology

According to the WHO, 2.5 billion people today are living in over 100 endemic countries with 50 to 100 million dengue infections occurring annually. These numbers represent a 30-fold increase in the incidence of dengue over a relatively short period of 50 years. The number of countries experiencing dengue infections has also expanded at an explosive pace from only nine in the early 1900s to the current number. This number is expected to continue to increase due to the resilient nature of the *Aedes* mosquito, increasing urbanisation which is outpacing public health facilities in endemic countries and accelerating international movement of infected passengers and of goods which may carry the *Aedes* larva [1].

The incidence of dengue-related ocular disease has been reported to vary from 7 % in patients with dengue fever to 60 % in those with dengue haemorrhagic fever/dengue shock syndrome [2, 3]. However, its true incidence is difficult to ascertain as there were only few scattered reports prior to the 1900s [4], and even today, there are very few large series with the majority of publications consisting of single case reports or small case series. This paucity of reported cases could be related to variations in ocular

S.-P. Chee, M. Khairallah (eds.), *Emerging Infectious Uveitis*, DOI 10.1007/978-3-319-23416-8_13

manifestations with different serotypes as during an epidemic involving dengue serotype 1, dengue maculopathy was observed in 10 % of patients as compared to none during an epidemic caused by dengue serotype 2 [5, 6].

This difference in ocular manifestations with different serotypes is further supported by the finding that although dengue is the commonest cause of infectious posterior uveitis in Singapore, there has been a decrease in the number of cases seen over the years due to a shift in the predominant serotype responsible for the outbreaks [7].

Another cause for the scarcity of epidemiological data regarding dengue eye disease is the lack of systematic screening for ocular involvement especially in patients with mild systemic disease. Furthermore, in a study by Kapoor et al., while ocular findings were seen in 54 hospitalised dengue patients (40 %) and ten (7.5 %) had fundal changes, none of these patients had any visual symptoms as the macula was not involved in all these cases [8]. On the contrary, Seet et al. noted that while 28 (18 %) of their hospitalised patients had at least two ocular symptoms including 16 (10 %) with blurring of vision, which triggered a full ophthalmic examination, in fact only two patients had retinal pathology [9]. Hence, since most authors screen only hospitalised or symptomatic patients, due to these discrepancies between symptoms and signs, the incidence of ocular involvement is probably underestimated.

13.3 Pathophysiology

The dengue virus is an RNA virus belonging to the *Flaviviridae* family and consists of four main serotypes, DENV-1 to DENV-4, with a fifth serotype having been recently discovered whose true impact in humans remains to be seen but which may further hinder the development of a dengue vaccine [10].

The pathogenesis of dengue is multifactorial involving a complex interplay between viral virulence [5, 7, 11] and host susceptibility [12–14], many aspects of which remain unclear. Both humoral and cellular immunity responses are activated following the viremia resulting in complement activation with a reduction particularly of plasma complement C3 components being seen in patients with severe dengue. The consequent release of cytokines and increase in vascular permeability are responsible for the fluid extravasation seen in dengue haemorrhagic fever/dengue shock syndrome [15–17].

The majority of patients with ocular manifestations present about 1 week after the onset of fever usually when the platelet count is at the lowest with a range of 5–77 x 10^9 cells/l. Hence the haemorrhagic lesions such as subconjunctival and retinal haemorrhages are possibly a result primarily of the thrombocytopenia. On the other hand, the mean timing of the onset of symptoms at 1 week after the onset of the fever as well as the finding of low complement C3 and C4 as well as microalbuminuria in some of these patients suggest that immune-mediated mechanisms rather the viremia itself are responsible for manifestations such as uveitis, vasculitis, maculopathy and optic neuropathy [6, 18–22].

13.4 Clinical Features

1. Systemic disease

There is a wide spectrum of systemic manifestations in dengue. The symptoms generally come on about a week after being bitten by an infected female *Aedes* mosquito. In classic dengue fever, typically, there is high fever with headache, retro-orbital pain, arthralgia, myalgia, skin rashes, nausea and vomiting and perhaps epistaxis or bleeding gums. However, it may be asymptomatic, and in young children and those with a first episode of dengue, the symptoms may be mild and non-specific, and the diagnosis of dengue may be missed. At the other end of the spectrum is what used to be termed dengue haemorrhagic fever and the dengue shock syndrome with multi-organ involvement which are potentially fatal due to the accompanying increase in vascular permeability and thrombocytopenia. In order to facilitate the diagnosis and management of these life-threatening aspects of dengue infection, the WHO has reclassified dengue in 2009 to dengue

Table 13.1 WHO revised criteria for dengue case classification 2009

Probable dengue without warning signs
Live in/travel to dengue endemic area with fever and two of the following:
Nausea, vomiting
Rash
Aches and pains
Leukopenia
Positive tourniquet test
Dengue with warning signs[a]
Dengue as defined above with any of the following:
Abdominal pain or tenderness
Persistent vomiting
Clinical fluid accumulation (ascites, pleural effusion)
Mucosal bleeding
Lethargy, restlessness
Liver enlargement >2 cm
Laboratory: increase in HCT concurrent with rapid decrease in platelet count
Severe dengue
Dengue with at least one of the following criteria:
Severe plasma leakage leading to:
Shock (DSS)
Fluid accumulation with respiratory distress
Severe bleeding as evaluated by clinician
Severe organ involvement
Liver: AST or ALT ≥ 1000
CNS: impaired consciousness
Heart and other organs

[a]Requires strict observation and medical intervention

with and without warning signs and severe dengue (Table 13.1) [23].

In addition to encephalopathy, other neurological changes seen in dengue include encephalitis, meningitis, Guillain-Barré syndrome, myelitis, acute disseminated encephalomyelitis, polyneuropathy, mononeuropathy, hypokalaemic paralysis, cerebromeningeal haemorrhage as well as neuro-ophthalmic signs which will be discussed below [20, 24–39].

2. Ocular disease

13.4.1 Symptoms

Pain is the commonest symptom and its severity ranges from a feeling of eye strain (30 %) or foreign body sensation (3 %) to a retro-orbital pain (20 %) [9]. In the majority of patients, it is a non-specific and benign symptom. However, in certain patients, ocular pain in dengue may represent a sight-threatening event such as acute angle closure [40]. In this particular patient though, who was female with fairly short axial length of 22 mm and normal posterior segments on B scan ultrasonography, it is uncertain if the angle closure was a direct complication of dengue infection or a coincidental occurrence. Of greater significance is a 6-year-old child who presented with what was thought to be acute angle closure initially and was subsequently diagnosed as panophthalmitis which resulted in permanent visual loss [41]. Hence, although pain in dengue often has no detrimental outcome, a high index of suspicion needs to be maintained for potentially blinding causes.

Other symptoms commonly reported include blurring of vision (10 %), diplopia (3 %) and floaters and flashes (3 %) [9]. However, a significant proportion of patients with maculopathy may be asymptomatic, and although an abnormal Amsler chart test has high specificity of 95 % for maculopathy, nonetheless its sensitivity is only 30 % [6, 8]. Therefore, the absence of visual symptoms does not exclude the presence of ocular involvement, and systematic screening especially in patients with severe dengue remains the main means of detection.

13.4.2 Signs

13.4.2.1 Anterior Segment

Anterior segment lesions in the form of subconjunctival haemorrhage are the commonest reported ocular manifestation of dengue, occurring in about 40 % of all patients [2, 8] and in up to 60 % in patients with severe dengue haemorrhagic fever, usually in association with severe thrombocytopenia [3]. As a consequence of the thrombocytopenia, haemorrhages have also been noted to occur in the periocular tissues, including the retrobulbar space where it may be of such severity as to result in globe perforation [42, 43].

In addition, there have also been sporadic case reports of corneal involvement which is often mild in the form of superficial punctate erosions, but corneal ulceration with hypopyon which was attributed to exposure has also been reported [4, 44, 45].

13.4.2.2 Uveitis

Uveitis occurring as an isolated event is rare in dengue [2, 41, 46], and it is more commonly described in association with the occurrence of dengue maculopathy [19, 22, 45, 47]. The series of patients with isolated uveitis described by Gupta is unusual for a number of reasons. Firstly, these patients were noted to have no ocular lesions during the acute phase and only presented 3 to 5 months later with progressive loss of vision. Secondly, four of the six patients did not experience pain, and ciliary injection was absent or mild in all six patients despite the presence of significant cellular reaction. Only one eye had bilateral involvement. Five patients (six eyes) had only anterior segment involvement with fine to large keratic precipitates and 2 to 4 + anterior chamber cells and flare. The intraocular pressure was normal, and posterior synechiae was absent in all but one patient who also had concomitant vitritis, vasculitis, retinal haemorrhages and macula oedema. The inflammation in all these patients resolved with corticosteroid therapy [2].

The other two cases of uveitis reported in the literature presented within 1 week of onset of fever with pain and blurring of vision. Both had shallowing of the anterior chambers. In one patient the shallowing was due to bilateral iridocyclitis with choroidal effusions, and the intraocular pressures were low. This patient recovered well following treatment with topical corticosteroids [46]. The other patient was the 6-year-old child mentioned above who was initially diagnosed as having acute angle closure glaucoma in the left eye due to the presence of ciliary injection, hazy cornea and shallow anterior chamber and who had in fact severe panophthalmitis with periocular extension resulting in visual loss [41].

13.4.2.3 Fundal Changes in Dengue

There is a wide spectrum of fundal changes that have been described in patients with dengue including vitreous haemorrhage, retinal haemorrhages, peripapillary haemorrhages, optic disc hyperaemia, Roth spots, cotton wool spots, intraretinal precipitates, retinal oedema, maculopathy and retinal vasculopathy. There may be a concomitant anterior uveitis and vitritis [3, 18, 19, 21, 22, 35, 45, 47–53].

13.4.3 Dengue Maculopathy

Although macula changes such as cotton wool spots, oedema and haemorrhages may be observed together in association with major changes in the peripheral retina or with an optic neuritis [3, 18, 19, 21, 22, 31, 37, 45, 53], a predominant involvement of the macula with none or minimal peripheral changes is increasingly being reported as a cause of visual symptoms in patients with dengue, occurring in up to 10 % of patients hospitalised with dengue. It is usually a bilateral condition (73 to 80 %), although it may be asymmetrical, manifesting about 1 week after the onset of fever, when the platelet counts are generally at their lowest. Blurring of vision (18 to 100 %) and central scotoma (7 to 90 %) are the most common complaints. Less commonly, the patients may complain of floaters or metamorphopsia (5 %). The presenting visual acuity varied from 20/25 to count fingers closely, corresponding to the extent of macula oedema. In addition to oedema, other features of dengue maculopathy include foveolitis, small white or yellow subretinal dots, intraretinal haemorrhages, retinal epithelial swelling, vascular sheathing, optic disc hyperaemia and vitritis [6, 19, 21, 22, 35, 47, 54, 55] (Figs. 13.1, 13.2 and 13.3).

13.4.4 Foveolitis

The term foveolitis is used to describe a small, well-circumscribed yellow-orange subretinal lesion localised to the fovea (Fig. 13.4a, b). These lesions measure between 0.2 and 0.5 mm and may be seen as an isolated lesion or in combination with the other findings described above such as retinal haemorrhages and vascular sheathing. Optical coherence tomography (OCT) of these lesions shows a disruption of the outer sensory retina with or without any

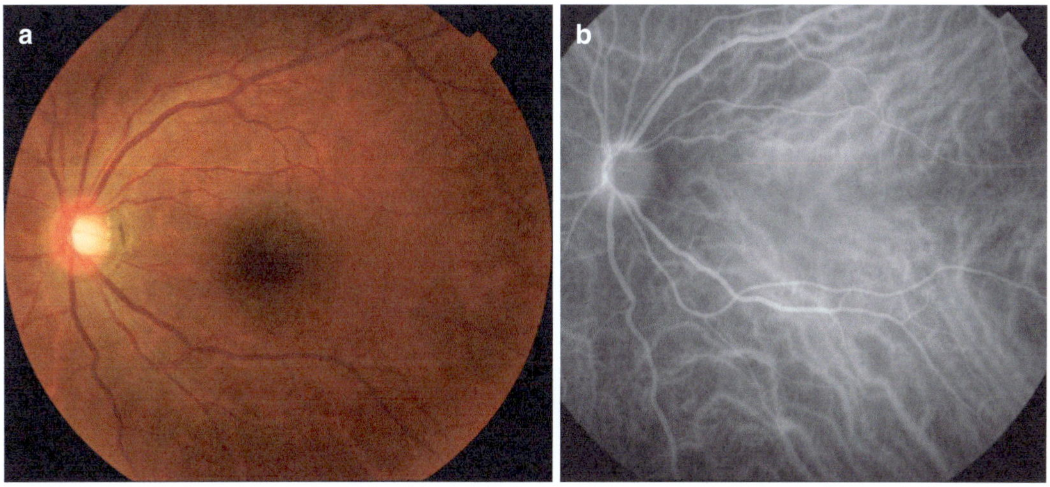

Fig. 13.1 (**a**) Fundal photograph showing small *yellow dots* and mild sheathing of perifoveal vessels. (**b**) Indocyanine green angiography of the same eye showing mild large vessel hyperfluorescence in the early phase

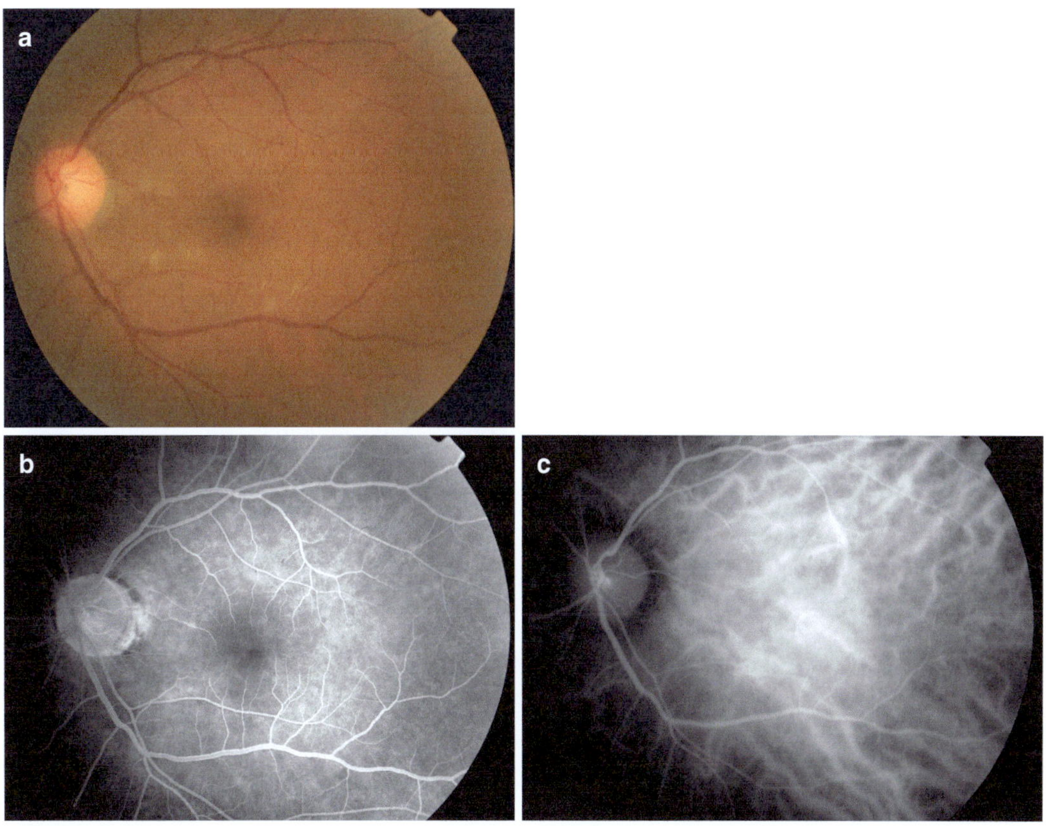

Fig. 13.2 (**a**) Fundal photograph showing sheathing of perifoveal venules. (**b**) Fundal fluorescein angiography of the same eye showing mild staining of the venules in the mid phase. (**c**) Indocyanine green angiography of the same eye showing large vessel hyperfluorescence in the early phase

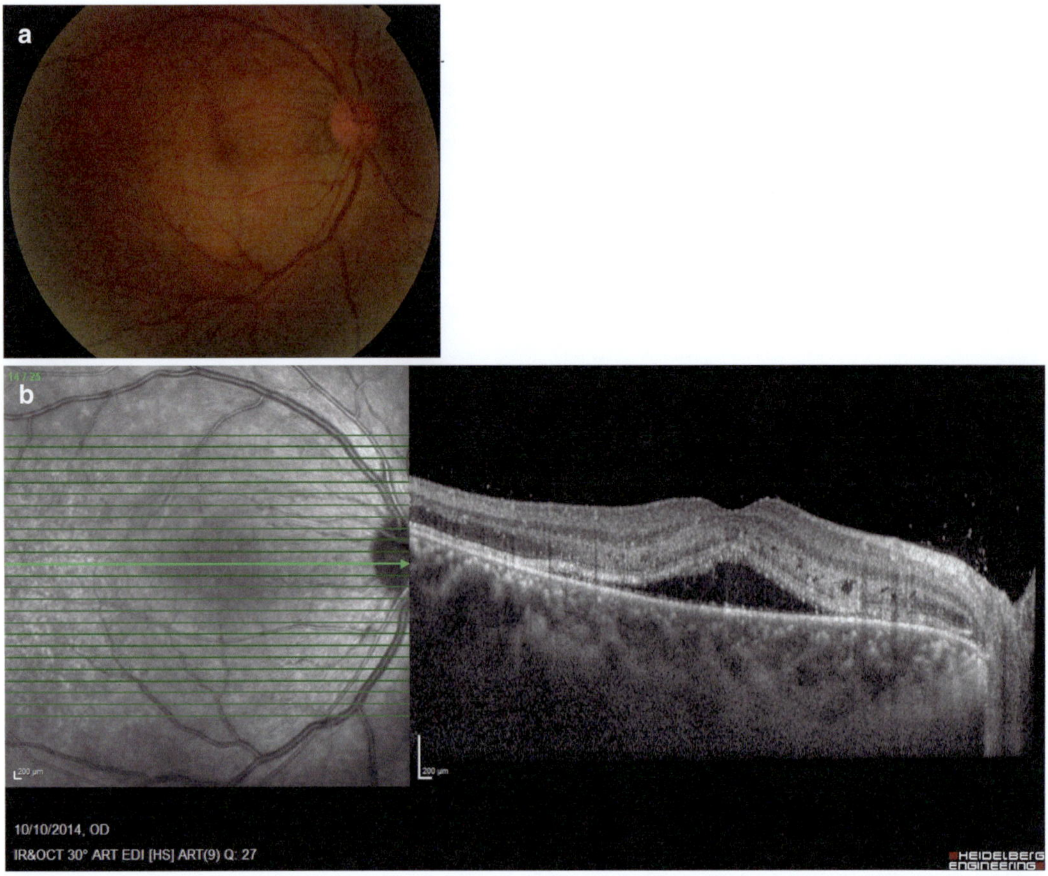

Fig. 13.3 (**a**) Fundal photograph showing exudative detachment of the macula with striae, retinal haemorrhages, small *yellow dots* and perivascular cuffing. (**b**) Optical coherence tomography of the same eye showing the presence of subretinal as well as intraretinal fluid

accompanying elevation of adjacent retina [54, 55]. In addition to foveolitis, other OCT changes that have been seen in eyes with dengue maculopathy include diffuse retinal thickening, cystoid macular oedema and exudative detachment [19, 22, 56]. All these changes resolved within a month, but the visual function was not always similarly restored. Teoh et al. showed that the different types of OCT changes were useful predictors of visual outcome at 2 years. Patients with diffuse retinal thickening had the least visual disturbance at presentation with more than 85 % having 20/40 or better vision and the best visual outcome. Only 30 % had a residual scotoma and all had 20/40 or better vision. In contrast, the majority of eyes with foveolitis (96 %) presented with 20/80 or worse vision, and although the Snellen acuity improved to 20/40 or better in at least 60 %, all eyes still had a visually disturbing scotoma. While 80 % of eyes with cystoid oedema also had poor visual at presentation and extremely swollen maculae, 81 % regained 20/40 or better vision with only 56 % still experiencing a residual scotoma [56].

Fundus fluorescein angiography (FFA) may be normal in up to 70 % of eyes with dengue maculopathy. FFA changes that have been described include the presence of early hyperfluorescence that persists to the late phase, blocked fluorescence, small vessel occlusion or leakage, capillary non-perfusion, knobbly hyperfluorescence of perifoveal arterioles and early pinpoint hyperfluorescence.

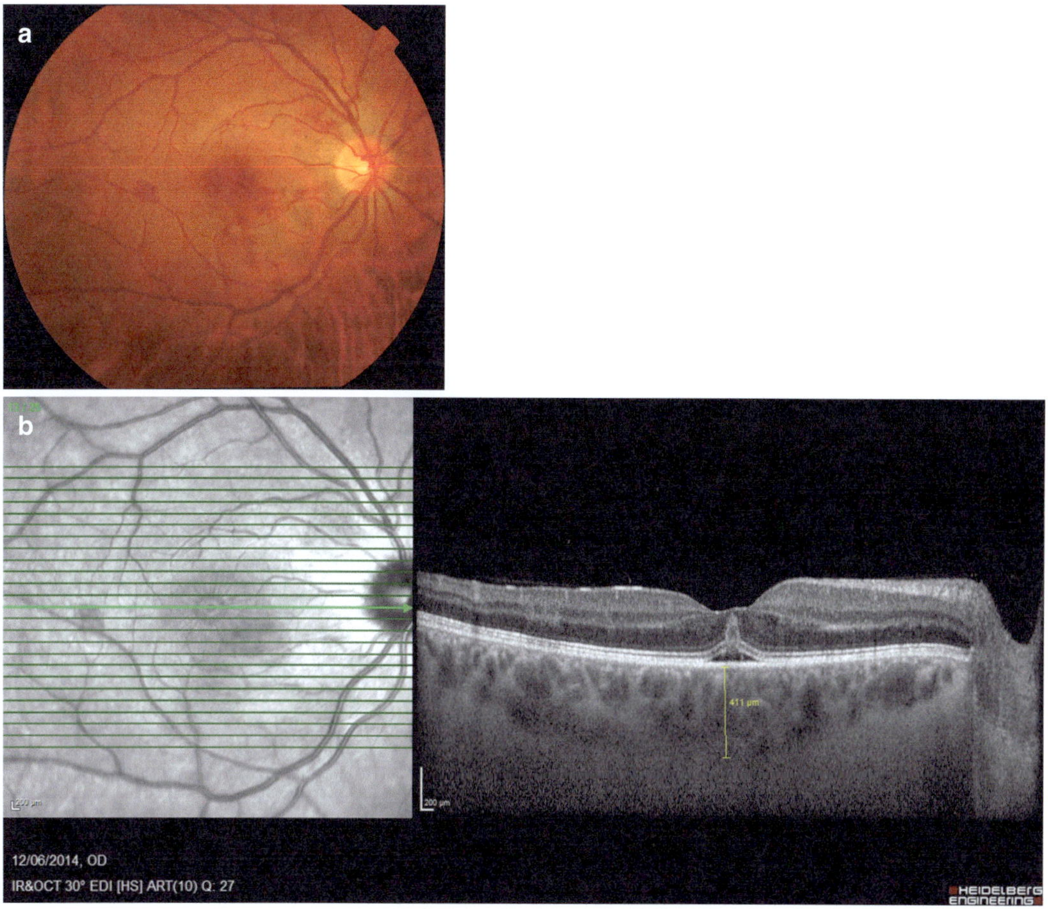

Fig. 13.4 (**a**) Fundal photograph showing macula haemorrhages with a small yellow elevated lesion at the fovea. (**b**) Optical coherence tomography of the same eye showing focal thickening of subfoveal outer retina with underlying subretinal fluid. The foveal contour is slightly elevated

Similarly, indocyanine green angiography (ICGA) may be normal in about 60 % of eyes or show mid- or late phase hypofluorescent spots or large vessel hyperfluorescence suggesting that there may be an underlying choroidopathy as well. The predictive value of angiography is uncertain as in the series from Loh et al., although FFA changes were seen only in eyes that had poor presenting visual acuity of 20/400 or worse, all recovered to 20/40 or better vision. Similarly, other authors also found that despite the presence of severe leakage or non-perfusion on angiography, the retinal changes resolved with visual acuity of 20/40 or better in the majority of eyes [19, 22, 47, 54].

The vasculopathy in dengue affects mainly the venules and arterioles and is usually evident clinically as sheathing of the involved vessels. In a few cases, however, the vasculopathy may only be obvious on FFA (Fig. 13.5a, b and c) [22]. Occlusion of the main retinal arteries have also been described with the patients presenting clinically as a branch or central retinal arterial occlusion with corresponding changes FFA [57, 58].

13.4.4.1 Neuro-Ophthalmic Involvement

Optic nerve involvement in dengue is a rare event, and of the 14 patients reported, ten (70 %) had bilateral disease with visual loss being the main presenting complaint [20, 30–37]. The initial visual acuity may range from 6/6 to no light perception, and colour vision and visual field defects

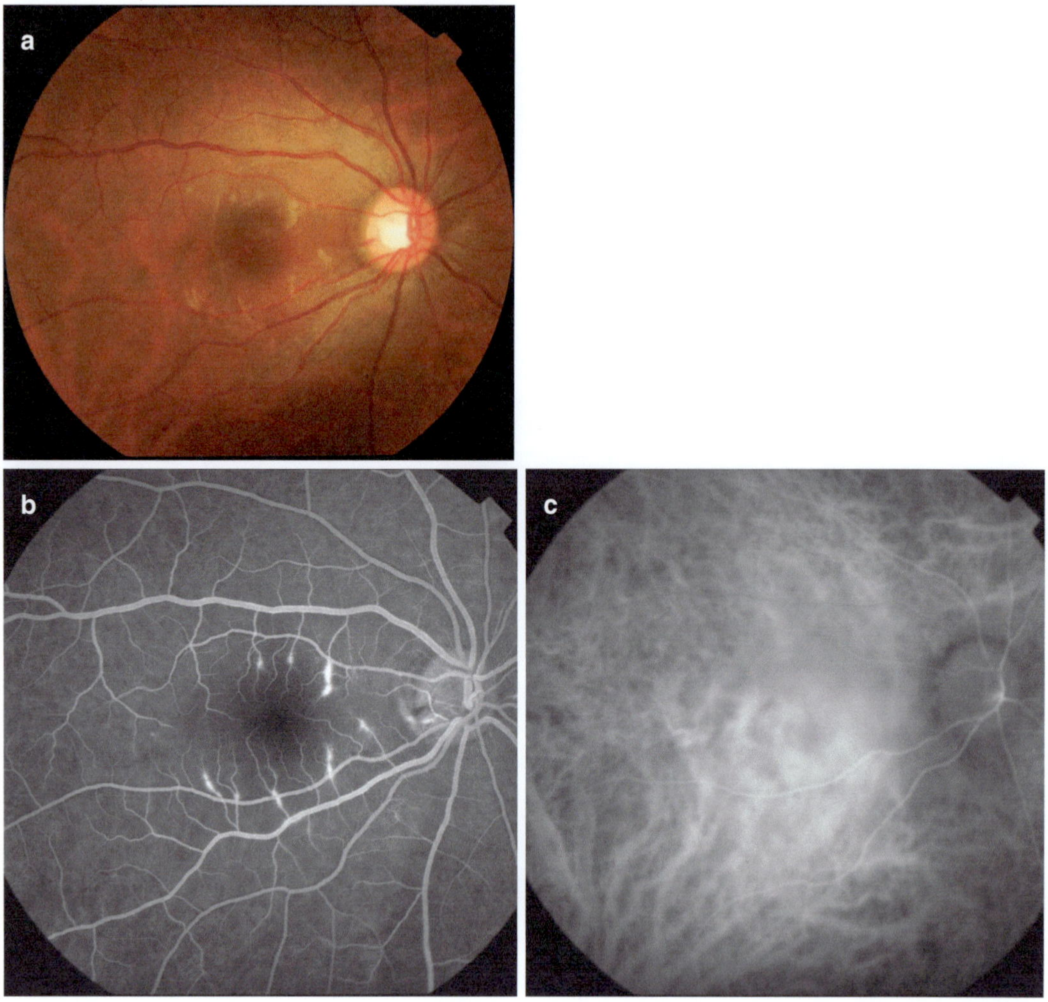

Fig. 13.5 (**a**) Fundal photograph showing swelling of the macula with cotton wool spots. (**b**) Fundal fluorescein angiography of the same eye showing leakage from perifoveal venules in the mid phase. (**c**) Indocyanine green angiography of the same eye showing large vessel hyperfluorescence in the early phase

are present unless the visual loss was too profound to permit their recording together with a relative afferent pupillary defect in unilateral cases. The optic nerve involvement is usually in the form of a papillitis with disc swelling and accompanying peripapillary haemorrhages and cotton wool spots. It may also appear as a retrobulbar neuritis with a normal fundal examination with only the observation of dilated sluggishly reactive pupils in the presence of poor vision to suggest an optic nerve lesion [20, 33]. Seventy percent of the eyes eventually regained 20/40 or better vision, but some patients may have persistent colour vision and field defects, and disc pallor may be seen [20, 30–37]. One of the patients with optic neuropathy also had bilateral exudative retinal detachment. Although the disc and retinal swellings are resolved, there were residual intraretinal lipid deposits which limited her visual recovery from an initial 20/250 in both eyes to 20/100 in one eye and 20/30 in the other [31]. Another of these patients presented as a neuroretinitis with macular star exudates. However, this patient had complete resolution with no residual visual deficits [37]. Three eyes (12.5 %) continued to progress to an eventual hand movement or worse vision.

Optic disc hyperaemia has also been observed in eyes with maculopathy [22], and in these cases, it can be difficult to exclude a concomitant neuropathy without ancillary tests such as FFA and electrophysiological tests as a severe maculopathy can also give rise to colour vision deficits, visual field defects as well as a relative afferent pupil defect [59]. There have also been sporadic cases of isolated palsies of the cranial nerves supplying the external ocular muscles all of which resolved spontaneously by 3 months [33, 38, 39].

13.4.5 Investigations

In addition to OCT, FFA and ICGA, ancillary tests that may be required include perimetry and electrophysiology.

13.4.5.1 Perimetry

Conventional perimetry with kinetic or static perimeter is useful in documenting the field defects in dengue optic neuropathy as well as the scotomas seen in eyes with maculopathy. However, as the maculopathy resolves, the subsequent changes in the scotomas may be subtle, and microperimetry may better able to monitor these changes [60].

13.4.5.2 Electrophysiology

Various modalities of electroretinography (ERG) may be used in combination with the visual evoked potential (VEP) to distinguish between retinal and optic nerve dysfunction in cases where the causes of poor vision are not clinically apparent.

1. ERG

The full-field ERG reflects the global retinal response and hence may be normal even when maculopathy is present with a reduction in scotopic b-wave amplitude, maximal b-wave implicit time delay or amplitude reduction being seen in only 50 % of patients with dengue maculopathy [59]. The pattern ERG which measures macular function specifically showed a decrease in the P50 amplitude with preservation of the N95:P50 ratio in 57 % of the eyes in the series by Chia et al. and in both patients studied by Mendes et al. [59, 61]. The N95 component of the pattern ERG is selectively decreased in eyes with retina ganglion cell dysfunction and hence an abnormal N95:P50 ratio serves as an indicator of optic nerve involvement. The multifocal ERG provides a topographical map of central retinal function and was found to be abnormal in 73 % of Chia et al.'s eyes [59] and is also useful in the evaluation of macular function when clinical examination, OCT, FFA and ICGA are normal [62].

2. VEP

A delay in the P100 latency is non-specific and may occur as a result of both optic nerve and macular pathology. However, a delayed P100 in the presence of a normal pattern ERG or fundal examination serves to support a diagnosis of optic neuropathy in eyes with poor vision and abnormal pupillary response [33].

13.5 Diagnosis

The laboratory tests used to confirm a diagnosis of dengue fever are determined by the timing as well as local availability of the tests. Prior to day 5, when the patient is still febrile, the virus may be detected by means of polymerase chain reaction for viral RNA, ELISA or rapid tests for viral antigen, in particular the nonstructural protein 1 (NS1) antigen, or virus cell culture. Subsequently, as the fever settles when the viral load decreases in tandem with an increase in antibodies production, immunoglobulin (Ig)M or a rise in paired sera IgG immunoassays is preferred. Although NS1 antigen levels are highest during the first week, it may still be detectable in some patients even up to the second week of onset [63, 64].

13.6 Differential Diagnosis

The differential diagnosis for dengue fever include numerous other febrile illnesses especially viral fevers such as chikungunya, West Nile virus as well as other infections such as malaria, leptospirosis and rickettsial infections as these are also common in the tropical countries. Although travel history is a vital component in the diagnosis of dengue fever as its diagnosis may be made on clinical grounds alone in patients from endemic areas, laboratory tests described above may be required to establish the diagnosis in other cases.

A number of the ocular manifestations of dengue may also be seen in other infectious as well as non-infectious conditions. Subconjunctival haemorrhages in particular are non-specific and may be spontaneous. Optic neuritis may be related to demyelinating disease as well as infectious diseases such as *Bartonella* especially when there is accompanying neuroretinitis. Retinal haemorrhages, cotton wool spots and vasculitis may also occur as a result of non-infective conditions such as diabetes mellitus and hypertension or in viral fevers such as chikungunya and human immunodeficiency virus infections. Foveolitis however has not thus far been described in association with any other conditions.

13.7 Management

There is no specific treatment for the systemic disease and management consists of supportive measures such as intravenous fluid resuscitation and platelets transfusions. Similarly there is no specific treatment required for subconjunctival haemorrhage, the commonest manifestations of ocular dengue. Corticosteroids have been used in situations where an immune-mediated mechanism has been postulated.

13.7.1 Dengue Uveitis

Seven of the eight reported cases that presented with uveitis were treated with topical, periocular and/or systemic corticosteroids according to the severity and extent of the inflammation with supplemental cycloplegics and glaucoma medications as required with good response. The management and outcome of the child with panophthalmitis was not described [2, 41, 46].

13.7.2 Dengue Maculopathy

In general, patients who were asymptomatic had good presenting vision, and/or rapid recovery was managed conservatively. On the other hand, those that had poor presenting visual acuity or progressive visual loss and/or severe vasculitis on angiography were treated with corticosteroids.

However, there are considerable variations in the regimen used for including induction with intravenous methylprednisolone at 1 g/day for 3 days followed by a tapering dose of oral prednisolone, oral corticosteroids alone and periocular corticosteroids alone especially in eyes with unilateral disease or where systemic therapy was contraindicated as well as combinations of various modalities of corticosteroids. Intravenous immunoglobulins with intravenous hydrocortisone were also administered if there was no response to the initial corticosteroid therapy or if there was further deterioration of the visual acuity. Eighty to 100 % of eyes regained at least 20/40 vision with resolution of the fundal changes although a slight scotoma may persist in a significant proportion of eyes with foveolitis [18, 19, 22, 47, 54, 65, 66].

One patient with bilateral occlusive vasculopathy and vitreous haemorrhage was treated with oral anti-platelet therapy, panretinal photocoagulation to one eye and pars plana vitrectomy in the worse eye but lost vision in that eye due to macula ischemia [53]. Vitrectomy was also required in a young girl who presented with light perception vision in one eye due to an organised vitreous haemorrhage and had a resolving vitreous haemorrhage in the fellow eye. At 3 months postoperatively, her vision had recovered to 20/40. The fellow eye was observed and remained stable at 20/40 vision as well [48].

13.7.3 Dengue Optic Neuropathy

The indications for immunosuppressive therapy were similar to those for maculopathy with almost all patients receiving intravenous methylprednisolone at 1 g/day for 3 days followed by a tapering dose of oral prednisolone. Of the 13 treated eyes, the vision in three eyes (23 %) remained poor at hand movement or worse vision due to optic atrophy, and seven (54 %) recovered 20/40 or better vision [20, 30, 32–35].

However, the benefits of therapy in dengue maculopathy and optic neuropathy are uncertain as fairly rapid, spontaneous recovery of Snellen acuity may also occur even in eyes that had poor initial acuity [8, 19–21, 35, 37, 54–56, 60, 67, 68]. Furthermore regardless of whether the patients were actively managed or not and despite clinical improvement, residual scotoma with ERG abnormalities was perceived by almost all the patients.

13.8 Prognosis

Most patients with dengue maculopathy regained good Snellen acuity with considerable variation in recovery rates, ranging from days to years. However, despite normalisation of the retinal profile on OCT, 30 to 100 % of patients may still notice a scotoma especially in eyes that had foveolitis [8, 18, 19, 21, 22, 47, 54–56, 60]. Unfortunately, recurrent maculopathy may occur with subsequent dengue infection by a different serotype resulting in an increase in size of the previous residual scotoma [68].

The majority of patients with optic neuritis similarly recover well although the recovery again may be over years and there may be residual colour vision and visual field defects despite a good Snellen acuity. However, about 10 % of eyes sustained severe visual loss of hand movement or worse [20, 30–37].

Conclusion

Dengue can affect any of the structures in the eye and orbit as well as the cranial nerves either via a thrombocytopenia-related event such as a subconjunctival haemorrhage or an immune-mediated process as in dengue maculopathy and neuropathy. Many of these signs and symptoms are non-specific, and the patients may be asymptomatic unless the macula or optic nerve is involved. The only finding that is pathognomonic for dengue is a foveolitis. Some of the posterior segment changes may be subtle and may be missed unless there is a high index of suspicion and may require electrophysiology to establish a diagnosis. The management of dengue-related ocular disease is also unclear as the majority of patients recover spontaneously as their blood counts normalise, and even with treatment, most patients with maculopathy or neuropathy still continue to have a persistent scotoma.

Core Messages

Dengue remains a major cause of morbidity in tropical countries and is also of increasing concern even in previously non-endemic areas due to the resilience of its host vector as well as the lack of a vaccine. In view of the non-specific nature of its clinical features, a detailed travel history is an important element in any person presenting with fever and visual symptoms.

References

1. WHO Global Alert and Response Impact of Dengue. Available from http://www.who.int/csr/disease/dengue/impact/en/
2. Gupta A, Srinivasan R, Setia S, Soundravally R, Pandian DG (2009) Uveitis following dengue fever. Eye (Lond) 23(4):873–876
3. Mehta S (2005) Ocular lesions in severe dengue hemorrhagic fever (DHF). J Assoc Physicians India 53:656–657
4. Richardson S (1933) Ocular symptoms and complications observed in dengue. Trans Am Ophthalmol Soc 31:450–477
5. Chee E, Sims JL, Jap A, Tan BH, Oh H, Chee SP (2009) Comparison of prevalence of dengue maculopathy during two epidemics with differing predominant serotypes. Am J Ophthalmol 148(6):910–913
6. Su DH, Bacsal K, Chee SP, Flores JV, Lim WK, Cheng BC, Jap AH, Dengue Maculopathy Study Group (2007) Prevalence of dengue maculopathy in patients hospitalized for dengue fever. Ophthalmology 114(9):1743–1747
7. Mi H, Ho SL, Lim WK, Wong EP, Teoh SC (2014) Trends in patterns of posterior uveitis and panuveitis in a tertiary institution in Singapore. Ocul Immunol Inflamm 20:1–10

8. Kapoor HK, Bhai S, John M, Xavier J (2006) Ocular manifestations of dengue fever in an East Indian epidemic. Can J Ophthalmol 41(6):741–746
9. Seet RC, Quek AM, Lim EC (2007) Symptoms and risk factors of ocular complications following dengue infection. J Clin Virol 38(2):101–105
10. Mustafa MS, Rasotgi V, Jain S, Gupta V (2015) Discovery of fifth serotype of dengue virus (DENV-5): a new public health dilemma in dengue control. Med J Armed Forces India 71(1):67–70
11. Fried JR, Gibbons RV, Kalayanarooj S, Thomas SJ, Srikiatkhachorn A, Yoon IK, Jarman RG, Green S, Rothman AL, Cummings DA (2010) Serotype-specific differences in the risk of dengue hemorrhagic fever: an analysis of data collected in Bangkok, Thailand from 1994 to 2006. PLoS Negl Trop Dis 4(3):e617
12. Appanna R, Ponnampalavanar S, Lum Chai See L, Sekaran SD (2010) Susceptible and protective HLA class 1 alleles against dengue fever and dengue hemorrhagic fever patients in a Malaysian population. PLoS One 28:5(9)
13. Nguyen TP, Kikuchi M, Vu TQ, Do QH, Tran TT, Vo DT, Ha MT, Vo VT, Cao TP, Tran VD, Oyama T, Morita K, Yasunami M, Hirayama K (2008) Protective and enhancing HLA alleles, HLA-DRB1*0901 and HLA-A*24, for severe forms of dengue virus infection, dengue hemorrhagic fever and dengue shock syndrome. PLoS Negl Trop Dis 2(10):e304
14. Monteiro SP, Brasil PE, Cabello GM, Souza RV, Brasil P, Georg I, Cabello PH, De Castro L (2012) HLA-A*01 allele: a risk factor for dengue haemorrhagic fever in Brazil's population. Mem Inst Oswaldo Cruz 107(2):224–230
15. Pathogenetic mechanisms in dengue haemorrhagic fever: report of an international collaborative study (1973). Bull World Health Organ 48(1):117–133.
16. An J, Zhou DS, Zhang JL, Morida H, Wang JL, Yasui K (2004) Dengue-specific CD8+ T cells have both protective and pathogenic roles in dengue virus infection. Immunol Lett 95(2):167–174
17. Friberg H, Burns L, Woda M, Kalayanarooj S, Endy TP, Stephens HA, Green S, Rothman AL, Mathew A (2011) Memory CD8+ T cells from naturally acquired primary dengue virus infection are highly cross-reactive. Immunol Cell Biol 89(1):122–129
18. Chang PE, Cheng CL, Asok K, Fong KY, Chee SP, Tan CK (2007) Visual disturbances in dengue fever: an answer at last? Singapore Med J 48(3):e71–e73
19. Chan DP, Teoh SC, Tan CS, Nah GK, Rajagopalan R, Prabhakaragupta MK, Chee CK, Lim TH, Goh KY, Eye Institute Dengue-Related Ophthalmic Complications Workgroup (2006) Ophthalmic complications of dengue. Emerg Infect Dis 12(2):285–289
20. Sanjay S, Wagle AM, Au Eong KG (2008) Optic neuropathy associated with dengue fever. Eye (Lond) 22(5):722–724
21. Chlebicki MP, Ang B, Barkham T, Laude A (2005) Retinal hemorrhages in 4 patients with dengue fever. Emerg Infect Dis 11(5):770–772
22. Bacsal KE, Chee SP, Cheng CL, Flores JV (2007) Dengue-associated maculopathy. Arch Ophthalmol 125(4):501–510
23. WHO (2009) Dengue guidelines for diagnosis, treatment, prevention and control, 3rd edn. World Health Organization, Geneva
24. Verma R, Sahu R, Holla V (2014) Neurological manifestations of dengue infection: a review. J Neurol Sci 346(1–2):26–34
25. Gupta M, Nayak R, Khwaja GA, Chowdhury D (2013) Acute disseminated encephalomyelitis associated with dengue infection: a case report with literature review. J Neurol Sci 335(1–2):216–218
26. Carod-Artal FJ, Wichmann O, Farrar J, Gascón J (2013) Neurological complications of dengue virus infection. Lancet Neurol 12(9):906–919
27. Koshy JM, Joseph DM, John M, Mani A, Malhotra N, Abraham GM, Pandian J (2012) Spectrum of neurological manifestations in dengue virus infection in Northwest India. Trop Doct 42(4):191–194
28. Puccioni-Sohler M, Orsini M, Soares CN (2012) Dengue: a new challenge for neurology. Neurol Int 4(3):e15
29. Araújo FM, Araújo MS, Nogueira RM, Brilhante RS, Oliveira DN, Rocha MF, Cordeiro RA, Araújo RM, Sidrim JJ (2012) Central nervous system involvement in dengue: aemic area. Neurology 78(10):736–742
30. Beral L, Merle H, David T (2008) Ocular complications of dengue fever. Ophthalmology 115(6):1100–1101
31. Haritoglou C, Dotse SD, Rudolph G, Stephan CM, Thurau SR, Klauss V (2002) A tourist with dengue fever and visual loss. Lancet 360(9339):1070
32. Miranda de Sousa A, Puccioni-Sohler M, Dias Borges A, Fernandes Adorno L, Papais Alvarenga M, Papais Alvarenga RM (2006) Post-dengue neuromyelitis optica: case report of a Japanese-descendent Brazilian child. J Infect Chemother 12(6):396–398
33. Weeratunga PN, Caldera MC, Gooneratne IK, Gamage R, Perera P (2014) Neurological manifestations of dengue: a cross sectional study. Travel Med Infect Dis 12(2):189–193
34. Preechawat P, Poonyathalang A (2005) Bilateral optic neuritis after dengue viral infection. J Neuroophthalmol 25(1):51–52
35. Wen KH, Sheu MM, Chung CB, Wang HZ, Chen CW (1989) The ocular fundus findings in dengue fever. Gaoxiong Yi Xue Ke Xue Za Zhi 5(1):24–30
36. Aragão RE, Barreira IM, Lima LN, Rabelo LP, Pereira FB (2010) Bilateral optic neuritis after dengue viral infection: case report. Arq Bras Oftalmol 73(2):175–178
37. de Amorim Garcia CA, Gomes AH, de Oliveira AG (2006) Bilateral stellar neuroretinitis in a patient with dengue fever. Eye (Lond) 20(12):1382–1383
38. Shivanthan MC, Ratnayake EC, Wijesiriwardena BC, Somaratna KC, Gamagedara LK (2012) Paralytic squint due to abducens nerve palsy: a rare consequence of dengue fever. BMC Infect Dis 12:156

39. Donnio A, Béral L, Olindo S, Cabie A, Merle H (2010) Dengue, a new etiology in oculomotor paralysis. Can J Ophthalmol 45(2):183–184
40. Pierre Filho Pde T, Carvalho Filho JP, Pierre ET (2008) Bilateral acute angle closure glaucoma in a patient with dengue fever: case report. Arq Bras Oftalmol 71(2):265–268
41. Saranappa SBS, Sowbhagya HN (2012) Panophthalmitis in dengue fever. Indian Pediatr 49(9):760
42. Kumar V, Ghosh B, Raina UK, Goel N (2009) Bilateral periorbital ecchymosis in a case with dengue fever. Indian J Ophthalmol 57(3):242–243
43. Nagaraj KB, Jayadev C, Yajmaan S, Prakash S (2014) An unusual ocular emergency in severe dengue. Middle East Afr J Ophthalmol 21(4):347–349
44. Chhavi N, Venkatesh C, Soundararajan P, Gunasekaran D (2013) Unusual ocular manifestations of dengue fever in a young girl. Indian J Pediatr 80(6):522–523
45. Mehta S, Mehta S, Jaindani P (2006) Ocular features of dengue septic shock (DSS). J Assoc Physicians India 54:866
46. Cruz-Villegas V, Berrocal AM, Davis JL (2003) Bilateral choroidal effusions associated with dengue fever. Retina 23(4):576–578
47. Lim WK, Mathur R, Koh A, Yeoh R, Chee SP (2004) Ocular manifestations of dengue fever. Ophthalmology 111(11):2057–2064
48. Nainiwal S, Garg SP, Prakash G, Nainiwal N (2005) Bilateral vitreous haemorrhage associated with dengue fever. Eye (Lond) 19(9):1012–1013
49. Gupta S, Das D (2013) Subhyaloid haemorrhage in dengue fever. J Indian Med Assoc 111(9):623–624
50. Gupta P, Jain C, Aggarwal A, Gupta SC (2011) Dengue fever presenting with macular hemorrhages. Retin Cases Brief Rep 5(3):213–218
51. Sumardi U, Nelwan EJ (2011) Retinal hemorrhage in dengue hemorrhagic fever. Acta Med Indones 43(1):66–67
52. Tabbara K (2012) Dengue retinochoroiditis. Ann Saudi Med 32(5):530–533
53. Siqueira RC, Vitral NP, Campos WR, Oréfice F, de Moraes Figueiredo LT (2004) Ocular manifestations in dengue fever. Ocul Immunol Inflamm 12(4):323–327
54. Loh BK, Bacsal K, Chee SP, Cheng BC, Wong D (2008) Foveolitis associated with dengue fever: a case series. Ophthalmologica 222(5):317–320
55. Juanarita J, Azmi MN, Azhany Y, Liza-Sharmini AT (2012) Dengue related maculopathy and foveolitis. Asian Pac J Trop Biomed 2(9):755–756
56. Teoh SC, Chee CK, Laude A, Goh KY, Barkham T, Ang BS, Eye Institute Dengue-related Ophthalmic Complications Workgroup (2010) Optical coherence tomography patterns as predictors of visual outcome in dengue-related maculopathy. Retina 30(3):390–398
57. Sadiq N, Naqaish T, Arif A, Mohammad K, Jalis M (2014) Central retinal artery occlusion secondary to dengue fever. J Ayub Med Coll Abbottabad 26(1):98–99
58. Kanungo S, Shukla D, Kim R (2008) Branch retinal artery occlusion secondary to dengue fever. Indian J Ophthalmol 56(1):73–74
59. Chia A, Luu CD, Mathur R, Cheng B, Chee SP (2006) Electrophysiological findings in patients with dengue-related maculopathy. Arch Ophthalmol 124(10):1421–1426
60. Tan MH, Tan PE, Wong EN, Chen FK (2014) Structure and function correlation in a patient with dengue-associated maculopathy. Clin Experiment Ophthalmol 42(5):504–507
61. Mendes TS, Sobrinho EF, Rosa AA, dos Anjos LM, da Costa GM, Souza Gda S, Gomes BD, Saito CA, da Silva FM, Silveira LC (2009) Dengue maculopathy: visual electrophysiology and optical coherence tomography. Doc Ophthalmol 119(2):145–155
62. Lai TY, Mohamed S, Chan WM, Lai RY, Lam DS (2007) Multifocal electroretinography in dengue fever-associated maculopathy. Br J Ophthalmol 91(8):1084–1085
63. Dengue: guidelines for diagnosis, treatment, prevention and control: new edition. World Health Organization, Geneva, 2009. 4, Laboratory Diagnosis and Diagnostic Tests. Available from: http://www.ncbi.nlm.nih.gov/books/NBK143156/
64. Wang SM, Sekaran SD (2010) Evaluation of a commercial SD dengue virus NS1 antigen capture enzyme-linked immunosorbent assay kit for early diagnosis of dengue virus infection. J Clin Microbiol 48(8):2793–2797
65. Tan SY, Kumar G, Surrun SK, Ong YY (2007) Dengue maculopathy: a case report. Travel Med Infect Dis 5(1):62–63
66. Yamamoto K, Takahashi H, Kanno M, Noda Y, Fujino Y (2013) Changes in parafoveal retinal thickness and subfoveal choroidal thickness in a patient with dengue fever-associated maculopathy. J Ophthalmic Inflamm Infect 3(1):63
67. Luk FO, Chan CK, Lai TY (2013) A case of dengue maculopathy with spontaneous recovery. Case Rep Ophthalmol 4(2):28–33
68. Quek DT, Barkham T, Teoh SC (2009) Recurrent bilateral dengue maculopathy following sequential infections with two serotypes of dengue virus. Eye (Lond) 23(6):1471–1472

14 Rift Valley Fever

Rim Kahloun, Imen Ksiaa, and Sonia Zaouali

14.1 Introduction

Rift Valley fever (RVF) is an emerging arthropod-borne zoonotic disease caused by RVF virus, which belongs to the *Bunyaviridae* family and the genus *Phlebovirus* [1]. RVF virus infection in humans usually causes a self-limiting, acute and febrile illness, but severe potentially lethal forms may occur [2, 3]. Macular or paramacular retinitis that may lead to severe visual impairment is the most common ocular complication of RVF [4–10].

14.2 Epidemiology

RVF virus was first isolated in Kenya in 1930. It has been responsible of outbreaks in Egypt in 1977, in Kenya and Somalia from 1997 through 1998 and in 2006–2007, in the southwestern region of Saudi Arabia in 2000 [5], in Tanzania in 2007, in Sudan in 2007–2008 [11], and in Mauritania in 2012 [12]. From the recent outbreaks, RVF appears to have great potential for spreading into new areas and with huge impact on human and animal health [11].

14.3 Pathophysiology

The RVF virus is an RNA virus with a diameter of 94 to 100 nm that is transmitted to humans mainly through direct contact with blood, excreta, meat, or secretions of infected animals, consumption of raw milk, and through mosquito bites that belong to the genera *Anopheles*, *Aedes*, and *Culex* [11]. Virus replication in the cattle gives high rates of mortality and abortion. RVF virus infection in humans usually causes a self-limiting, acute and febrile illness; however, a small number of cases progress to neurological disorders, partial or complete blindness, hemorrhagic fever, or thrombosis [13].

The timing of onset of RVF retinitis suggests an autoimmune origin. A recent study shows that serum samples from patients with RVF retinitis were slightly more likely to have antibodies against retinal tissue than control populations [14].

14.4 Clinical Features

14.4.1 Systemic Disease

The incubation period is generally from 3 to 7 days in humans [2, 3]. After the incubation period, RVF virus is often responsible for influenza-like symptoms including fever, headache, arthralgias, myalgias, and gastrointestinal disturbances [2, 3]. The temperature curve usually shows a biphasic pattern, with an initial

R. Kahloun (✉) • I. Ksiaa • S. Zaouali
Department of Ophthalmology, Fattouma Bourguiba University Hospital, Faculty of Medicine, University of Monastir, Monastir, Tunisia
e-mail: rim.korbaa@gmail.com; khay.imen@yahoo.fr; soniazaoualiletaief@gmail.com

S.-P. Chee, M. Khairallah (eds.), *Emerging Infectious Uveitis*, DOI 10.1007/978-3-319-23416-8_14

elevation lasting 2 to 3 days, followed by a remission and then a second febrile episode [2, 3]. Convalescence is typically rapid within few days.

Severe life-threatening clinical presentations may rarely occur including a hemorrhagic fever with liver involvement, thrombocytopenia, icterus and bleeding tendencies, and a neurologic involvement with encephalitis following a febrile episode with confusion and coma [2, 3]. Death is infrequent but there may be some residual damage.

14.4.2 Ocular Disease

Ocular involvement has been reported to occur in 1 % to 20 % of RVF infections, usually 4 to 15 days after onset of RVF [4, 5]. Prevalent symptoms at presentation include blurred vision, floaters, and scotomas. Unilateral or bilateral retinitis is the most common finding [4–10]. It typically presents in the form of a large, single area of necrotizing retinitis, macular or paramacular in location (Figs. 14.1a and 14.2a). Retinal lesions show early hypofluorescence and late staining on fluorescein angiography. Associated posterior segment changes include severe retinal vasculitis, retinal hemorrhages (Fig. 14.2a), vitritis, and optic disc edema [4–10]. Nongranulomatous anterior uveitis has also been described in association with posterior uveitis in patients with RVF [4]. Anterior chamber inflammation resolves spontaneously within 2 to 3 weeks from the onset of systemic symptoms, and is unlikely to result in complications such as glaucoma, posterior synechiae, or cataract. On the other hand, retinitis usually recovers within 10 to 12 weeks. Permanent visual loss is common, mainly due to macular or paramacular scarring (Fig. 14.2b), retinal vascular occlusion, or optic atrophy (Fig. 14.1b) [4–10].

14.5 Diagnosis

Once an outbreak is recognized and early cases are diagnosed, it becomes easier to suspect further cases of RVF. The most common method of laboratory diagnosis is based on serologic testing

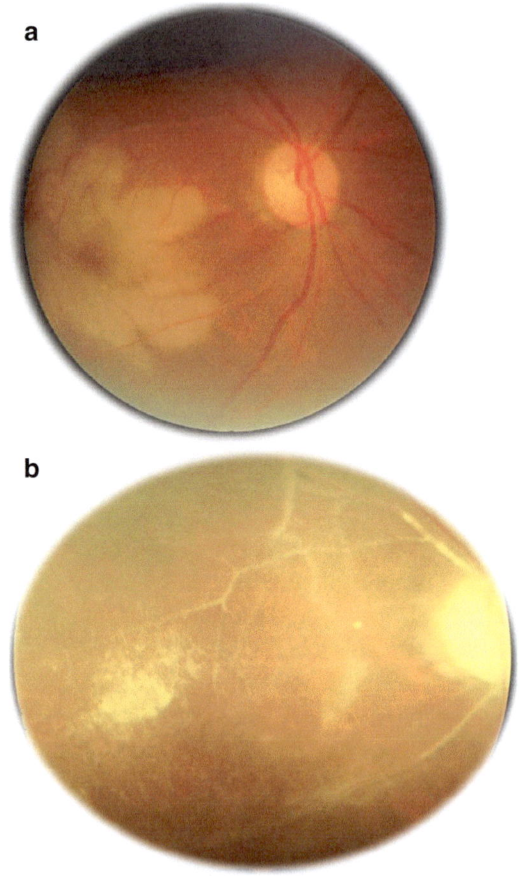

Fig. 14.1 (**a**) Fundus photograph of the right eye of a patient with Rift Valley fever shows a large active geographic retinitis involving the macula. (**b**) Six months later, the focus of retinitis healed leading to severe sheathing with optic disc atrophy (Courtesy, E. Abboud)

to detect anti-RVF virus IgM antibodies or a rising titer of IgG antibodies in the serum by ELISA technique. Furthermore, viral RNA by RT-PCR in serum or other tissue samples confirms the diagnosis of RVF [15, 16].

14.6 Differential Diagnosis

The differential diagnosis for RVF retinitis includes other infectious entities such as measles, rubella, influenza, cytomegalovirus, varicella zoster virus, herpes simplex virus, Chikungunya, Dengue fever, rickettsial infection, Lyme disease, syphilis, and cat scratch

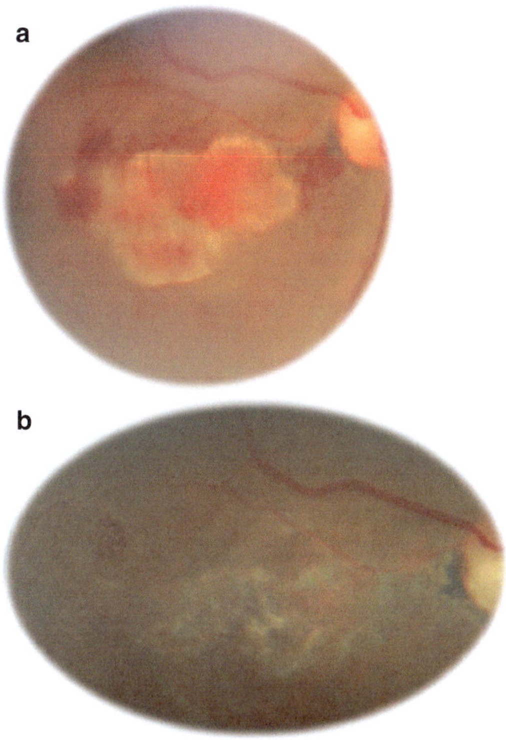

Fig. 14.2 (**a**) Fundus photograph of the right eye of a patient with Rift Valley fever shows a large active geographic retinitis involving the macula associated to retinal hemorrhages. (**b**) Fundus photograph of the same eye four months later shows resolution of the focus of retinitis leading to an atrophic macular retinochoroidal scar (Courtesy, E. Abboud)

disease [8]. Other hemorrhagic fever viruses have been reported to have ocular involvement such as Hantaan virus, Puumala, Marburg, and Ebola viruses [8]. The differential diagnosis of RVF retinitis may also include non-infectious entities like Behçet's retinitis.

These diseases can be differentiated from RVF by clinical history and serologic testing.

14.7 Management

The current treatment of RVF is entirely supportive with intravenous fluids and when indicated, blood transfusion, hemodialysis, or mechanical ventilation. There is no antiviral therapy with proven efficacy in this setting [11]. Preventive measures are recommended including intensified mosquito control, and protection against mosquito bites in areas of epizootic and human RVF activity [17, 18]. Education regarding modes of disease transmission and necessary precautions, especially protection against mosquito bites is vital. Vaccination of livestock may be a key element in breaking the chain of human epidemics, and could lead to control of this significant public health threat [19].

14.8 Prognosis

Prognosis of RVF virus infection systemic disease is good in most patients. However, severe cases may result in death [11]. Ocular involvement is frequently associated with permanent visual loss resulting from macular and paramacular scarring, vascular occlusion, or optic atrophy [4–10].

Conclusion

RVF infection should be considered in the differential diagnosis of macular or paramacular retinitis in a patient living in or returning from a specific endemic area, especially during confirmed outbreaks of the disease. Systemic involvement in RVF infection is usually self-limited; however, ocular involvement may lead to severe permanent visual impairment in most cases.

Core Messages

- Systemic disease: influenza-like symptoms with a biphasic-pattern fever, life-threatening hemorrhagic fever.
- Ocular disease: macular or paramacular necrotizing retinitis, anterior uveitis, occlusive retinal vasculitis, retinal hemorrhages, vitritis, optic disc edema.
- Diagnosis: primarily based on epidemiologic data and systemic symptoms, and confirmed by serologic testing or PCR.
- Treatment: entirely supportive, with prevention the mainstay of RVF infection control.

- Prognosis:
  Systemic disease: usually self-limited.
  Ocular involvement: persistent severe visual loss due to macular scarring, vascular occlusion, and/or optic atrophy.

References

1. Ikegami T (2012) Molecular biology and genetic diversity of Rift Valley fever virus. Antiviral Res 95:293–310
2. Isaäcson M (2001) Viral hemorrhagic fever hazards for travelers in Africa. Clin Infect Dis 33:1707–1712
3. Madani TA, Al-Mazrou YY, Al-Jeffri MH, Mishkhas AA, Al-Rabeah AM, Turkistani AM, Al-Sayed MO, Abodahish AA, Khan AS, Ksiazek TG, Shobokshi O (2003) Rift Valley fever epidemic in Saudi Arabia: epidemiological, clinical, and laboratory characteristics. Clin Infect Dis 37:1084–1092
4. Siam AL, Meegan JM, Gharbawi KF (1980) Rift Valley fever ocular manifestations: observations during the 1977 epidemic in Egypt. Br J Ophthalmol 64:366–374
5. Al-Hazmi A, Al-Rajhi AA, Abboud EB, Ayoola EA, Al-Hazmi M, Saadi R, Ahmed N (2005) Ocular complications of Rift Valley fever outbreak in Saudi Arabia. Ophthalmology 112:313–318
6. Khairallah M, Kahloun R, Ben Yahia S, Jelliti B, Messaoud R (2013) New infectious etiologies for posterior uveitis. Ophthalmic Res 49:66–72
7. Khairallah M, Kahloun R (2013) Ocular manifestations of emerging infectious diseases. Curr Opin Ophthalmol 24:574–580
8. Khairallah M, Jelliti B, Jenzeri S (2009) Emergent infectious uveitis. Middle East Afr J Ophthalmol 16:225–238
9. Khairallah M, Chee SP, Rathinam SR, Attia S, Nadella V (2010) Novel infectious agents causing uveitis. Int Ophthalmol 30:465–483
10. Khairallah M, Ben Yahia S, Attia S (2010) Arthropod vector-borne uveitis in the developing world. Int Ophthalmol Clin 50:125–144
11. Himeidan YE, Kweka EJ, Mahgoub MM, El Rayah e A, Ouma JO (2014) Recent outbreaks of Rift Valley fever in East Africa and the Middle East. Front Public Health 6(2):169
12. Sow A, Faye O, Ba Y, Ba H, Diallo D, Faye O, Loucoubar C, Boushab M, Barry Y, Diallo M, Sall AA (2014) Rift Valley fever outbreak, southern Mauritania, 2012. Emerg Infect Dis 20:296–299
13. Ikegami T, Makino S (2011) The pathogenesis of Rift Valley fever. Viruses (3):493–519
14. Newman-Gerhardt S, Muiruri S, Muchiri E, Peters CJ, Morrill J, Lucas AH, King CH, Kazura J, LaBeaud AD (2013) Potential for autoimmune pathogenesia of Rift Valley fever virus retinitis. Am J Trop Med Hyg 89:495–497
15. Maquart M, Temmam S, Héraud JM, Leparc-Goffart I, Cêtre-Sossah C, Dellagi K, Cardinale E, Pascalis H (2014) Development of real-time RT-PCR for the detection of low concentrations of Rift Valley fever virus. J Virol Methods 195:92–99
16. Wilson WC, Romito M, Jasperson DC, Weingartl H, Binepal YS, Maluleke MR, Wallace DB, van Vuren PJ, Paweska JT (2013) Development of a Rift Valley fever real-time RT-PCR assay that can detect all three genome segments. J Virol Methods 193:426–431
17. Dar O, McIntyre S, Hogarth S, Heymann D (2013) Rift Valley fever and a new paradigm of research and development for zoonotic disease control. Emerg Infect Dis 19:189–193
18. LaBeaud AD, Kazura JW, King CH (2010) Advances in Rift Valley fever research: insights for disease prevention. Curr Opin Infect Dis 23:403–408
19. Weingartl HM, Nfon CK, Zhang S, Marszal P, Wilson WC, Morrill JC, Bettinger GE, Peters CJ (2014) Efficacy of a recombinant Rift Valley fever virus MP-12 with NSm deletion as a vaccine candidate in sheep. Vaccine 32:2345–2349

Human T-Cell Leukemia Virus Type 1

15

Koju Kamoi and Manabu Mochizuki

15.1 Introduction

A retrovirus is an RNA virus encoding for a reverse transcriptase, which translates the viral RNA into a DNA provirus that is rapidly incorporated into the host's genome [1]. Retrovirus infections affect the systemic immune status and cause various diseases, including ocular diseases [2]. Retroviruses are currently classified as either oncoviruses or lentiviruses. Oncoviruses are associated with hematological proliferations and tumors of the connective tissues [3]. Human T-cell leukemia viruses (HTLVs) are representative oncoviruses, and HTLV-1 was the first retrovirus described as being a causative agent of human disease [4, 5]. Lentiviruses induce chronic and progressive pulmonary and/or neurological diseases. Human HIV is a representative of such viruses and is the causative agent of acquired immune deficiency syndrome [1].

After the discovery of the association between HTLV-1 and adult T-cell leukemia (ATL) in the early 1980s, other HLTV-1-related diseases that were identified included HTLV-1-associated myelopathy/tropical spastic paraparesis (HAM/TSP) [6, 7] and HTLV-1 uveitis (HU) [8–11]. By the 1990s, clinical and laboratory data including seroepidemiology, clinical features, detection of proviral DNA and mRNA of HTLV-1 from ocular tissues, and detection of viral particles from T-cell clones (TCC) derived from the aqueous humor of the patient helped establish that uveitis was significantly related to HTLV-1 [10–15]. In addition to HU which is the most common ocular finding, HTLV-1-associated ocular disease may also include opportunistic infections/malignant infiltrations of the eye in ATL patients and keratoconjunctivitis sicca [2].

This chapter is going to focuses on HU.

15.2 Epidemiology

HTLV-1 is known to have a unique geographic distribution, with an extremely high prevalence in the southern part of Japan, Melanesia, the Caribbean islands, Central and South America, as well as in central Africa. Worldwide, there are 20 million people estimated to be carrying the virus [16].

Recent surveys in Japan have indicated that the seroprevalence of HTLV-1 is decreasing in the general population. The reason for this reduction is thought to be due to serological screening for HTLV-1 in blood donors that was started 30 years ago. These screenings have successfully cut routes of the viral transmission, such as blood transfusion and breast-feeding from mother to child in endemic areas [17]. In contrast, a recent metropolitan area survey showed that there has been a significant increase in the number of

K. Kamoi (✉) • M. Mochizuki
Department of Ophthalmology & Visual Science, Graduate School of Medical and Dental Sciences, Tokyo Medical and Dental University, 1-5-45 Yushima, Bunkyo-ku, Tokyo 113-8519, Japan
e-mail: koju.oph@tmd.ac.jp

S.-P. Chee, M. Khairallah (eds.), *Emerging Infectious Uveitis*, DOI 10.1007/978-3-319-23416-8_15

HTLV-1 carriers due to the migration from endemic areas to metropolitan areas in Japan [18].

Although HU incidence has clearly decreased, it remains the most common cause of uveitis in endemic areas in Japan, coming before Vogt–Koyanagi–Harada disease, sarcoidosis, and toxoplasmosis [19]. HTLV-1 infection should also be considered as a possible cause of uveitis in other regions of the world, even though incidences appear to be higher in Japan [13, 19–23].

The prevalence rate of HU among the HTLV-1 carrier population was studied in the southern part of Japan. Independent clinical surveys conducted on the island of Kyushu reported and estimated 90–110 per 100,000 HTLV-1 carriers, which indicates there are approximately 1.0 HU cases per 1000 HTLV-1 carriers [24]. This prevalence is slightly higher than that reported for HAM/TSP [25].

HTLV-1 seroprevalence in patients with uveitis appears to be correlated with older age [15, 19, 20]. In addition to that, higher prevalences are found in women, especially after the age of 40 years. Since HTLV-1 is known to be transmitted by infected lymphocytes in the sperm, this may be a contributing factor for the higher prevalence of the disease in women versus men [15, 19, 20]. It is also of note that 25 % of the HU female patients had a previous medical history of Graves' disease [26].

15.3 Pathophysiology

The majority of the infiltrating cells in eyes with HU have been identified as CD3 T cells, and not malignant or leukemic cells [27, 28]. HTLV-1 proviral DNA, HTLV-1 protein, and viral particles have been detected in the infiltrating cells. HTLV-1-infected CD4 TCCs are able to produce various inflammatory cytokines in the eye, including interleukin (IL)-1, IL-6, IL-8, tumor necrosis factor (TNF-α), and interferon (IFN)-γ, which results in ocular inflammation [29] (Fig. 15.1).

The amount of integrated virus in the host genome is referred to as the provirus load and is involved in the HTLV-1 disease pathogenesis. Previous studies have shown that peripheral blood of HU patients contains a significantly higher provirus load compared to HTLV-1 asymptomatic carriers [28]. HTLV-1 provirus load in the peripheral blood mononuclear cells was also found to be correlated with intensity of the intraocular inflammation and with history of Graves' disease [30]. In addition to that, a greater HTLV-1 provirus load in the eye, as compared to peripheral blood

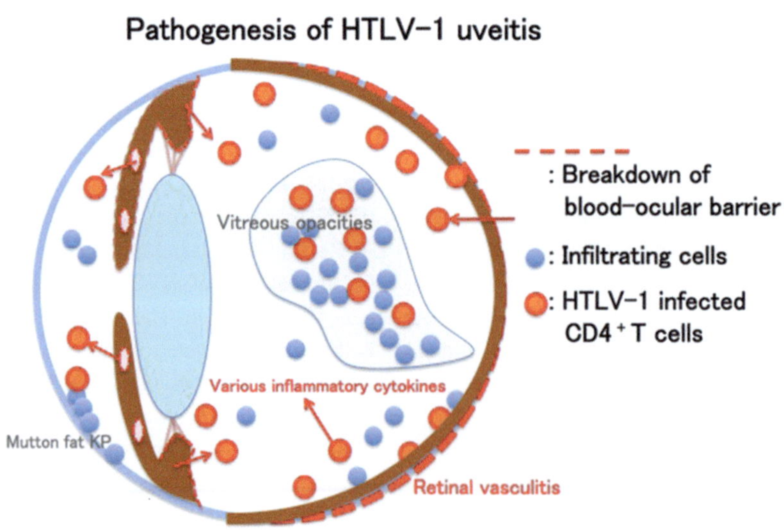

Fig. 15.1 Schema for the pathogenesis of HTLV-1 uveitis
HTLV-1 uveitis is caused by inflammatory cytokines produced by HTLV-1-infected CD4+ T cells that significantly accumulate in the eyes of patients

suggests a significant accumulation of HTLV-1-infected lymphocytes in eyes with HU [28].

15.4 Clinical Features

15.4.1 Systemic Disease

Most HTLV-1-infected persons are considered to be asymptomatic carriers. HTLV-1 causes HAM/TSP and ATL in a small percentage of infected individuals. HTLV-1-infected subjects, without a diagnosis of HAM/TSP, may also report subjective neurological symptoms such as paresthesia and weakness, or rheumatologic complaints mainly arthralgia. They may also develop oral disorders including gingivitis, periodontitis, and dry oral mucosa, or dermatitis [31]. Interval between HTLV-1 infection and disease manifestations remains unclear.

15.4.2 Ocular Disease

HTLV-1-associated ocular disease includes HU, opportunistic infections/malignant infiltrations of the eye in ATL patients, and keratoconjunctivitis sicca.

HU is usually characterized by a sudden onset with floaters, foggy vision, or moderate visual disturbance, with half of the affected patients developing bilateral HU [20]. HU typically presents with moderate to severe vitreous inflammation accompanied by mild anterior chamber cells and mild retinal vasculitis without any chorioretinal lesions (Fig. 15.2). Fluorescein angiography shows mild dye leakage from the retinal blood vessels (Fig. 15.3).

In most individuals, HU presents as an intermediate uveitis. Panuveitis, anterior uveitis and retinal vasculitis without vitreous

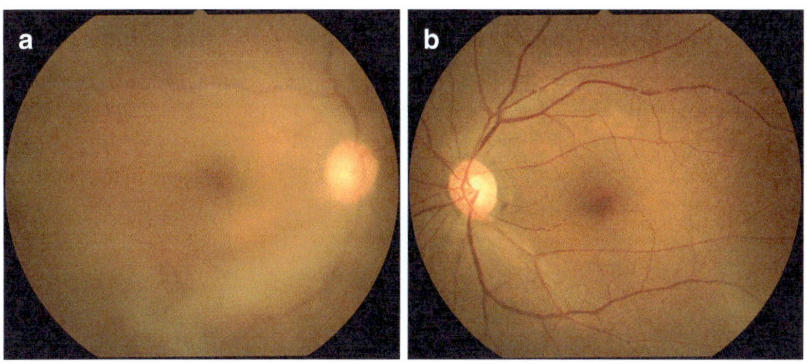

Fig. 15.2 Color fundus pictures in a typical patient with HTLV-1 uveitis. (**a**) Moderate vitreous opacities are seen in the right eye. (**b**) Inflammation is not seen in the left eye

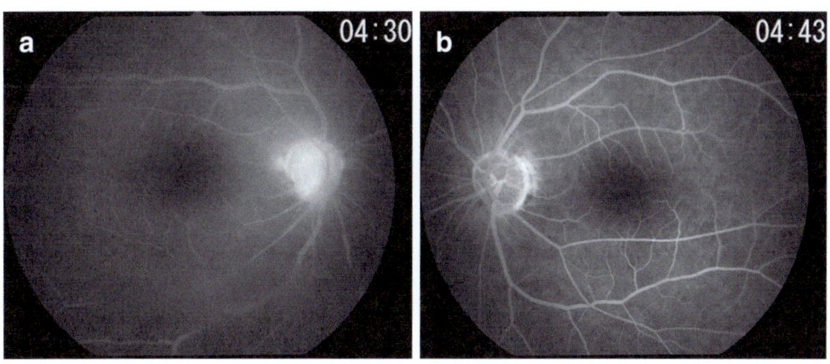

Fig. 15.3 Fluorescein angiographic pictures in a typical patient with HTLV-1 uveitis. (**a**) Mild dye leakage from the optic disc and retinal blood vessels is seen in the right eye. (**b**) Leakage is not seen in the left eye

opacities are less common. Mutton-fat KPs are often seen, but fibrin and hypopyon are extremely rare in the anterior chamber. Vitreous opacities are seen in more than 80 % of the patients, with more than half showing some form of vitreous membranous, lacework-like or dense opacities. Mild non-occlusive retinal vasculitis confirmed by fluorescein angiography is also seen in more than half of the patients. Although optic disc hyperemia may be observed in some patients, it disappears upon recovery from the intraocular inflammation and usually does not lead to atrophy. Cystoid macular edema has been reported to develop in less than 10 % of these patients [20].

15.5 Diagnosis

The diagnosis of HU should be based on seropositivity for HTLV-1 with no systemic evidence of HTLV-1-related diseases such as ATL and exclusion of other uveitis entities with defined causes such as ocular sarcoidosis, Behçet's disease, or candidiasis [2, 32]. Careful ophthalmic and systemic assessments and laboratory tests are needed. The polymerase chain reaction method on aqueous humor and peripheral blood samples may be used to detect the HTLV-1 provirus [33].

15.6 Differential Diagnosis

As previously mentioned, vitreous opacity and mild vasculitis are the major clinical features observed in HU. When diagnosing patients with vitreous opacities for potential HU, ocular sarcoidosis, Behçet's disease, pars planitis, and candidiasis must be excluded.

In ocular sarcoidosis, the nature of the vitreous opacities is clinically similar to that during HU. In HU, however, multiple snowball-like opacities are seen to a lesser degree, and typically punched-out-like multiple chorioretinal lesions in the peripheral retina are not seen.

In Behçet's disease, the vitreous opacity is denser than that observed in HU. Hypopyon, retinal hemorrhages, and infiltrates, which are typical features of Behçet's uveitis, are not seen in HU. Identification of systemic signs such as recurrent oral aphthous ulcers, and skin lesions are also helpful for differential diagnosis.

In addition to that, HU does not present "string of pearls" or "balls of fluff" patterns seen in candidiasis. The *Candida* antigens such as β-D-glucan in the peripheral blood will be negative in HU. Moreover, the snowbank-like changes seen in pars planitis are not observed in HU.

Venous sheathing, occlusion, and thrombosis of the retinal vessels typically seen in ocular sarcoidosis are not common in HU. In addition, the obstructive retinal vasculitis seen in Behçet's disease is not normally found in HU.

15.7 Management

Various inflammatory cytokines are produced by the HTLV-1-infected CD4+ T cells that significantly accumulate in the eyes of HU patients [32]. Therefore, corticosteroid treatment should be effective in treating the intraocular inflammation seen in these patients, as it will suppress the cytokine production of the HTLV-1-infected CD4+ T cells. The effectiveness of corticosteroid administration is supported by an in vitro study which found that addition of corticosteroids to a culture medium suppressed the cytokine production from the infiltrating cells [34].

A mild degree of anterior inflammation in HU can be managed by the use of topical nonsteroidal or corticosteroidal drugs together with mydriatics. A sub-Tenon's injection of corticosteroids such as triamcinolone acetonide may be an additional option when the patients have only moderate inflammatory activity in the vitreous cavity.

In patients with severe vitreous inflammatory activity and retinal vasculitis, oral corticosteroids should be better prescribed. It has been reported that an initial dosage of prednisolone started at 0.5 mg/kg daily followed by a tapering off of the drug is effective. However, long-term administration oral corticosteroids should be avoided [2, 32].

15.8 Prognosis

A good visual outcome is usually achieved with topical, and/or periocular, or systemic corticosteroids. However, approximately half of the patients experience recurrence of the uveitis [15]. Persistent visual impairment may result from secondary glaucoma, cystoid macular edema, or epiretinal membrane.

Conclusion

There have been clinical, seroepidemiological, molecular, biological, and virological evidence of HTLV-1-associated uveitis. Studies have allowed a better understanding of HU immunopathogenesis. However, many of the mechanisms of HU remain unclear, including how the HTLV-1-infected CD4+ cells are able to breakdown the ocular blood barrier and why the vitreous cavity is the major site of inflammation. Corticosteroids are the mainstay of HU treatment. They are able to suppress the cytokines produced by the infiltrating HTLV-1-infected cells. However, it remains unknown whether long-term corticosteroid treatment is safe or if it will adversely affect patients with HU.

Recent studies have shown new insights into the molecular functions of the HTLV-1 basic leucine zipper factor and Tax [35]. However, at the present time, there have been few studies undertaken to apply these new findings in further HU research. A better understanding of the mechanism of HU will make it possible to potentially find more effective treatments in the future.

Core Messages

- A better understanding of HTLV-1 uveitis is of more importance today for ophthalmologists as recent surveys have indicated that HTLV-1 carriers are now thought to be spreading the disease from local endemic areas to non-endemic metropolitan areas.
- The diagnosis of HTLV-1 uveitis is made based on positive serology for HTLV-1 and the exclusion of other uveitis entities, which include sarcoidosis, Behçet's disease, pars planitis, acute retinal necrosis, and candidiasis.
- A good prognosis is achieved following adequate treatment with topical and/or systemic corticosteroids, although the uveitis recurrence rate is high in these patients.

References

1. G DT (1989) HTLV-1 and chronic progressive encephalomyelopathies: an immunovirological perspective. Alan R Liss, New York
2. Kamoi K, Mochizuki M (2012) HTLV infection and the eye. Curr Opin Ophthalmol 23:557–561
3. Poiesz BJ, Ruscetti FW, Gazdar AF et al (1980) Detection and isolation of type C retrovirus particles from fresh and cultured lymphocytes of a patient with cutaneous T-cell lymphoma. Proc Natl Acad Sci U S A 77:7415–7419
4. Yoshida M, Seiki M, Yamaguchi K et al (1984) Monoclonal integration of human T-cell leukemia provirus in all primary tumors of adult T-cell leukemia suggests causative role of human T-cell leukemia virus in the disease. Proc Natl Acad Sci U S A 81:2534–2537
5. Gallo RC (2005) The discovery of the first human retrovirus: HTLV-1 and HTLV-2. Retrovirology 2:17
6. Gessain A, Barin F, Vernant JC et al (1985) Antibodies to human T-lymphotropic virus type-I in patients with tropical spastic paraparesis. Lancet 2:407–410
7. Osame M, Usuku K, Izumo S et al (1986) HTLV-I associated myelopathy, a new clinical entity. Lancet 1:1031–1032
8. Mochizuki M, Watanabe T, Yamaguchi K et al (1992) Uveitis associated with human T-cell lymphotropic virus type I. Am J Ophthalmol 114:123–129
9. Mochizuki M, Watanabe T, Yamaguchi K et al (1992) Uveitis associated with human T lymphotropic virus type I: seroepidemiologic, clinical, and virologic studies. J Infect Dis 166:943–944
10. Mochizuki M, Yamaguchi K, Takatsuki K et al (1992) HTLV-1 and uveitis. Lancet 399:1110
11. Ohba N, Matsumoto M, Sameshima M et al (1989) Ocular manifestations in patients infected with human T-lymphotropic virus type I. Jpn J Ophthalmol 33:1–12
12. Shirao M, Yoshimura K, Mochizuki M et al (1993) Uveitis in human T-lymphotropic virus type I (HTLV-I) carriers – 1. A seroepidemiological study. Nippon Ganka Gakkai Zasshi 97:726–732

13. Yoshimura K, Shimada N, Shirao M et al (1993) Uveitis in human T-lymphotropic virus type I (HTLV-I) carriers – 2. An analysis of clinical features. Nippon Ganka Gakkai Zasshi 97:733–740
14. Nakashima S, Shirao M, Mochizuki M et al (1993) Uveitis in human T-lymphotropic virus type I (HTLV-I) carriers – 3. A molecular biological study. Nippon Ganka Gakkai Zasshi 97:741–746
15. Yoshimura K, Mochizuki M, Araki S et al (1993) Clinical and immunologic features of human T-cell lymphotropic virus type I uveitis. Am J Ophthalmol 116:156–163
16. Watanabe T (2011) Current status of HTLV-1 infection. Int J Hematol 94:430–434
17. Iwanaga M, Chiyoda S, Kusaba E et al (2009) Trends in the seroprevalence of HTLV-1 in Japanese blood donors in Nagasaki Prefecture, 2000–2006. Int J Hematol 90:186–190
18. Uchimaru K, Nakamura Y, Tojo A et al (2008) Factors predisposing to HTLV-1 infection in residents of the greater Tokyo area. Int J Hematol 88:565–570
19. Miyanaga M, Shimizu K, Kawaguchi T et al (2009) A clinical survey of uveitis in HTLV-1 endemic region. Ocul Immunol Inflamm 17:335–341
20. Takahashi T, Takase H, Urano T et al (2000) Clinical features of human T-lymphotropic virus type 1 uveitis: a long-term follow-up. Ocul Immunol Inflamm 8:235–241
21. Merle H, Cabre P, Olindo S et al (2002) Ocular lesions in 200 patients infected by the human T-cell lymphotropic virus type 1 in martinique (French West Indies). Am J Ophthalmol 134:190–195
22. Pinheiro SR, Martins-Filho OA, Ribas JG et al (2006) Immunologic markers, uveitis, and keratoconjunctivitis sicca associated with human T-cell lymphotropic virus type 1. Am J Ophthalmol 142:811–815
23. Yamamoto JH, Segurado AA, Hirata CE et al (1999) Human T-cell lymphotropic virus type 1 infection and ocular manifestations in Sao Paulo, Brazil. Arch Ophthalmol 117:513–517
24. Ikeda E, Ono A, Hikita N et al (1998) Estimated prevalence rate of HTLV-I uveitis in Chikugo. Nippon Ganka Gakkai Zasshi 102:327–332
25. Osame M, Janssen R, Kubota H et al (1990) Nationwide survey of HTLV-I-associated myelopathy in Japan: association with blood transfusion. Ann Neurol 28:50–56
26. Yamaguchi K, Mochizuki M, Watanabe T et al (1994) Human T lymphotropic virus type 1 uveitis after Graves' disease. Br J Ophthalmol 78:163–166
27. Mochizuki M, Sugita S, Kamoi K (2013) Immunological homeostasis of the eye. Prog Retin Eye Res 33:10–27
28. Ono A, Mochizuki M, Yamaguchi K et al (1997) Immunologic and virologic characterization of the primary infiltrating cells in the aqueous humor of human T-cell leukemia virus type-1 uveitis. Accumulation of the human T-cell leukemia virus type-1-infected cells and constitutive expression of viral and interleukin-6 messenger ribonucleic acids. Invest Ophthalmol Vis Sci 38:676–689
29. Sagawa K, Mochizuki M, Masuoka K et al (1995) Immunopathological mechanisms of human T cell lymphotropic virus type 1 (HTLV-I) uveitis. Detection of HTLV-I-infected T cells in the eye and their constitutive cytokine production. J Clin Invest 95:852–858
30. Ono A, Ikeda E, Mochizuki M et al (1998) Provirus load in patients with human T-cell leukemia virus type 1 uveitis correlates with precedent Graves' disease and disease activities. Jpn J Cancer Res: Gann 89:608–614
31. Poetker SK, Porto AF, Giozza SP et al (2011) Clinical manifestations in individuals with recent diagnosis of HTLV type I infection. J Clin Virol: the official publication of the Pan American Society for Clinical Virology 51:54–58
32. Kamoi K, Mochizuki M (2012) HTLV-1 uveitis. Front Microbiol 3:270
33. Sugita S, Ogawa M, Shimizu N et al (2013) Use of a comprehensive polymerase chain reaction system for diagnosis of ocular infectious diseases. Ophthalmology 120:1761–1768
34. Sagawa K, Mochizuki M, Katagirl K et al (1996) In vitro effects of immunosuppressive agents on cytokine production by HTLV-I-infected T cell clones derived from the ocular fluid of patients with HTLV-I uveitis. Microbiol Immunol 40:373–379
35. Yasunaga J, Matsuoka M (2011) Molecular mechanisms of HTLV-1 infection and pathogenesis. Int J Hematol 94:435–442

HHV6, HHV7, and HHV8

16

Sunao Sugita and Tomoyuki Inoue

16.1 Introduction

The virus, particularly herpes virus family, has a particular propensity for infecting ocular tissues. Human herpes virus type 6 (HHV6), type 7 (HHV7), and type 8 (HHV8) are members of the herpes virus family [1–3]. Recent diagnostic techniques have indicated that infection/reactivation of these viruses is implicated in ocular inflammatory diseases. In this era of readily available polymerase chain reaction (PCR) examination, the viruses causing ocular inflammatory diseases, as well as HHV6, HHV7, and HHV8 can be identified. Here we describe HHV6, HHV7, and HHV8 infection in the eye and associated ocular diseases.

16.2 Epidemiology

HHV6 is a widespread virus. HHV6 may infect virtually almost all children during the early years of life, and this virus establishes latency after primary infection. It is difficult to be certain whether HHV6 is the causative agent of intraocular inflammation in patients. As shown in our previous report [4], PCR analyses indicated that 7/350 ocular inflammatory patients (2 %) were positive for HHV6 genomic DNA. In addition, the corneal tissue samples of 1/65 patients (1.5 %) tested positive for HHV6. The study of another group also reported that HHV6 DNA was detected in approximately 1 % of vitreous samples from patients with ocular inflammation [5].

HHV7, like HHV6, is ubiquitous with transmission occurring early in childhood although initial infection appears to occur later than for HHV6 [6, 7]. HHV7 that was isolated from the peripheral blood lymphocytes of a healthy individual could replicate and produce progeny viruses in T cells [8]. Little is known about the epidemiological characteristics and manifestation of HHV7 infection. HHV7-related ocular manifestation was first reported as a unilateral corneal endotheliitis in a healthy individual [9]. In our unpublished results, HHV7 genomic DNA was detected in the aqueous humor of approximately 1 % of cases with anterior uveitis or corneal endotheliitis associated with anterior segment ocular inflammation due to unknown cause.

HHV8, the newest human herpes virus, was identified using a molecular biological method in tissues with Kaposi's sarcoma of patients with AIDS. This sarcoma is a rare malignant tumor of the endothelia and vascular smooth muscle cells [3]. HHV8 is also known under the alias of Kaposi's

S. Sugita, MD, PhD (✉)
Laboratory for Retinal Regeneration, Center for Developmental Biology, RIKEN, 2-2-3 Minatojima-minamimachi, Chuo-ku, Kobe 650-0047, Japan
e-mail: sunaoph@cdb.riken.jp

T. Inoue
Tane Memorial Eye Hospital, Osaka, Japan

Department of Ophthalmology, Ehime University School of Medicine, Ehime, Japan

S.-P. Chee, M. Khairallah (eds.), *Emerging Infectious Uveitis*, DOI 10.1007/978-3-319-23416-8_16

sarcoma-associated herpes virus. The DNA sequence of HHV8 was detected in most of this neoplastic lesions in AIDS patients; however, HHV8 is present in all forms of this disease whether the patients are HIV infected or not [10]. HHV8 is associated with the neoplastic disease. HHV8-related ocular manifestation was reported in ocular adnexa, conjunctival Kaposi's sarcoma, and other neoplasms [11]. Apart from its presence in neoplasms, we were the first to report the presence of HHV8 in unilateral corneal endotheliitis with anterior segment eye inflammation in a healthy individual after keratoplasty [12]. In our unpublished results, HHV8 genomic DNA was detected in the aqueous humor in several cases with anterior uveitis or corneal endotheliitis due to unknown cause.

16.3 Pathophysiology

HHV6 can reactivate from its latent form after primary infection. HHV6 can be classified into two groups: variant A (HHV6-A) and variant B (HHV6-B). HHV6 mRNA was detected in intraocular samples from HHV6 genomic DNA-positive patients with active intraocular inflammation, suggesting that viral replication or reactivation may occur in the eye [4].

HHV6 can reside in a latent form in cells of the lymphoid (e.g., T cells/B cells) and myeloid lineage (e.g., monocytes), and it may enter the inflamed eye via immune cells. Once in the eye, HHV6 can infect human retinal pigment epithelial cells [13]. The majority of HHV6 DNA in intraocular fluids of inflamed eyes might be a consequence of the release of HHV6 DNA from resident ocular cells and infiltrating immune cells caused by intraocular inflammation.

HHV7 has strong homology with HHV6 and belongs to the beta-herpes virus subfamily. HHV7 uses the CD4 of $CD4^+$ T cells as its cellular receptor and competes with HIV infection [14]. The association of HHV7 with human diseases has not been almost recognized, although HHV7 is also known to cause exanthema subitum in children [15]. HHV7 is reactivated from latently infected peripheral blood mononuclear cells by T-cell activation, and HHV7 can provide a transacting function(s) mediating HHV7 reactivating from latency [16].

The HHV8 DNA sequence is closely related to that of the Epstein-Barr virus (EBV) and to that of a member of the gamma-herpes virus subfamily [17]. These viruses infect lymphocytes and are associated with cell immortalization and transformation, which would lead to HHV8-related neoplastic disease and could be associated with ocular inflammatory diseases [6].

16.4 Clinical Features

HHV6 is associated with immunodeficiency disorders and neurological diseases [18, 19]. HHV6-B is a widely known causative agent of exanthema subitum in children [19]. In addition, HHV6 type A is a known causative agent of neurological diseases [18, 19]. In the case of eye diseases, HHV6 has been implicated in infectious uveitis [4, 20] and other inflammatory diseases. According to the previous reports regarding HHV6 [4, 20], almost all patients with uveitis and endophthalmitis have active ocular inflammation; that is, there are anterior chamber cells, keratic precipitates, vitreous opacity, and fresh retinal exudates/necrosis. On the other hand, this virus is also associated with ocular surface inflammation. In a patient with HHV6 DNA-positive keratitis (Fig. 16.1), corneal infection (corneal epithelial ulcer and ciliary injection) was indicated. Since the clinical findings for different viruses are virtually indistinguishable, the diagnosis is based on PCR of ocular samples.

Patients with HHV7-related ocular diseases have active inflammation of the anterior segment of the eye; that is, there are anterior chamber cells, keratic precipitates, ocular hypertension, and/or corneal edema that initiates from corneal periphery and gradually progresses to total corneal area [9].

HHV8-related ocular neoplastic diseases such as Kaposi's sarcoma of the ocular adnexa or conjunctival Kaposi's sarcoma include a vascular-like lesion composed of spindle-shaped cells [21]. In AIDS patients with Kaposi's sarcoma, many more patients might have some form of

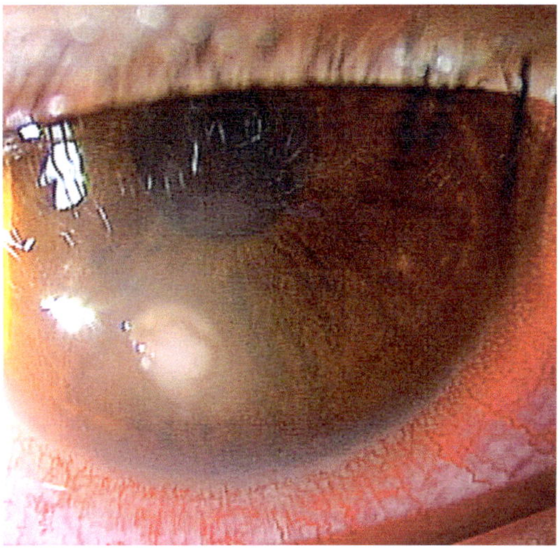

Fig. 16.1 Slit-lamp photograph of HHV6 DNA-positive keratitis

ocular involvement. A case with bilateral Kaposi's sarcoma was reported for a HIV-positive homosexual male with histological, DNA and serological evidence of HHV8 [11]. Patients with HHV8-related ocular inflammatory disease similar to those with HHV7 disease have active inflammation of the anterior segment of the eye and/or corneal edema [12]. We have summarized the systemic and ocular diseases associated with HHV6, HHV7, and HHV8 infection (Table 16.1).

16.5 Diagnosis

The diagnosis of HHV6 can be challenging due to the high prevalence of infection and viral persistence. Detection of the viral genome indicates active or latent infections in the ocular samples. PCR tests have been established in order to detect active HHV6 infections [4, 22, 23]. Using these PCR techniques, HHV6 genomic DNA was found in ocular inflammatory diseases. For example, high copy numbers of HHV6 DNA can be detected in ocular samples using quantitative PCR examination (Fig. 16.2). For such diagnosis, ocular samples (aqueous humor, vitreous fluids, cornea tissues, and other ocular samples) need to be collected.

HHV7 or HHV8 genomic DNA has also been detected by PCR in ocular samples. For the diagnosis of corneal endotheliitis, an aqueous humor sample is prepared for examination. A case of HHV7-related corneal endotheliitis after Descemet's stripping endothelial keratoplasty is shown in Fig. 16.3.

Table 16.1 Summary of systemic and ocular diseases with HHV6-, HHV7-, HHV8-associated infection

Virus	Systemic disease	Ocular disease
HHV6	Exanthema subitum	AIDS-associated retinitis
	Pneumonitis	Iritis (uveitis)
	Infections of CNS	Endophthalmitis
		Corneal inflammation (keratitis)
		Optic neuropathy
HHV7	Exanthema subitum	Iritis (uveitis)
		Corneal endotheliitis
HHV8	Kaposi's sarcoma	Iritis (uveitis)
	Multicentric Castleman disease	Corneal endotheliitis
	Primary effusion lymphoma	Conjunctival Kaposi's sarcoma
		Kaposi's sarcoma of the ocular adnexa

CNS central nervous system

16.6 Differential Diagnosis

Differential diagnosis of viral involvement in ocular disease is not yet possible because the involvement of HHV6, HHV7, or HHV8 in ocular infections has not yet been clearly demonstrated. In particular, it is necessary to differentiate HHV7- or HHV8-related corneal endotheliitis from other viral causes including herpes simplex, varicella zoster virus, and cytomegalovirus. In cases after corneal transplantation, specific viral involvement in allograft rejection needs to be differentiated.

16.7 Management

It is still controversial whether antiviral medication should be used or not for the treatment of HHV6-related ocular diseases. However, in our

Fig. 16.2 Detection of HHV6 DNA using quantitative real-time PCR

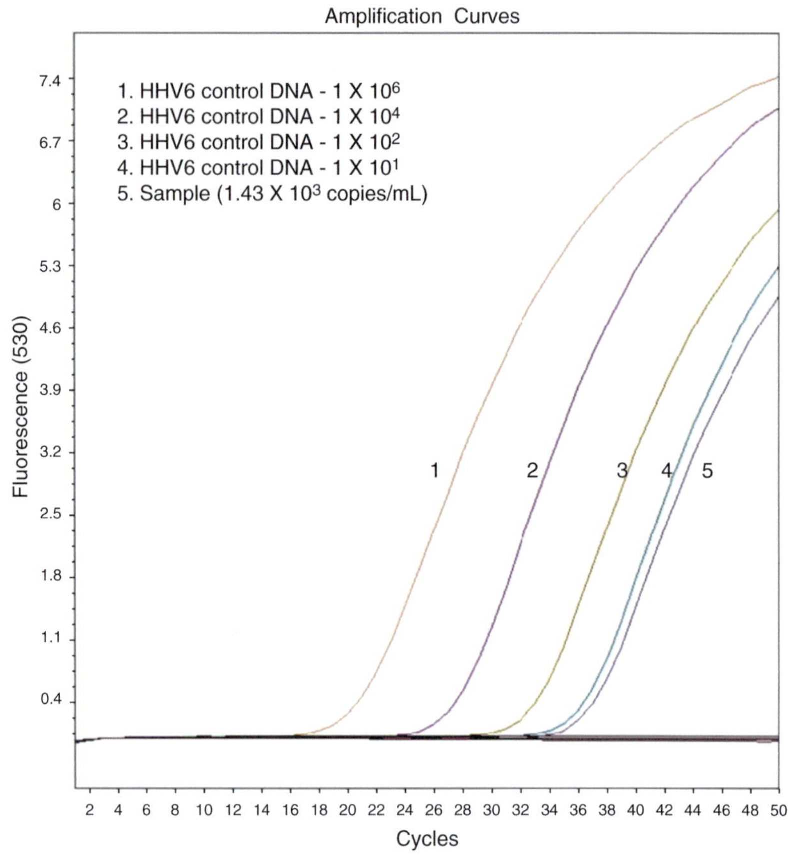

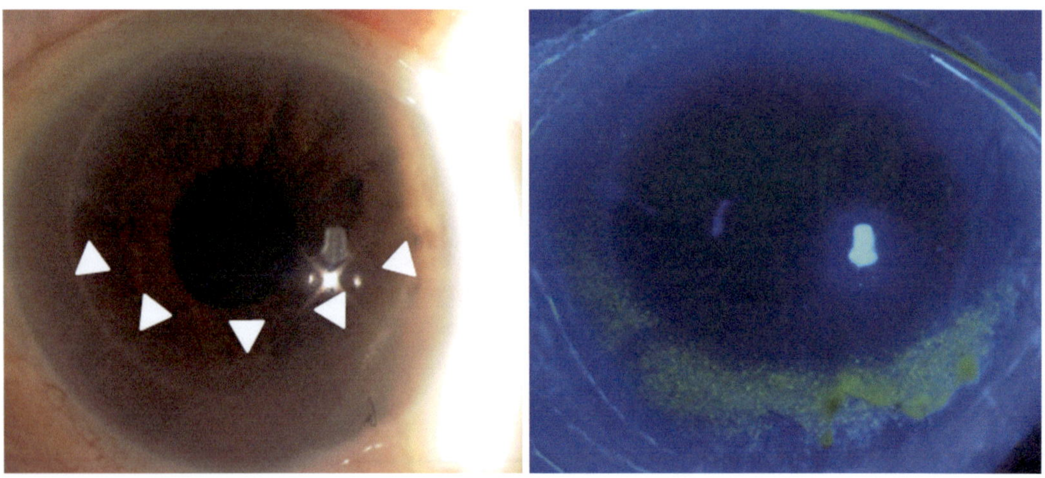

Fig. 16.3 Slit-lamp photograph(*left*) and fluorescein stain (*right*) of HHV7-positive corneal endotheliitis. Localized corneal edema in the inferior peripheral area is shown by the white arrowheads in a slit-lamp photograph (*left*), and epithelial edema is stained by fluorescein staining (*right*) with keratic precipitates and mild anterior chamber inflammation

experience, the intraocular viral DNA level and intraocular inflammation decreased in response to an antiviral agent plus systemic steroids [20]. Antiviral agents such as valaciclovir or valganciclovir should be used for such treatment. These results suggest that HHV6 has some role in the pathological physiology of ocular inflammation.

Treatment for HHV7-related corneal endotheliitis, like that of HHV6 treatment, remains controversial. For the treatment of HHV7-related corneal endotheliitis, local and/or systemic ganciclovir, an antiviral agent for cytomegalovirus or HHV7, and topical steroid were used [9]. In mild cases, the ocular inflammatory symptoms related to HHV7 were healed with topical ganciclovir alone. However, the cases with severe ocular inflammation related to HHV7 need to treat with the systemic administration of ganciclovir in addition to the topical ganciclovir.

Since anti-HHV8 therapy has not been established and is therefore unavailable, there is no treatment option for specific HHV8-related corneal endotheliitis, and general anti-inflammatory treatment using an agent such as a steroid can be used. In a previous report, HHV8-positive corneal endotheliitis was found in patients after penetrating keratoplasty. Allograft rejection and viral corneal endotheliitis can present with a similar appearance. This case positive for HHV8 in the aqueous humor received only topical and systemic steroid treatment as a unique therapeutic option; however, graft finally failed [12].

16.8 Prognosis

The prognosis depends on the extent of ocular inflammation. For example, in corneal endotheliitis, prognosis depends on the remaining normal corneal endothelial cell number after acute inflammation.

Conclusion

HHV6 infection may have a role as a causative agent of severe intraocular inflammation. The clinical relevance of HHV7 or HHV8 in corneal endotheliitis remains to be elucidated, because detection of HHV7 or HHV8 using PCR does not necessarily mean that HHV7 or HHV8 caused the clinical manifestations of corneal endotheliitis. However, in a previous report of HHV7 corneal endotheliitis, confirmation of HHV7 presence using real-time PCR allowed confident initiation of the appropriate ganciclovir treatment and subsequent clinical improvement [9]. This topical antiviral therapy that was effective for HHV7 improved the clinical status along with decreasing the HHV7 load, which validated the possibility that HHV7 is a causative agent of corneal endotheliitis. On the other hand, there is no therapeutic validation regarding HHV8-related corneal endotheliitis because anti-HHV8 therapy has not yet been established. However, in a published report of HHV8 corneal endotheliitis, HHV8 DNA expression was high in the aqueous humor in the active inflammatory phase but not in the stable phase [12]. Thus, since other human herpes viruses are related with corneal endotheliitis, HHV8 can also be considered a candidate virus related with corneal endotheliitis. These findings suggested that HHV7 or HHV8 infection can play a role in corneal endotheliitis. The observed cases of HHV7 or HHV8 corneal endotheliitis presented unilaterally in the same manner as other types of herpetic keratitis such as HSV, VZV, or CMV [24]. A previous report indicated that HHV7 appears to be closely related to CMV and is found in similar clinical situations. We recently reported that we detected CMV in about 25 % of cases with corneal endotheliitis of unknown etiology [25]. The causes of the other 75 % of the endotheliitis cases are unknown.

Core Messages

Since these virus-positive cases are found to have the viral genome in the inflamed eye, HHV6, HHV7, and HHV8 infection is implicated in ocular inflammatory diseases. Thus, the ocular samples collected from patients with infectious/inflammatory ocular disorders contain HHV6, HHV7, and HHV8 genomic DNA.

References

1. Salahuddin SZ, Ablashi DV, Markham PD et al (1986) Isolation of a new virus, HBLV in patients with lymphoproliferative disorders. Science 23:596–601
2. Frenkel N, Schirmer EC, Wyatt LS et al (1990) Isolation of a new herpesvirus from human CD4+ T cells. Proc Natl Acad Sci USA 87:748–752
3. Chang Y, Cesarman E, Pessin MS et al (1998) Identification of herpesvirus-like DNA sequences in AIDS-associated Kaposi's sarcoma. Science 266:1865–1869
4. Sugita S, Shimizu N, Watanabe K et al (2012) Virological analysis in patients with human herpes virus 6-associated ocular inflammatory disorders. Invest Ophthalmol Vis Sci 53:4692–4698
5. Cohen JI, Fahle G, Kemp MA et al (2010) Human herpesvirus 6-A, 6-B, and 7 in vitreous fluid samples. J Med Virol 82:996–999
6. Lavy JA (1997) Three new human herpesviruses (HHV6, 7, and 8). Lancet 349:558–562
7. Caserta MT, Hall CB, Schnabel K et al (1998) Primary human herpes 7 infection: a comparison of human herpesvirus 7 and human herpesvirus 6 infection in children. J Pediatr 133:386–389
8. Frenkel N, Schirmer EC, Wyatt LS et al (1990) Isolation of a new herpesvirus from human CD4+ T cells. Proc Natl Acad Sci USA 87:748–752
9. Inoue T, Kandori M, Takamatsu F et al (2010) Corneal endotheliitis with quantitative polymerase chain reaction positive for human herpesvirus 7. Arch Ophthalmol 128:502–503
10. Levy JA (1995) A new human herpesvirus: is it KSHV or HHV8? Lancet 345:786
11. Minoda H, Usui N, Sato T et al (2006) Human herpesvirus-8 in Kaposi's sarcoma of the conjunctiva in a patient with AIDS. Jpn J Ophthalmol 50:7–11
12. Inoue T, Takamatsu F, Kubota A et al (2011) Human herpesvirus 8 in corneal endotheliitis resulting in graft failure after penetrating keratoplasty refractory to allograft rejection therapy. Arch Ophthalmol 129:1629–1630
13. Arao Y, Soushi S, Sato Y et al (1997) Infection of a human retinal pigment epithelial cell line with human herpesvirus 6 variant A. J Med Virol 53:105–110
14. Lusso P, Secchiero P, Crowley RW et al (1994) CD4 is a critical component of the receptor for human herpesvirus 7: interference with human immunodeficiency virus. Proc Natl Acad Sci USA 91:3872–3876
15. Abrashi DV, Berneman ZN, Kramarsky B et al (1995) Human herpesvirus-7 (HHV-7): current status. Clin Diag Virol 4:1–13
16. Katasafanas GC, Schirmer EC, Wyatt LS et al (1996) In vivo activation of human herpesvirus 6 and 7 from latency. Proc Natl Acad Sci USA 93:9788–9792
17. Moore PS, Gao S-J, Dominguez G et al (1996) Primary characterization of a herpesvirus agent associated with Kaposi's sarcoma. J Virol 70:549–558
18. Schirmer EC, Wyatt LS, Yamanishi K et al (1991) Differentiation between two distinct classes of viruses now classified as human herpesvirus 6. Proc Natl Acad Sci USA 88:5922–5926
19. Zerr DM (2006) Human herpesvirus 6: a clinical update. Herpes 13:20–24
20. Sugita S, Shimizu N, Kawaguchi T et al (2007) Identification of human herpesvirus 6 in a patient with severe unilateral panuveitis. Arch Ophthalmol 125:1426–1427
21. Boshoff C, Schultz TF, Kennedy MM et al (1995) Kaposi's sarcoma-associated herpesvirus infects endothelial and spindle cells. Nat Med 1:1274–1278
22. Huang LM, Kuo PF, Lee CY et al (1992) Detection of human herpesvirus-6 DNA by polymerase chain reaction in serum or plasma. J Med Virol 38:7–10
23. Suga S, Yazaki T, Kajita Y et al (1995) Detection of human herpesvirus 6 DNAs in samples from several body sites of patients with exanthem subitum and their mothers by polymerase chain reaction assay. J Med Virol 46:52–55
24. Inoue T, Ohashi Y (2013) Utility of real-time PCR analysis for appropriate diagnosis for keratitis. Cornea 32:S71–S76
25. Kandori M, Inoue T, Takamatsu F et al (2010) Prevalence and features of keratitis with quantitative polymerase chain reaction positive for cytomegalovirus. Ophthalmol 117:216–222

Part III

Emerging Parasitic Infections

Cysticercosis

17

Kalpana Babu, Moupia Mukhopadhyay, and Krishna R. Murthy

17.1 Introduction

Cysticercosis is the most common ocular tapeworm infection. It is caused by *Cysticercus cellulosae*, the larval form of the pork tapeworm, *Taenia solium*. Man becomes infected by drinking contaminated water or eating food containing the eggs of *Taenia solium* [1]. Cysticercosis was first reported by Semmering in 1830 from the anterior chamber of the human eye, and the larva was isolated by Schott in 1836 [2, 3]. The most common form of systemic involvement is neurocysticercosis. Ocular and adnexal cysticercosis represents 13–46 % of systemic disease [2, 3]. Cysticerci can remain quiescent in the eye for up to 5 years.

17.2 Epidemiology

Cysticercosis has a worldwide distribution [3, 4]. It is common in India, South and Central America, Mexico, Southeast Asia and Sub-Saharan Africa. It is rare in Great Britain and the United States. Risk factors include poverty and poor sanitation, both of which promote fecal-oral transmission of disease. Although there is no gender or racial predilection, patients are relatively young, and the disease is usually unilateral. Involvement of the left eye seems to be more common than the right eye [4, 5].

17.3 Pathophysiology

Taenia solium passes its life cycle in two hosts: humans are the definitive hosts and the adult parasites live in the small intestine for several years. The pig is the intermediate host and is also the main host of the larva.

Human cysticercosis is caused by the ingestion of the pork tapeworm, *T. solium*, when contaminated food such as contaminated vegetables, fruits or water is consumed. The consumed eggs behave as if they are within the intermediate host and hatch in the upper intestines of humans. The embryo penetrates the gut, invades lymphatics and bloodstream, and travels to various organs like the central nervous system, eyes and skeletal muscles. The embryo discards the hooks and forms a head or the scolex by invagination of its wall, transforms into larvae and encysts in these tissues which have a high metabolic turnover and good glycogen supply. They may remain quiescent or die inciting an immunological reaction due to the chemical toxins they release [1, 2].

Autoinfection can also occur from faecal-oral contamination. In this case, man becomes the definitive host of the adult tapeworm, and eggs are released into the feces. Sometimes, man acquires the parasite by ingestion of undercooked

K. Babu (✉) • M. Mukhopadhyay • K.R. Murthy
Prabha Eye Clinic & Research Centre, Vittala International Institute of Ophthalmology, Bangalore, India
e-mail: kalpanababumurthy@gmail.com

S.-P. Chee, M. Khairallah (eds.), *Emerging Infectious Uveitis*, DOI 10.1007/978-3-319-23416-8_17

pork containing the larval cysts. The larval cyst develops in the intestine as the adult tapeworm. Thus a patient can harbor both the larval cyst and the adult forms of *T. solium.* It has been speculated that the cysticercosis enters the eye via the choroidal circulation, where the vessels have a larger flow rate. From the choroid, it migrates into the subretinal space and then into the vitreous cavity through a hole in the retina. This passage probably incites inflammation and results in the formation of a chorioretinal scar [6].

17.4 Clinical Features

Ocular cysticercosis may affect any portion of the visual pathway from the orbit to the visual cortex. The common sites of ocular involvement include retina/subretinal space (41 %), vitreous cavity (27 %), subconjunctival space (21 %), anterior segment (8 %) and lids/orbit (4 %) [7]. The symptoms depend on the location and the problems caused due to the mass effect of the cyst or inflammation due to the dying parasite. Review of symptoms may reveal a history of epilepsy [6, 7].

Intraocular cysticercosis may be asymptomatic or present with poor or blurring of vision, floaters, pain, photophobia or red eye. Cysts may be present in the anterior segment and vitreous, subretinal and submacular locations (Figs. 17.1, 17.2, and 17.3) [8–11]. Symptoms may occur for a few weeks or months before presentation. Visual acuity varies from slight blur in vision in peripheral subretinal cysticercosis to hand movements in submacular cysticercosis. If the cyst is alive within the eye, it often induces a mild to moderate inflammatory reaction in the anterior chamber and/ or the vitreous. It is spherical, translucent with a scolex that undulates with evagination or invagination in response to the examining light. A dying parasite can lead to intense inflammatory reaction due to the liberated chemical toxins, which can even lead to blindness and phthisis (Fig. 17.4). Oedema, haemorrhages, subretinal exudates, sheathing of retinal vessels, exudative retinal detachment, retinal pigment epithelial disturbances and optic disc hyperaemia may also be seen. Optic nerve involvement is a very rare presentation. It usually presents

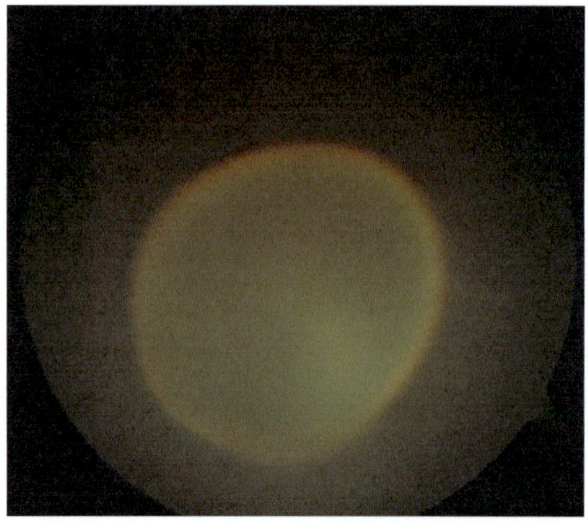

Fig. 17.1 Fundus photograph showing a cysticercus cyst in the vitreous

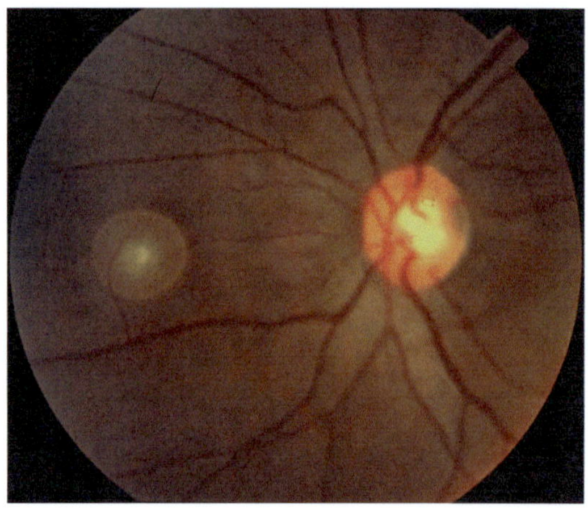

Fig. 17.2 Fundus photograph showing subretinal cyst

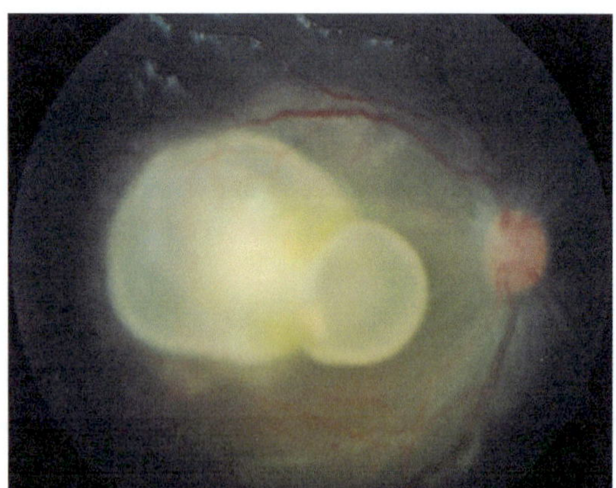

Fig. 17.3 Fundus photograph showing mushrooming of the cyst from the subretinal layer into the vitreous

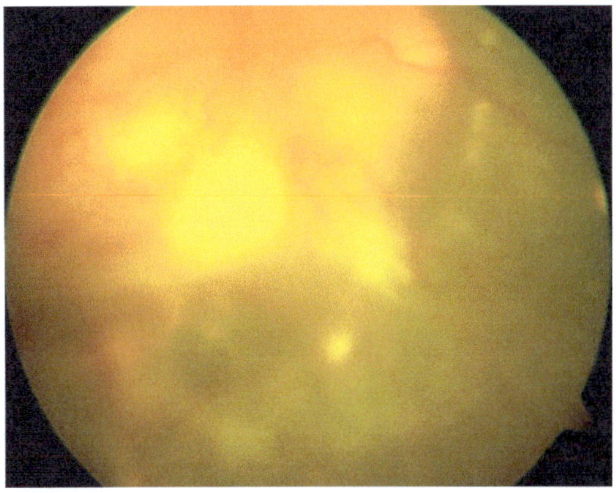

Fig. 17.4 Fundus photograph showing severe inflammation in a dead cyst

with marked diminution of vision and field loss with or without proptosis. Papilledema and papillitis with a relative afferent papillary defect are common presenting signs [12] (Fig. 17.5).

Subconjunctival involvement may be asymptomatic, present as recurrent conjunctivitis not responsive to topical antibiotics or a painful or painless swelling of the conjunctiva. The most common symptoms associated with orbital cysticercosis are diplopia (due to restrictive ophthalmopathy), recurrent pain and redness. Other presentations include gradually increasing nonaxial proptosis, ptosis and lid nodules. Infection of the extraocular muscles usually causes problems due to the mass effect or

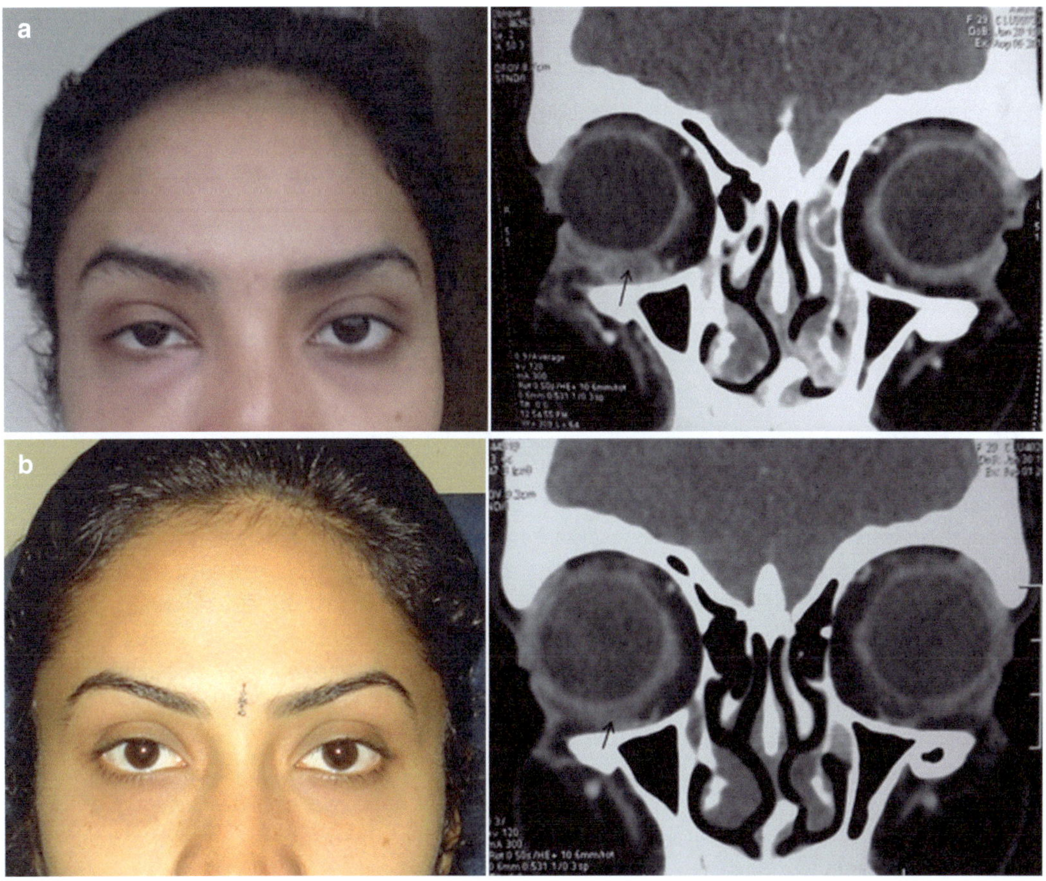

Fig. 17.5 External photograph and CT scan orbits showing ptosis and restriction of elevation in the right eye before medical treatment (**a**) and improvement after medical treatment (**b**). *Arrow* showing the location of cyst

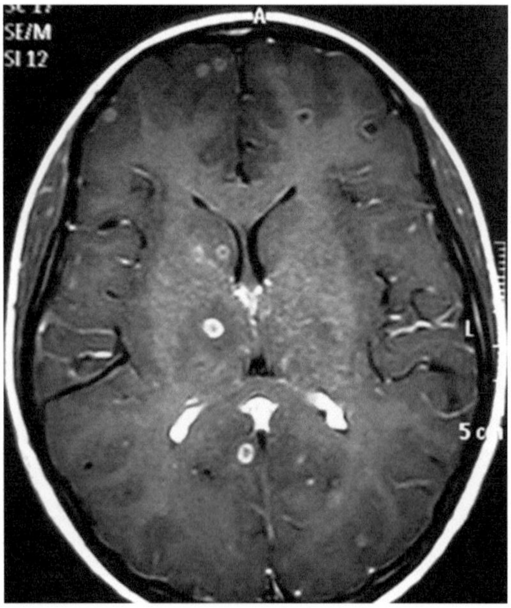

Fig. 17.6 CT scan of the brain showing multiple ring lesions in neurocysticercosis

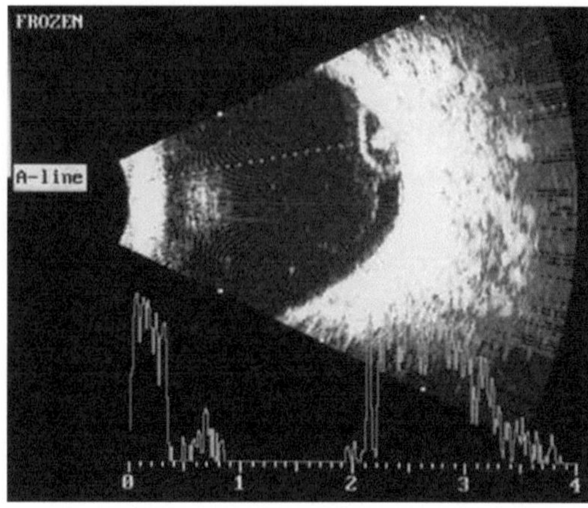

Fig. 17.7 Ultrasonography of the eye showing a globular cyst with high reflectivity inner wall and a high reflective echo corresponding to the scolex in the centre

the inflammatory response. The most common muscle to be infected is the medial rectus (42 %) followed by the superior rectus (18 %), lateral rectus (15 %), inferior rectus (13 %), superior oblique and levator palpebral superioris (5 % each) and inferior oblique (1 %) [7].

17.5 Systemic Cysticercosis

The most common systemic manifestation is neurocysticercosis (Fig. 17.6). It is the cause of epilepsy in 50 % of partial seizures in adults. The patients may present with seizures, recurrent headaches, increased intracranial pressure or as a psychiatric disorder. Signs of meningoencephalitis may occur in case of multiple cysts. Subcutaneous nodules and inflammatory cells in the muscles may be seen [1, 2, 6].

17.6 Diagnosis

The diagnosis is usually on the basis of history including travel to endemic regions of the world, ingestion of raw or undercooked pork or known previous infections with this tapeworm. A history of relapsing inflammations, subcutaneous nodules or neurologic symptoms may indicate infection with this parasite [7]. Laboratory findings include eosinophilia in 71 % cases. Enzyme-linked immunosorbent assay (ELISA) for the cysticercosal antigen is available. It has sensitivities of 65–98 % and specificities of 67–100 % in neurocysticercosis depending on the specific test, cyst burden, location and phase of the infection. A positive test needs to be interpreted in the context of the clinical picture [7, 13, 14].

Imaging is the most useful test because of the highly specific appearance of the encysted parasites. The characteristic "hanging drop" sign of a sonolucent cyst with well-defined margins in orbital cysticercosis is characteristic. A central circular and highly reflective scolex within the cyst is highly supportive of the diagnosis of cysticercosis. It can also be used for follow-up examinations to note the regression following medical treatment [7, 15, 16].

On CT scans, it appears isodense to the vitreous humour, while on MRI, it appears isointense to CSF on T1- and T2-weighted images. A live cyst does not enhance with contrast, while the dying cyst enhances in contrast due to the surrounding inflammatory reaction. CT scan cranium shows multiple ring lesions in neurocysticercosis.

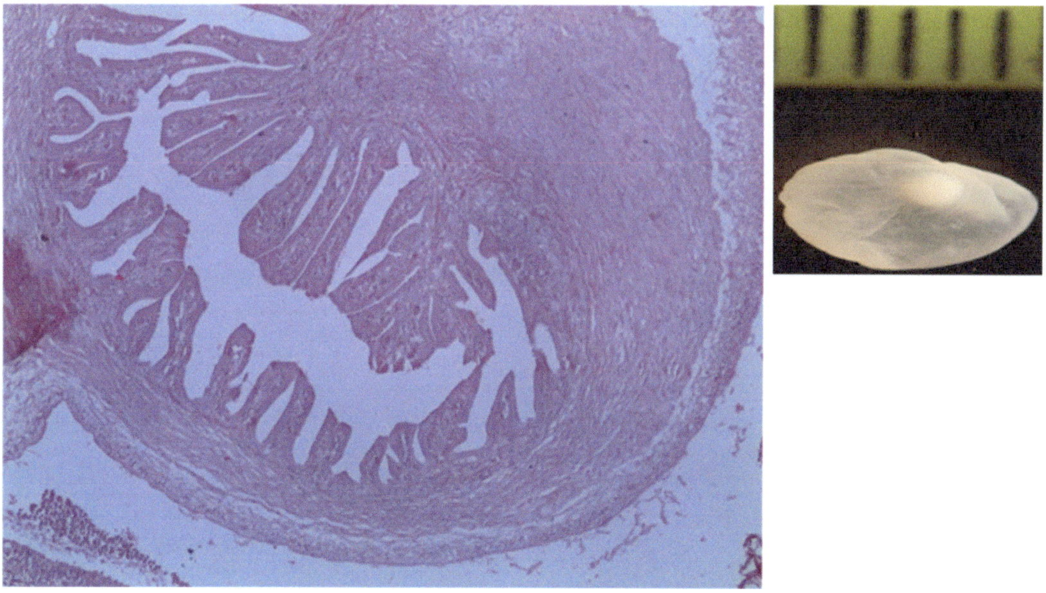

Fig. 17.8 Photograph of the excised cyst with pearly white scolex (*inset*) and microphotograph showing the cyst wall and branching body cavity of the *Cysticercus cellulosae*

Ultrasonography of the eye reveals a cyst-like structure with a high amplitude echo corresponding to the inner wall of the cyst and the overlying retina. A dot-like echo corresponding to the scolex may be seen in the cyst (Figs. 17.7 and 17.8).

17.7 Differential Diagnosis

Cysticercosis can mimic focal chorioretinitis as in toxoplasmosis in hazy media, retinoblastoma and coats disease in children, diffuse unilateral subacute neuroretinitis and a choroidal tumour [6, 17].

17.8 Management

The type of treatment used for cysticercosis should be tailored to the symptoms and location of the cyst. For orbital cysticercosis, medical treatment is very useful [7]. The first line of therapy includes oral albendazole given at the rate of 15 mg/kg body weight/day for a month, although different randomized clinical trials mention 1 month, 15 days and even 1 week [18]. This broad-spectrum antihelminthic acts by inhibiting glucose uptake of the parasite and interferes with its ATP production. Due to lack of energy production, the parasite becomes immobilized and eventually dies. An alternative is praziquantel but has an inferior cyst elimination rate compared to albendazole [18]. It is recommended that oral corticosteroids at a dose of 1 mg/kg body weight along with cysticidal drugs are given to suppress the associated inflammatory response from the dying cyst. Surgical removal is usually contraindicated because of the extensive resections needed, the posterior location of most of the lesions and the likelihood of inducing a fibrotic reaction further restricting the movement of the eye. The treatment of intraocular cysticercosis is usually surgical removal of the intact cyst. Recent reports show more favorable visual outcome with extraction of subretinal cysts with vitrectomy rather than via a sclerotomy [8, 9]. Sharma et al. reported relative good postoperative outcomes with final visual acuity of 20/200 or better achieved in more than half of eyes in their series [9]. The treatment guidelines of optic nerve cysticercosis are not well established due to the paucity of literature. Though cysticidal therapy with oral steroids is the treatment of choice in most cases, the treatment needs to be individualised [12]. Cysticidal therapy may not be very useful in calcified lesions.

17.9 Prognosis

A successful outcome from treatment of ocular cysticercosis requires death and removal of the organism and effective suppression of any inflammation. Cysts elimination rates of 92–95 % have been reported in orbital cysticercosis. Complete recovery of ocular motility usually occurs within 3–6 months but may take longer [7]. It depends on the chronicity of the disease and the sequelae of inflammation. Barring few reports, good visual recovery has been reported even with optic nerve involvement [12]. Visual outcomes due to intraocular cysticercosis have been quite poor in the past. More favourable visual outcomes have been reported in recent years due to early presentation and diagnosis, improved surgical techniques of cyst removal and extraction of subretinal cysts with vitrectomy rather than sclerotomy [9].

Core Messages
Cysticercosis is a parasitic infection caused by *Cysticercus cellulosae*, the larval form of *Taenia solium*. It can involve any part of the visual pathway including the orbits and adnexa. Diagnosis needs to be considered in patients coming from endemic regions and history of seizures. Diagnosis is confirmed by imaging and does not routinely require tissue biopsy. Treatment needs to be individualized and includes medical treatment with antihelminthic drugs and oral steroids and surgically excision of an intact cyst.

References

1. Chatterjee KD (1976) Helminthology. In: Chatterjee KD (ed) Parasitology, 11th ed. Chatterjee medical Publishers, Calcutta, p 107–206
2. Duke-Elder S (1978) Cysticerosis, system of ophthalmology. CV Mosby, St.Louis, p 40.
3. Kaliaperumal S, Rao VA, Parija SC (2005) Cysticercosis of the eye in South India-A case series. Ind J Med Microbiol 23:227–230
4. Madigubba S, Vishwanath K, Reddy GBKG, Vemuganti GK (2007) Changing trends in ocular cysticercosis over two decades: an analysis of 118 surgically excised cysts. Indian J Med Microbiol 25(3):214–219
5. Atul K, Kumar TH, Mallika G, Sandip M (1995) Socio-demographic trends in ocular cysticercosis. Acta Ophthalmol Scand 73(5):438–441
6. Foster CS, Vitale A (2001) Diagnosis and treatment of uveitis, 1st edn. W.B.Saunders, Philadelphia, pp. 468–473
7. Ziaei M, Elgohary M, Bremner FD (2011) Orbital cysticercosis, case report and review. Orbit 30(5):230–235
8. Wender JD, Rathinam S, Shaw RE, Cunnningham ET (2011) Intraocular cysticercosis: case series and comprehensive review of the literature. Ocul Immunol Inflamm 19(4):240–245
9. Sharma T, Sinha S, Shah N, Gopal L, Shanmugam MP, Bhende P et al (2003) Intraocular cysticercosis: clinical characteristics and visual outcome after vitreoretinal surgery. Ophthalmol 110(5):996–1004
10. Mahendradas P, Biswas J, Khetan V (2007) Fibrinous anterior uveitis due to cysticercus cellulosae. Ocul Immunol Inflamm 15(6):451–454
11. Kruger-Leite E, Jalkh AE, Quiroz H, Schepens CL (1985) Intraocular cysticercosis. Am J Ophthalmol 99(3):252–257
12. Sudan R, Muralidhar R, Sharma P (2005) Optic nerve cysticercosis - case report and review of current management. Orbit 24:159–162
13. Coken-Vann MR, Subianto DB, Brown P, Diwan AR, Desowitz R, Garruto RM et al (1981) ELISA antibodies of cysticerci of *Taenia solium* in human populations in New Guinea, Oceania and South East Asia. Southeast Asian J Trop Med Public Health 12:499–505
14. Rosas N, Sotelo J, Nieto D (1986) ELISA in the diagnosis of neurocysticercosis. Arch Neurol 43:353–356
15. Honavar SG, Sekhar CG (1998) Ultrasonological characteristics of extraocular cysticercosis. Orbit 17(4):271–284
16. Murthy H, Kumar A, Verma L (1990) Orbital cysticercosis – an ultrasonic diagnosis. Acta Ophthalmol 68:612–614
17. Agarwal B, Vemuganti GK, Honavar SG (2003) Intraocular cysticercosis simulating retinoblastoma in a 5-year-old child. Eye (Lond) 17(3):447–449
18. García HH, Evans CA, Nash TE, Takayanagui OM, White AC Jr, Botero D et al (2002) Current consensus guidelines for treatment of neurocysticercosis. Clin Microbiol Rev 15(4):747–756 Review

18 Intraocular Nematode

Jyotirmay Biswas and Nishat Bansal

18.1 Nematodes

18.1.1 Introduction

Nematodes are complex multicellular worms approximately 5–100 μm thick and 0.1 mm to less than 2.5 mm long [1]. After entering the body, the nematode can localize to any part of the eye: lids, extraocular tissue, lacrimal gland, anterior chamber, vitreous, retina and subretinal space creating visual problems and destroying the various structures in the eye by mechanical, immunological or allergic reaction or a combination of all these.

Ocular diseases caused by nematodes:

1. Toxocariasis
2. Gnathostomiasis
3. Onchocerciasis
4. Loiasis
5. Diffuse unilateral subacute neuroretinitis (DUSN)
6. Dirofilariasis
7. Angiostrongyliasis
8. Bancroftian and Brugian filariasis

J. Biswas, MS, FAMS, FIC Path, FAICO (✉)
Uveitis & Ocular Pathology Department, Medical Research Foundation, Sankara Nethralaya, Chennai, India
e-mail: drjb@snmail.org

N. Bansal, MBBS, DNB
Shri Bhagwan Mahavir Vitreoretinal Services, Sankara Nethralaya, Chennai, India
e-mail: docnish82@yahoo.co.in

18.2 Toxocariasis

Toxocariasis in humans is caused accidentally by ingesting infected eggs from soil or eating food contaminated with faeces. Direct contact with infected animal can be another mode of infection though it occurs less frequently. Most commonly children who have the habits of pica, geophagia or coprophagia are more prone for contracting toxocariasis [2].

18.2.1 Epidemiology

Toxocariasis cases are found worldwide and are found both in rural and urban parts of the world. High prevalence has been reported from the United States, Japan and Argentina [3–5]. Low prevalence reported from rural areas can be due to diagnostic challenges. There is an increased trend in tropical regions than in temperate regions [6]. The prevalence of toxocariasis ranges from 2.8 % to 92.8 % [7].

18.2.2 Parasitology/Life Cycle (Table 18.1)

Toxocara larva is one of the smallest larvae that is encountered in the eye [8]. It is caused by organism *Toxocara canis*, which occurs from infected dog or less frequently from *Toxocara catis*, where cat is infected by the organism [1]. It has a complex life

S.-P. Chee, M. Khairallah (eds.), *Emerging Infectious Uveitis*, DOI 10.1007/978-3-319-23416-8_18

Table 18.1 Ocular nematode, their host and infective stage

Parasite/disease	Definite host	Intermediate host	Accidental host	Infective stage in man
Toxocariasis	Cats and dogs	Birds and rodents	Humans	Cyst, migrating larvae
Onchocerciasis	Human	Black fly (*Simulium*)	–	Third-stage larvae
Loiasis	Human	Deer fly (*Chrysops*)	–	Third-stage larvae
Gnathostomiasis	Dogs, cats, wild carnivores	Cyclops (first), fish, snakes, frog (second)	Human	Third-stage larvae
Dirofilariasis	Dog, cats	Mosquito – *Aedes, Anopheles, Culex*	Humans	Larvae
Angiostrongyliasis	Rodents	Snails, prawns, crabs	Humans	Third-stage larvae
Bancroftian and Brugian filariasis	Humans	Mosquito – *Aedes, Anopheles, Culex Anopheles, Mansonia*		Adult worm or microfilariae

cycle. Humans are the paratenic host (unsuitable host – in which no transformation in the larval stage takes place). The second stage larva enters in the systemic circulation and reaches up to the terminal arterioles and form granuloma wherever they lodge.

18.2.3 Clinical Features

Toxocara larvae can be found in any organ in humans, and many cases are discovered accidentally. Clinically the disease occurs in two forms: systemic toxocariasis and ocular toxocariasis. Both the forms rarely coexist [2, 9].

18.2.3.1 Systemic

It is also known as *visceral larva migrans (VLM)* and occurs in children aged between 2 and 3 years, who have history of pica. They develop symptoms of fever, anorexia, weakness, failure to gain weight, myalgia and arthralgia. These symptoms are due to host immune response to *toxoplasma* larvae. There can be allergic pulmonary symptoms and other symptoms of pneumonitis, pneumonia, hepatomegaly, splenomegaly, lymphadenopathy, eosinophilia, hypergammaglobulinaemia, elevated level of IgE, neurological involvement with seizures and myocarditis [9].

18.2.3.2 Ocular

It is also known as ocular larva migrans (OLM). Ocular involvement usually occurs in children older than 3 years and in young adults. The symptoms occur due to weak host immune response. Children may present with strabismus, decreased vision and leukocoria which is an important differential diagnosis for retinoblastoma [2]. Ocular involvement occurs in five ways. **Anterior segment** involvement is very rarely involved. Only few case reports are available in literature [10]. In **peripheral variant** a fibrovascular band may be seen running from a whitish granuloma in the periphery to the optic nerve or posterior pole (Fig. 18.1). It can lead to tractional or rhegmatogenous retinal detachment [2, 9]. Sometimes a well-defined mass of variable size of ¼–4 disc diameter may be seen in the **posterior pole** associated with vitreous haze. It may masquerade as retinoblastoma. In the later stage, there may be either atrophy or hyperplasia of the retinal pigment epithelium in the macula [2, 11]. **Optic nerve** involvement is a rare entity, and when present it has the clinical features of optic neuritis/papillitis [12]. The most common presentation of *Toxocara* is as **endophthalmitis**. Dense vitreous haemorrhage may be present, and a yellowish-whitish mass may be faintly visible through vitreous haze. Externally the eye may look quiet or may sometimes have a granulomatous reaction with mutton

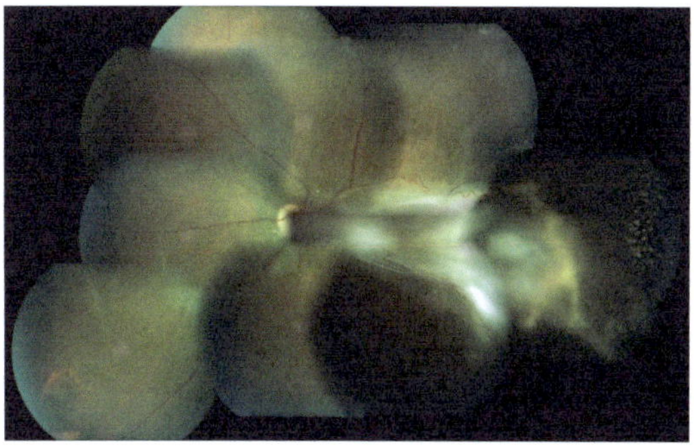

Fig. 18.1 Fundus image showing peripheral form of toxocariasis

fat keratic precipitates. Hypopyon may be seen in very severe cases [12].

The various differential diagnosis of toxocariasis includes retinoblastoma, Coats' disease, persistent hyperplastic primary vitreous (PHPV), familial exudative vitreoretinopathy (FEVR) and retinopathy of prematurity (ROP).

18.2.4 Diagnosis

The clinical diagnosis of *Toxocara* is quite obvious, but still a confirmatory diagnosis is required in suspicious cases or for documentation. The larvae or its fragments may be directly visible under the microscope from tissue sections, but it's extremely cumbersome and risky to collect samples from ocular tissues. In a Wilder's classic study, only one larva was detected in 2300 cases examined [1]. Eosinophilia is noted in the blood of patients with systemic toxocariasis; however, the eosinophil count can be normal in patients with ocular toxocariasis [2]. The diagnosis of *Toxocara* can be clinched by indirect enzyme-linked immunosorbent assay (ELISA) which detects the immunogenic proteins known as *Toxocara* excretory-secretory (TES) antigens that are shed from the larvae [13]. A titre of 1:8 or more of ELISA along with signs and symptoms of *Toxocara* is sufficient to aid the diagnosis of *Toxocara* [2, 14]. However, there are few case reports of negative ELISA in *Toxocara* [15]. In literature the sensitivity for ELISA for *Toxocara* is variable with a range between as low as 33 % and as high as 92.2 % (depending upon the cutoff value of the titres) [2]. Detecting rising titres of anti-TES-Ag immunoglobulin E (IgE) antibody indicates acute toxocariasis. The titres return to normal after treatment and help in monitoring treatment therapy [13]. Increased IgG titres confirm a past or present infection without significant inflammation. Ultrasonography (USG) is important to differentiate it from retinoblastoma, where *Toxocara* appears as mass lesion and multiple vitreous membranes can be seen running from mass to disc, some of which are highly reflective. Intraocular calcification has been reported in some cases, and in that case other imaging modalities and serological test differentiate it from retinoblastoma [16]. The role of ultrasound biomicroscopy (UBM) is synergetic with USG as demonstrated by Zhou et al., where they could identify 95 % of the peripheral subtypes of toxocariasis [17]. Typical pseudocystic degeneration of the vitreous was picked up on UBM by Tran et al. [18].

18.2.5 Treatment

Treatment of *Toxocara* depends upon the severity of disease. Oral steroids in a dose of 0.5–1 mg/kg body weight or periocular steroids may be required in cases of posterior uveitis along with topical steroids and cycloplegics for associated anterior uveitis [2]. The role of anthelmintic drugs (diethylcarbamazine, thiabendazole, mebendazole, albendazole) is controversial due unavailability of ocular pharmacodynamics and pharmacokinetics of these drugs. However, Barisani AT et al. [19] have treated seven eyes of five patients with oral albendazole along with steroids and have shown promising results. Ahn SJ et al. demonstrated that albendazole with steroids could reduce the recurrence to 17.4 % as compared to 54.5 % in patients who were administered only steroids by the end of 6 months, though the vision and inflammation improvement was the same in both the groups [2]. In majority of cases at the time of presentation, the parasite is dead and can be treated with steroids alone due to the inflammation caused by the dead parasite;

however, in cases of live parasite, systemic albendazole can be tried/recommended (adult dose 800 mg BID, children 400 mg BID for 7–14 days) [2]. Surgical intervention is required for associated tractional or rhegmatogenous retinal detachment or endophthalmitis [20].

18.3 Gnathostomiasis

Gnathostomiasis is a food-borne disease caused by infection with larvae of *Gnathostoma* species. Intraocular infection by *Gnathostoma* species is quite rare but can be devastating [21].

18.3.1 Epidemiology

Around 12 species of *Gnathostoma* are known till now; however, only four species (*Gnathostoma spinigerum, Gnathostomiasis hispidum, Gnathostoma doloresi, Gnathostoma nipponicum*) have been reported to be zoonotic. Among these *Gnathostoma spinigerum* is a well-studied species and was discovered in Thailand in 1889. The cases of infection with G. *spinigerum* are mostly reported from Thailand, Japan, Malaysia, China, India, Java, Israel, Vietnam and the Philippines [22–24]. The total 74 cases of gnathostomiasis were reported worldwide, and about 83.5 % of the cases have been reported from Asian countries or among people travelling from these endemic countries [25].

18.3.2 Parasitology/Life Cycle (Table 18.1)

Dogs/cats are the definitive host parasitizing the adult worms in their stomach; the eggs are released from the animal's stools. Cyclops are the first intermediate host, and freshwater fish, eel, frog or snake are the second intermediate host. Pigs, ducks and chicken are the paratenic hosts. Humans acquire infection by eating the second intermediate host or the paratenic hosts. The third-stage larvae migrate in the internal organs, eyes and subcutaneous tissues; however, they do not mature into adult in humans. In humans a third larval stage, immature worms and adult worms can be found [1].

18.3.3 Clinical Features

18.3.3.1 Systemic

Skin and mucous membrane involvement is known as *Gnathostoma externa*. The classical cutaneous lesions are migratory where the larvae can travel a centimetre or more within an hour under the skin producing local oedema and haemorrhage. The patient will have painless, non-pitting oedema with associated erythema and pruritus [26]. Internal organ involvement is also known as *Gnathostoma interna.* The patient presents with nausea, vomiting, pruritus, urticaria and abdominal pain. High mortality in gnathostomiasis is due to invasion of parasite to the brainstem and medulla oblongata or due to subarachnoid haemorrhage. Initially, the patient may present with symptoms of meningitis or meningoencephalitis [27–29].

18.3.3.2 Ocular

It occurs due to third larval stage of the parasite. The ocular involvement is due to migration of worm from the brain to the eye via optic nerve or directly through the scleral invasion. Two most striking forms of ocular involvement are of eyelid and the intraocular migration of the parasite (Fig. 18.2). The cornea and conjunctiva can also be

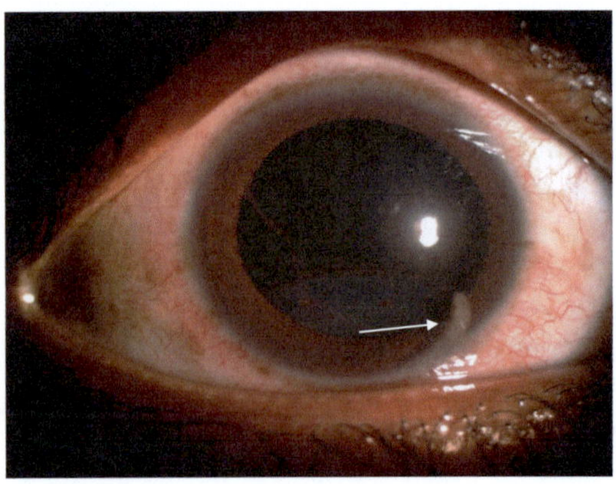

Fig. 18.2 Showing *Gnathostoma* worm in the anterior chamber

involved. The patient may present with corneal ulceration, orbital cellulites like picture, hyphema, vitreous haemorrhage, central retinal artery occlusion, secondary glaucoma, traumatic retinal hole (due to larva migration) and retinal detachment [25, 30–34].

18.3.4 Diagnosis

The diagnosis of gnathostomiasis can be reached by this classical triad of patients travelling from endemic countries, history of consuming raw fish and peripheral eosinophilia, though reports in literature have shown that patients may present without eosinophilia and eosinophils are increased only during the migratory phase of the parasite [27]. Eosinophil count can also be used as a marker for treatment response [32]. Microscopic identification of the parasite is the only way of making the definitive diagnosis, though it's challenging due to the migratory nature of the parasite. ELISA test is a more recent and reliable methodology for diagnosis [31]. However, ELISA test for both *Gnathostoma* and *Angiostrongylus* species should be performed together as both of them show cross sensitivity for each other [25, 31, 32]. Elevated levels of immunoglobulin E (IgE) antibodies are noted in acute infections. Ultrasonography (USG) and ultrasound biomicroscopy (UBM) have been reported to be a useful entity for the diagnosis of nematode, where the parasite is not clinically visible. Bhende et al. [28] have shown the nematode to move from the iris root to the posterior segment through zonules over 6-min time span on UBM [30].

18.3.5 Treatment

Surgical removal of the parasite from the skin, anterior chamber and vitreous cavity of the eye is preferred because if the parasite migrates to the brain, the outcomes are fatal [30, 33, 34]. The role of anthelmintic medicine is controversial, though in literature there are case reports of successful treatment of *Gnathostoma* with oral albendazole 400 mg/day for 21 days [22, 24, 25].

18.4 Onchocerciasis

Onchocerciasis is an infection of humans caused by filarial nematode *Onchocerca* species, transmitted to human beings by the bite of infected black fly of the genus *Simulium* [11]. Of lately there has been increasing reports of zoonotic *Onchocerca*, and many reports have been with infections in and around the eye [8]. It may also manifest as dermatitis, subcutaneous nodules and sclerosing lymphadenitis [35–37].

Synonyms: River blindness, sowda [38, 39].

18.4.1 Epidemiology

About 37 million people are infected with onchocerciasis worldwide, and most of the cases (99 %) of onchocerciasis have been reported from Africa [40]. It has also been reported from Eastern Mediterranean, the United States, Hungary, Turkey and India [41–43]. The '*Onchocerca* Control Programme' started by WHO in 1974 in Africa has been successful in interrupting the transmission of onchocerciasis to near zero level [44, 45].

18.4.2 Parasitology/Life Cycle (Table 18.1)

The species reported to cause ocular infection are *O. volvulus*, *O. gutturosa or O. cervicalis*, *O. reticulata and O. lupi* [1, 8]. Adult worm is present in the skin of the host (man); it may produce half to one million microfilariae, which migrate to the skin or eyes of the host. When a black fly bites these infected humans (only female fly can bite), they suck blood with microfilariae and are then released to the skin of other hosts when it bites [1].

18.4.3 Clinical Features

18.4.3.1 Systemic

The clinical features include dermatitis, subcutaneous nodules, sclerosing lymphadenitis and ocular lesions. There is intense pruritus and depigmentation of the skin along the track of the worm. 'Onchocercomas' are painless fibrous nodules that are predominantly seen on the head and face and on the body involving the skin, periosteum or bone [35, 36]. These are due to female worms and microfilaria encapsulated in fibrous coat. The lymph nodes draining the affected area show granulomatous inflammation [37].

18.4.3.2 Ocular Features

The ocular features are mainly due to dead microfilaria. The corneal involvement is in the form of punctate keratitis (dead microfilaria) and sclerosing keratitis (live microfilaria). The peripheral cornea is most commonly involved with snowflake-like opacities which gradually progress towards the centre of the cornea leading to blindness. Microfilaria can also be seen in the iris stroma or anterior chamber causing granulomatous or non-granulomatous uveitis leading to iris atrophy, synechia and occlusio pupillae. There is involvement of the retina, or choroid is in the form of bilateral and symmetrical focal areas of atrophy and eventually progresses to large areas of atrophy. This chorioretinitis progresses to involve the optic disc leading to optic neuritis and secondary optic atrophy leading to blindness [35, 38, 42, 43, 45–49].

18.4.4 Diagnosis

Microfilaria can be demonstrated in the dermis or epidermis on skin biopsy [36]. Mazzotti test is an allergic reaction to oral administration of diethylcarbamazine (DEC), which causes intense pruritus, fever, swollen and tender lymph nodes and can be life threatening. This allergic reaction occurs due to death of the microfilaria. ELISA test and polymerase chain reaction (PCR) are the other tests for detection of microfilaria.

18.4.5 Treatment

The most effective drug against *Onchocerca* is ivermectin; it is administered orally as a single dose of 150 mg/kg/day and repeated every 6–12 months. It is microfilaricidal and is not effective against the adult worm [43, 45, 48]. Diethylcarbamazine (DEC), in a dose of 25 mg/day for 3 days, 50 mg/day for 5 days, 100 mg/day for 3 days and 150 mg/day for 12 days, is given. However, this regimen does not kill all the microfilaria; besides it is also associated with high recurrence of onchocerciasis. An allergic reaction (Mazzotti reaction) is also common with it [48]. Doxycycline is a microfilaricidal and well-tolerated drug. It has also been tried effectively for treatment of *O. volvulus* in co-infection with *Loa loa* [11]. Surgical removal of the onchocercomas can be done, but it's challenging in deep-seated nodules.

18.5 Loiasis

Loiasis is caused by 'eye worm' *Loa loa* and is transmitted by an insect vector deer fly of genus *Chrysops*. It has predilection for ocular tissue [50].

18.5.1 Epidemiology

It is endemic in Africa and its prevalence is reported to be 50 % [51]. There has been spread of loiasis to other countries like Spain. There are few case reports of loiasis from Italy and London [51–53]. Choi SU et al. studied 320 cases of parasitic infections from 2004 to 2011 and reported the incidence of *Loa loa* to 0.3 % [54].

18.5.2 Parasitology/Life Cycle (Table 18.1)

It is the adult worm that affects the eye as against the *Onchocerca volvulus* which is caused by microfilaria. *Chrysops* fly when it bites human beings (hosts) sucks the blood with microfilaria. This fly then inoculates the larvae into another host it bites. In host these microfilariae mature into adults in the subcutaneous area. The adult worm migrates to the eyes of the host. The adult worms live for 12–15 years [1].

18.5.3 Clinical Features

18.5.3.1 Systemic

The patient has intense pruritus of the limbs, chest, back and face. There is oedema of the limbs and face [55]. Later on in the disease, there can be involvement of the heart, kidney and CNS leading to death ultimately.

18.5.3.2 Ocular

The most interesting manifestation is seeing the worm move across the conjunctiva: it is pathognomonic for loiasis [55]. The patient may present with decreased vision, conjunctival injection and pain on ocular movement. There are numerous case reports of microfilaria migrating in the eyelids, anterior chamber, vitreous and retina (*Loa*-induced retinopathy) [56]. Obstruction of the retinal and choroidal vessels leads to aneurysmal dilation and haemorrhages in superficial layers of the retina [51].

18.5.4 Diagnosis

Diagnosis is mostly clinical in patients, who have travelled to endemic areas and are exhibiting symptoms suggestive of loiasis. Confirmatory diagnosis is made by seeing the worm under the microscope. The worm can be removed from subconjuctival space or subcutaneous space; however, the larvae may still be present in the blood after its removal [1]. Afternoon and midnight blood films help in the detection and quantification of microfilaraemia.

18.5.5 Treatment

Diethylcarbamazine is the mainstay of treatment. It is lethal to both adult worm and microfilaria. The standard regimen is Day 1, 50 mg; Day 2, 50 mg three times daily; Day 3, 100 mg three times daily; and from Day 4 to Day 21, constant dose of 3 mg/kg three times per day. Pretreatment with oral steroids should be considered before initiation of DEC therapy as it will take care of the severe immune reaction and encephalopathy caused by the death of microfilaria. Alternate treatment with ivermectin and albendazole can be considered [53, 57–59].

18.6 DUSN (Diffuse Unilateral Subacute Neuroretinitis)

Diffuse unilateral subacute neuroretinitis (DUSN) is a rare entity caused by a glistening white, motile nematode seen wandering in the subretinal space. It was initially known as 'unilateral wipe-out syndrome' [7]. The term DUSN was coined by Gass in 1978 [60].

18.6.1 Epidemiology

DUSN was initially reported from America and later from China, Brazil and India [61, 62].

18.6.2 Parasitology/Life Cycle (Table 18.1)

Two types of worms are said to cause DUSN: the small one, *Ancylostoma caninum* and *Toxocara*, and other larger worm – *Baylisascaris procyonis*. DUSN worm is tapered at both ends [7, 63, 64].

18.6.3 Clinical Features

18.6.3.1 Systemic

DUSN usually occurs in children and young adults. The patients may present with features of cutaneous larva migrans, which may precede the visual symptoms and the other devastating form of neural larva migrans [7].

18.6.3.2 Ocular

Gass demonstrated a non-granulomatous reaction. In early stages it manifests as vitritis, multifocal choroiditis and papillitis. Early diagnosis can aid in laser photocoagulation of the worm along the vicinity of grey white retinal lesions. In late stage it leads to secondary optic nerve atrophy (due to destructions of retinal layers), retinal

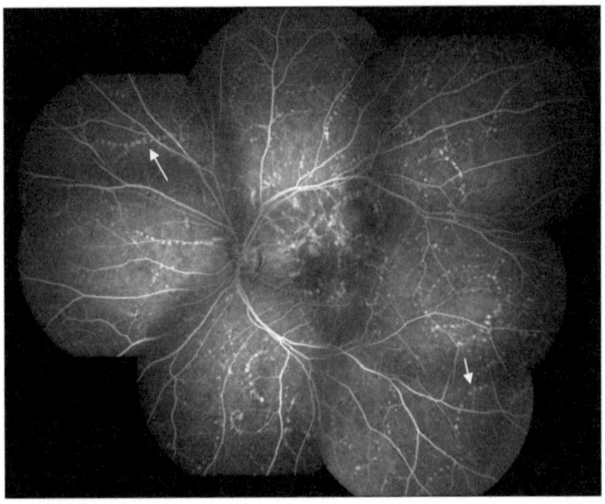

Fig. 18.3 Showing tracks of DUSN worm

vessel narrowing, diffuse changes in retinal pigment epithelium, peripheral RPE hypopigmentation and formation of various RPE tracks which are visible clinically (Fig. 18.3). These changes are caused due to toxic effect of the worm products on the outer retina [65]. DUSN though causes damage to all the layers of the retina, and it predominantly destroys the inner retina (nerve fibre layer) and retinal pigment epithelium [65, 66].

18.6.4 Diagnosis

Seeing a motile worm on biomicroscopy is the gold standard for diagnosis [61]. Berbel et al. have demonstrated that in cases where DUSN is suspected, optical coherence tomography (OCT) helps in the assessment of nerve fibre layer and areas of oedema [65]. This non-invasive test helps to differentiate it from other mimicking conditions like toxoplasmosis where the retinal nerve fibre layer is spared. Intraretinal worm can be picked up on enhanced depth imaging OCT, where it appears as a hyperreflective object of irregular shape, affecting all the layers of the retina [65].

18.6.5 Treatment

Laser photocoagulation can be used to treat the nematode in early disease with good visual prognosis. Oral albendazole 400 mg/day for 30 days has been tried [67–69]. High-dose systemic steroids are required to counter the severe inflammation caused by the worm and its by-products [69].

18.7 Dirofilariasis

Dirofilariasis is a zoonotic disease caused by the nematode *Dirofilaria* species. Mosquito is a vector responsible for the transmission from animal hosts to humans. Though it is a rare intraocular entity, many case reports across the globe are available [70].

18.7.1 Epidemiology

It is endemic in Mediterranean countries. Now various cases are reported from all across the globe; Europe, France, Greece, Spain, Russia, Dubai and South Asia [71–75]. The highest number of cases has been reported from Italy, Sri Lanka and Republic of ex-Soviet Union [76]. Off lately there has been an increase in case reports from South India, though it is a non-endemic country [76–79].

18.7.2 Parasitology/Life Cycle (Table 18.1)

The most common species infecting humans are *D. tenuis*, *D. immitis*, *D. repens*, *D. striata*, *D. ursi and D. spectans* [80]. It affects mostly the dogs, cats and other canines (wolves, foxes). Mosquito acts as a vector for dirofilariasis, which proliferates in warm and humid areas; therefore, the incidence of dirofilariasis is on the increase in hot and humid areas [1]. Man is an unsuitable host for *Dirofilaria* and the microfilaria dies before it gets mature in human.

18.7.3 Clinical Features

18.7.3.1 Systemic

The pulmonary and cutaneous manifestations are the most common presentation of dirofilariasis, followed by the cardiopulmonary manifestations. Ocular presentations are less common [71, 72].

18.7.3.2 Ocular

It can affect the various intraocular and periocular tissues [70, 81]. It can occur in subconjuctival space, in the Tenon's layer, lids, orbit and intraocular in the anterior chamber or vitreous (Fig. 18.4) [81, 82]. Subconjuctival is the most common location, seen in almost greater than 60 % of people, followed by orbital/eyelid seen approximately in 25 % [80]. Kalogeropoulos et al. have seen intravitreal dirofilariasis in two out of their eight cases (25 %) [80]. Mostly the cases are unilateral; recently Gupta et al. have reported bilateral intraocular dirofilariasis with a live motile worm in the anterior segment of one eye and a cystic lesion on the optic disc of the other eye [70]. Dirofilariasis can also present as multifocal choroiditis [83].

18.7.4 Diagnosis

Nematode can be expressed from the subcutaneous tissue and subconjunctival or after vitrectomy and examined under the microscope. High suspicion should be kept in endemic areas. Peripheral blood shows eosinophilia and the count returns to normal after the removal of parasite. Indirect hemagglutination test and ELISA test have also been used in the diagnosis of dirofilariasis. Ultrasound and magnetic resonance imaging can be non-invasive and quick diagnostic modalities [72, 81].

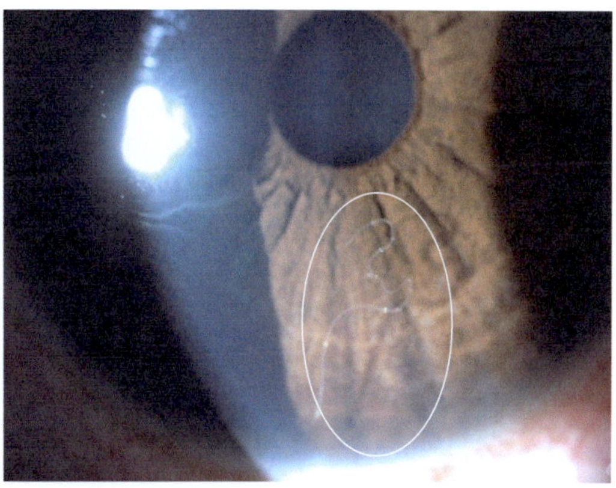

Fig. 18.4 Showing *Dirofilaria* worm in anterior chamber

18.7.5 Treatment

Parasite should be removed from the ocular tissues as suggested by Kalogeropoulos et al. [80]. No anthelmintic treatment was required as the parasite was reproductively inactive.

18.8 Angiostrongyliasis

Angiostrongyliasis is caused by nematode *Angiostrongylus cantonensis* species and is transmitted by rodents (Table 18.1). Ocular angiostrongyliasis is a rare entity affecting only 1.1 % of the patients affected with *Angiostrongylus* [84]. Ocular involvement is seen in the cerebral form of the disease [85]. Most of the cases were reported from Thailand, and few cases were reported from other countries like Sri Lanka, India, China, Taiwan, Japan and Vietnam [24, 86–88]. Human beings are the intermediate host, and they acquire the infection by eating prawns, crabs or snails (carriers of nematode). The worm can be isolated from the anterior chamber, vitreous, retina or subretinal space. Patients may have generalized retinal pigment alterations, subretinal tracks and macular oedema. Optic neuritis is another manifestation of *A. cantonensis*. Eosinophilia, ELISA test, Western blot and use of specific monoclonal antibodies aid in the diagnosis of angiostrongyliasis. Examining the nematode with its tapering ends is the most reliable diagnostic method. Surgical removal of the living nematode is the recommended therapeutic measure, and the worm has been removed even from the subretinal space. Oral steroids reduce the intraocular inflammation. There is no role of anthelmintics, because the dead parasite may create havoc inside the eye [89].

18.9 Bancroftian and Brugian Filariasis

Bancroftian filariasis is caused by the worm *Wuchereria bancrofti*, and Brugian filariasis is caused by the worm *Brugia malayi* or *Brugia timori* (Table 18.1). These are one of the oldest groups of parasitic infections occurring in the eye, which date back to several years [8, 90]. These infections are also known as 'lymphatic filariasis' as these worms harbor in the lymphatic system of the body. The obstruction of the lymphatics causes the classical symptoms of elephantiasis, chyluria and hydrocele. Though there is no lymphatic drainage for the ocular tissue, still *Wuchereria bancrofti* has been identified from intraocular tissues in humans. There are numerous case reports of *W. bancrofti* being identified from the conjunctiva and anterior chamber, but there are very few case reports of the worm being identified from the vitreous cavity [91–94]. The first case report was reported in 2005 [94]. Presumably *Wuchereria bancrofti* causing retinal pigment epithelium inflammation and retinal vasculitis is managed effectively by diethylcarbamazine citrate therapy [95]. Recently Rao NG et al. were successful in removing a live Brugian microfilaria from the vitreous by pars plana vitrectomy [96]. Microfilaria can invade any structure of the eye including the anterior chamber, iris, lens capsule, retina, choroid and lacrimal gland. Elephantiasis of the lid has also been reported in the literature [97].

Conclusion

Seeing a live worm in and around the eye is always a horrifying situation for the patient as well as the clinician. Though intraocular nematode is a rare entity, various nematodes have been isolated from the human eye. Prompt diagnosis with high index of suspicion in endemic areas and early identification of the worm on biomicroscopy can be sight saving for the patient. Appropriate removal of the live nematode from the eye and identification of its morphology under the microscope are the preferred treatment modality in most of the cases. The dead parasite itself in the eye can cause devastating immunologic reaction, which can be controlled to some extent with the use of steroids. Anthelmintics should be initiated whenever needed. Healthcare-based programmes, public health notifications and awareness among physicians help to curb these parasites and various parasite-related diseases at very early stage.

Core Messages

Parasitic infections pose a major health concern in both developed and developing countries, causing significant morbidity and mortality. There is variety of nematodes which may localize to any part of eye and may lead to significant visual loss. Hence necessary actions are required at Government level which can spread awareness among masses by organizing various awareness and eradication programmes. Efforts are also required at Individual level to help in proper sanitation and sticking to the treatment regimen can overcome this challenging situation.

Bibliography

1. Kean BH, Sun T, Ellsworth RM (1991) Color atlas/text of ophthalmic parasitology. Igaku-Shoin, New York
2. Ahn SJ, Ryoo N-K, Woo SJ (2014) Ocular toxocariasis: clinical features, diagnosis, treatment, and prevention. Asia Pac Allergy 4:134–141
3. Lee RM, Moore LB, Bottazzi ME, Hotez PJ (2014) Toxocariasis in North America: a systematic review. PLoS Negl Trop Dis 8:e3116
4. Rubinsky-Elefant G, Hirata CE, Yamamoto JH, Ferreira MU (2010) Human toxocariasis: diagnosis, worldwide seroprevalences and clinical expression of the systemic and ocular forms. Ann Trop Med Parasitol 104:3–23
5. Stewart JM, Cubillan LDP, Cunningham ET (2005) Prevalence, clinical features, and causes of vision loss among patients with ocular toxocariasis. Retina Phila Pa 25:1005–1013
6. Wilder HC (1950) Nematode endophthalmitis. Trans Am Acad Ophthalmol Otolaryngol 55:99–109
7. Gupta A (2009) Uveitis: text and imaging. Jaypee Bros. Medical Publishers, New Delhi
8. Otranto D, Eberhard ML (2011) Zoonotic helminths affecting the human eye. Parasit Vectors 4:41
9. Ahn SJ, Woo SJ, Jin Y et al (2014) Clinical features and course of ocular toxocariasis in adults. PLoS Negl Trop Dis 8:e2938
10. Baldone JA, Clark WB, Jung RC (1964) Nematode ophthalmitis report of two cases. Am J Ophthalmol 57:763–766
11. Rathinam SR, Ashok KA (2010) Ocular manifestations of systemic disease: ocular parasitosis. Curr Opin Ophthalmol 21:478–484

12. Yokoi K, Goto H, Sakai J, Usui M (2003) Clinical features of ocular toxocariasis in Japan. Ocul Immunol Inflamm 11:269–275
13. Majumder PD, Sudharshan S, Biswas J (2013) Laboratory support in the diagnosis of uveitis. Indian J Ophthalmol 61:269–276
14. Garweg JG, de Groot-Mijnes JDF, Montoya JG (2011) Diagnostic approach to ocular toxoplasmosis. Ocul Immunol Inflamm 19:255–261
15. Sharkey JA, McKay PS (1993) Ocular toxocariasis in a patient with repeatedly negative ELISA titre to Toxocara canis. Br J Ophthalmol 77:253–254
16. Bhende M, Sankara Nethralaya (Hospital) (2006) The Sankara Nethralaya atlas of ophthalmic ultrasound. Jaypee Brothers, New Delhi
17. Zhou M, Chang Q, Gonzales JA, Chen Q, Zhang Y, Huang X, Xu G, Wang W, Jiang R (2012) Clinical characteristics of ocular toxocariasis in eastern China. Graefes Arch Clin Exp Ophthalmol Albrecht Von Graefes Arch Für Klin Exp Ophthalmol 250:1373–1378
18. Tran VT, LeHoang P, Herbort CP (2001) Value of high-frequency ultrasound biomicroscopy in uveitis. Eye Lond Engl 15:23–30
19. Barisani-Asenbauer T, Maca SM, Hauff W, Kaminski SL, Domanovits H, Theyer I, Auer H (2001) Treatment of ocular toxocariasis with albendazole. J Ocul Pharmacol Ther Off J Assoc Ocul Pharmacol Ther 17:287–294
20. Maguire AM, Green WR, Michels RG, Erozan YS (1990) Recovery of intraocular Toxocara canis by pars plana vitrectomy. Ophthalmology 97:675–680
21. Biswas J, Gopal L, Sharma T, Badrinath SS (1994) Intraocular Gnathostoma spinigerum. Clinicopathologic study of two cases with review of literature. Retina Phila Pa 14:438–444
22. Sujata DN, Renu BS (2013) Intraocular gnathostomiasis from coastal part of Maharashtra. Trop Parasitol 3:82–84
23. Fernando D (2005) Intra-ocular nematode worms: rare but important. Ceylon Med J 50:141–143
24. Teekhasaenee C, Ritch R, Kanchanaranya C (1986) Ocular parasitic infection in Thailand. Rev Infect Dis 8:350–356
25. Pillai GS, Kumar A, Radhakrishnan N, Maniyelil J, Shafi T, Dinesh KR, Karim S (2012) Intraocular gnathostomiasis: report of a case and review of literature. Am J Trop Med Hyg 86:620–623
26. Kraivichian K, Nuchprayoon S, Sitichalernchai P, Chaicumpa W, Yentakam S (2004) Treatment of cutaneous gnathostomiasis with ivermectin. Am J Trop Med Hyg 71:623–628
27. Ramirez-Avila L, Slome S, Schuster FL, Gavali S, Schantz PM, Sejvar J, Glaser CA (2009) Eosinophilic meningitis due to Angiostrongylus and Gnathostoma species. Clin Infect Dis Off Publ Infect Dis Soc Am 48:322–327
28. Munkon W, Sawanyawisuth K Pongtipakorn K, Kongbunkiat K, Limpawattana P, Senthong V,Chindaprasirt J, Chotmongkol V, Kanpittaya J, M Intapan P, Maleewong W and Kitkhuandee A.(2014) Subarachnoid hemorrhage due to vascular causes and gnathostomiasis: clinical features and laboratory findings. Southeast Asian J Trop Med Public Health. Sep;45(5):984–9
29. Bunnag T, Comer DS, Punyagupta S (1970) Eosinophilic myeloencephalitis caused by gnathostoma spinigerum. Neuropathology of nine cases. J Neurol Sci 10:419–434
30. Bhende M, Biswas J, Gopal L (2005) Ultrasound biomicroscopy in the diagnosis and management of intraocular gnathostomiasis. Am J Ophthalmol 140:140–142
31. Herman JS, Chiodini PL (2009) Gnathostomiasis, another emerging imported disease. Clin Microbiol Rev 22:484–492
32. Moore DAJ, McCroddan J, Dekumyoy P, Chiodini PL (2003) Gnathostomiasis: an emerging imported disease. Emerg Infect Dis 9:647–650
33. Barua P, Hazarika NK, Barua N, Barua CK, Choudhury B (2007) Gnathostomiasis of the anterior chamber. Indian J Med Microbiol 25:276–278
34. Bhattacharjee H, Das D, Medhi J (2007) Intravitreal gnathostomiasis and review of literature. Retina Phila Pa 27:67–73
35. Coffeng LE, Fobi G, Ozoh G et al (2012) Concurrence of dermatological and ophthalmological morbidity in onchocerciasis. Trans R Soc Trop Med Hyg 106:243–251
36. Okulicz JF, Stibich AS, Elston DM, Schwartz RA (2004) Cutaneous onchocercoma. Int J Dermatol 43:170–172
37. Abdel-Hameed AA, Noah MS, Schacher JF, Taher SA (1987) Lymphadenitis in Sowda. Trop Geogr Med 39:73–76
38. Burki T (2013) River blindness elimination in Columbia. Lancet Infect Dis 13:922–923
39. Gasparini G (1962) "Sowda": a new disease or an unpublished type of onchocerciasis? Arch Ital Sci Med Trop Parassitol 43:635–646
40. Dunn C, Callahan K, Katabarwa M, Richards F, Hopkins D, Withers PC, Buyon LE, McFarland D (2015) The contributions of onchocerciasis control and elimination programs toward the achievement of the millennium development goals. PLoS Negl Trop Dis. doi:10.1371/journal.pntd.0003703
41. Centers for Disease Control and Prevention (CDC) (2013) Progress toward elimination of onchocerciasis in the Americas – 1993–2012. MMWR Morb Mortal Wkly Rep 62:405–408
42. Eberhard ML, Sims AC, Bishop HS, Mathison BA, Hoffman RS (2012) Ocular zoonotic onchocerca infection in a resident of Oregon. Am J Trop Med Hyg 87:1073–1075
43. Barua P, Sharma A, Hazarika NK, Barua N, Bhuyan S, Alam ST (2011) A rare case of ocular onchocerciasis in India. Southeast Asian J Trop Med Public Health 42:1359–1364
44. Coffeng LE, Stolk WA, Zouré HGM et al (2014) African programme for onchocerciasis control 1995–2015: updated health impact estimates based on new disability weights. PLoS Negl Trop Dis 8:e2759

45. Turner HC, Walker M, Churcher TS, Basáñez M-G (2014) Modelling the impact of ivermectin on River Blindness and its burden of morbidity and mortality in African Savannah: EpiOncho projections. Parasit Vectors 7:241
46. Ament CS, Young LH (2006) Ocular manifestations of helminthic infections: onchocerciasis, cysticercosis, toxocariasis, and diffuse unilateral subacute neuroretinitis. Int Ophthalmol Clin 46:1–10
47. Babalola OE (2012) Onchocerciasis as a risk factor for night blindness. Ophthalmic Epidemiol 19:204–210
48. Babalola OE (2011) Ocular onchocerciasis: current management and future prospects. Clin Ophthalmol Auckl NZ 5:1479–1491
49. Banla M, Tchalim S, Karabou PK, Gantin RG, Agba AI, Kére-Banla A, Helling-Giese G, Heuschkel C, Schulz-Key H, Soboslay PT (2014) Sustainable control of onchocerciasis: ocular pathology in onchocerciasis patients treated annually with ivermectin for 23 years: a cohort study. PLoS One 9:e98411
50. Bowler GS, Shah AN, Bye LA, Saldana M (2011) Ocular loiasis in London 2008–2009: a case series. Eye Lond Engl 25:389–391
51. Ocular loiasis in London 2008-2009: a case series. Bowler GS, Shah AN, Bye LA, Saldana M. Eye (Lond). 2011 Mar;25(3):389–91
52. Padgett JJ, Jacobsen KH (2008) Loiasis: African eye worm. Trans R Soc Trop Med Hyg 102:983–989
53. Aiello F, Palma S, Varesi C, Cerulli A, Valente R, Aiello L (2010) A rare case report of Loa loa ocular filariasis. Eur J Ophthalmol 20:237–239
54. Choi S-C, Lee S-Y, Song H-O, Ryu J-S, Ahn M-H (2014) Parasitic infections based on 320 clinical samples submitted to Hanyang University, Korea (2004–2011). Korean J Parasitol 52:215–220
55. Cho H-Y, Lee Y-J, Shin S-Y, Song H-O, Ahn M-H, Ryu J-S (2008) Subconjuctival Loa loa with calabar swelling. J Korean Med Sci 23:731–733
56. Toussaint D, Danis P (1965) Retinopathy in generalized loa-loa filariasis. A clinicopathological study. Arch Ophthalmol Chic Ill 74:470–476
57. Stemmle J, Markwalder KA, Zinkernagel AS, Wirth MG, Grimm F, Hirsch-Hoffmann S, Thiel MA (2005) Loa loa infection of the eye – a case series. Klin Monatsblätter Für Augenheilkd 222:226–230
58. Renard G (1978) Ocular manifestations of loaiasis. J Fr Ophtalmol 1:83–86
59. Moussala M, Fobi G, Ongolo Zogo P, Bella Hiag LA, Bengono G, McMoli TE (2004) Retinal hemorrhages after ivermectin treatment for onchocerciasis in a patient with Loa loa microfilaremia. J Fr Ophtalmol 27:63–66
60. Foster CS, Vitale AT (2002) Diagnosis and treatment of uveitis. W.B. Saunders, Philadelphia
61. Rosa AAM, Rodrigues Neto Tdos S (2013) Diffuse unilateral subacute neuroretinitis (DUSN): current update. Arq Bras Oftalmol 76:256–260
62. Venkatesh P, Sarkar S, Garg S (2005) Diffuse unilateral subacute neuroretinitis: report of a case from the Indian subcontinent and the importance of immediate photocoagulation. Int Ophthalmol 26:251–254
63. De Amorim Garcia Filho CA, Gomes AHB, de A Garcia Soares ACM, de Amorim Garcia CA (2012) Clinical features of 121 patients with diffuse unilateral subacute neuroretinitis. Am J Ophthalmol 153:743–749
64. Myint K, Sahay R, Mon S, Saravanan VR, Narendran V, Dhillon B (2006) "Worm in the eye": the rationale for treatment of DUSN in south India. Br J Ophthalmol 90:1125–1127
65. Berbel RF, Casella AMB, de Souza EC, Farah ME (2014) Evaluation of patients with diffuse unilateral subacute neuroretinitis by spectral domain optical coherence tomography with enhanced depth imaging. Clin Ophthalmol Auckl NZ 8:1081–1087
66. Vezzola D, Kisma N, Robson AG, Holder GE, Pavesio C (2014) Structural and functional retinal changes in eyes with DUSN. Retina Phila Pa 34:1675–1682
67. Malaguido MR, Casella AMB, Malaguido DRG (2007) Clinical treatment of diffuse unilateral subacute neuroretinitis with albendazole. Arq Bras Oftalmol 70:814–822
68. Souza EC, Casella AMB, Nakashima Y, Monteiro MLR (2005) Clinical features and outcomes of patients with diffuse unilateral subacute neuroretinitis treated with oral albendazole. Am J Ophthalmol 140:437–445
69. Sudharshan S, Ganesh SK, Biswas J (2010) Current approach in the diagnosis and management of posterior uveitis. Indian J Ophthalmol 58:29–43
70. Gupta V, Sankaran P, Mohanraj SJC, Menon V (2014) Bilateral intraocular dirofilariasis. Indian J Ophthalmol 62:357–358
71. Senanayake MP, Infaq MLM, Adikaram SGS, Udagama PV (2013) Ocular and subcutaneous dirofilariasis in a Sri Lankan infant: an environmental hazard caused by dogs and mosquitoes. Paediatr Int Child Health 33:111–112
72. Ilyasov B, Kartashev V, Bastrikov N, Morchón R, González-Miguel J, Simón F (2013) Delayed diagnosis of dirofilariasis and complex ocular surgery, Russia. Emerg Infect Dis 19:326–328
73. Argy N, Sabou M, Billing A, Hermsdorff C, Candolfi E, Abou-Bacar A (2011) A first human case of ocular dirofilariasis due to Dirofilaria repens in northeastern France. J Trop Med 2011:698647
74. Mittal M, Sathish KR, Bhatia PG, Chidamber BS (2008) Ocular dirofilariasis in Dubai, UAE. Indian J Ophthalmol 56:325–326
75. Tafti MF, Hajilary A, Siatiri H, Rokni M, Mobedi I, Mowlavi G (2010) Ocular dirofilariasis, a case report. Iran J Parasitol 5:64–68

76. Kini RG, Leena JB, Shetty P, Lyngdoh RH, Sumanth D, George L (2015) Human dirofilariasis: an emerging zoonosis in India. J Parasit Dis Off Organ Indian Soc Parasitol 39:349–354
77. Sahdev SI, Sureka SP, Sathe PA, Agashe R (2012) Ocular dirofilariasis: still in the dark in western India? J Postgrad Med 58:227–228
78. Sekhar HS, Srinivasa H, Batru RR, Mathai E, Shariff S, Macaden RS (2000) Human ocular dirofilariasis in Kerala southern India. Indian J Pathol Microbiol 43:77–79
79. Chopra R, Bhatti SM, Mohan S, Taneja N (2012) Dirofilaria in the anterior chamber: a rare occurrence. Middle East Afr J Ophthalmol 19:349–351
80. Kalogeropoulos CD, Stefaniotou MI, Gorgoli KE, Papadopoulou CV, Pappa CN, Paschidis CA (2014) Ocular dirofilariasis: a case series of 8 patients. Middle East Afr J Ophthalmol 21:312–316
81. Gopinath TN, Lakshmi KP, Shaji PC, Rajalakshmi PC (2013) Periorbital dirofilariasis-clinical and imaging findings: live worm on ultrasound. Indian J Ophthalmol 61:298–300
82. Nath R, Gogoi R, Bordoloi N, Gogoi T (2010) Ocular dirofilariasis. Indian J Pathol Microbiol 53:157–159
83. Agarwal M, Biswas J (2009) Live intraocular dirofilaria causing multifocal choroiditis. Retin Cases Brief Rep 3:228–229
84. Sinawat S, Yospaiboon Y, Sinawat S (2013) Subretinal angiostrongyliasis-induced optic neuritis. Clin Ophthalmol Auckl NZ 7:977–979
85. Kanchanaranya C, Punyagupta S (1971) Case of ocular angiostrongyliasis associated with eosinophilic meningitis. Am J Ophthalmol 71:931–934
86. Mattis A, Mowatt L, Lue A, Lindo J, Vaughan H (2009) Ocular angiostrongyliasis – first case report from Jamaica. West Indian Med J 58:383–385
87. Dissanaike AS, Ihalamulla RL, Naotunne TS, Senarathna T, Withana DS (2001) Third report of ocular parastrongyliasis (angiostrongyliasis) from Sri Lanka. Parassitologia 43:95–97
88. Nelson RG, Warren RC, Scotti FA, Call TG, Kim BS (1988) Ocular angiostrongyliasis in Japan: a case report. Am J Trop Med Hyg 38:130–132
89. Feng Y, Nawa Y, Sawanyavisuth K, Lv Z, Wu Z-D (2013) Comprehensive review of ocular angiostrongyliasis with special reference to optic neuritis. Korean J Parasitol 51:613–619
90. Stuckey EJ (1917) Circumocular filariasis. Br J Ophthalmol 1:542–546
91. Beaver PC (1989) Intraocular filariasis: a brief review. Am J Trop Med Hyg 40:40–45
92. Nanavaty MA, Nanavaty AJ, Lakhani JD, Lakhani SJ, Vasavada AR (2001) Subconjunctival adult bancroftian filarial worm. Indian J Ophthalmol 49:195–196
93. Bain O, Kusaladharma PIT, Weerasooriya MV, Ihalamulla R, Dissanaike AS (2002) An immature filarial worm, probably Wuchereria bancrofti, from the anterior chamber of the eye in a patient from Sri Lanka. Parasite Paris Fr 9:282–284
94. Samarasinghe S, Pathirana S (2005) A juvenile filarial worm, Wuchereria bancrofti, extracted from the vitreous of the eye: the first report in the world literature. Ceylon Med J 50:167–168
95. Gupta A, Agarwal A, Dogra MR (1992) Retinal involvement in Wuchereria bancrofti filariasis. Acta Ophthalmol 70:832–835
96. Rao NG, Mahapatra SK, Pattnayak S, Pattnaik K (2008) Intravitreal live adult Brugian filariasis. Indian J Ophthalmol 56:76–78
97. Anandakannan K, Gupta CP (1977) Microfilaria malayi in uveitis: case report. Br J Ophthalmol 61:263–264

Part IV

Emerging Fungal Infections

Emerging Infectious Uveitis: *Candida* 19

Julie Gueudry and Bahram Bodaghi

19.1 Introduction

Fungal endophthalmitis is a sight-threatening disease most commonly caused by *Candida* species [1–3]. *Candida* endophthalmitis can result from hematogenous dissemination or, more rarely, from direct inoculation following penetrating trauma, surgery to the eye, and intraocular extension of ocular surface infections. Endogenous infections range from isolated chorioretinitis to endophthalmitis with extension into the vitreous.

19.2 Epidemiology

Candida species are an important cause of nosocomial infections. In contrast to other types of endophthalmitis where bacteria are the most prevalent pathogens, patients with endogenous endophthalmitis are more likely to have fungal isolates, with a predominance of *Candida albicans* [1–3]. Although *Candida albicans* remains the most common pathogen, non-*albicans* species such as *C. tropicalis*, *C. parapsilosis*, and *C. stellatoidea* have also been identified [4]. The candidemia usually occurs in hospitalized patients. Historically, the rate of ocular involvement has been reported to be very high between 28 and 37 % of patients with candidemia [5–7]. However, some studies have suggested that the current prevalence of *Candida* chorioretinitis and endophthalmitis is significantly lower, ranging from 2 to 16 % [8–12]. In a recent study, the prevalence of definitive infectious chorioretinitis/endophthalmitis was less than 1 % in patients with fungemia [13]. The earlier recognition of infection and the use of prophylactic systemic antifungal therapy have been suggested as the main reason for the decrease in the prevalence of ocular involvement in fungemia [12–14]. Furthermore, outpatients may also present with endogenous *Candida* endophthalmitis. Some of these patients may have a recent history of hospitalization, gastrointestinal tract surgery, indwelling central venous catheter, or a history of illicit intravenous drug use [15]. For these patients, candidemia may be transient and visual acuity decrease may be their only complaint. Hence, endogenous fungal endophthalmitis represents a diagnostic challenge because they may be misdiagnosed as autoimmune uveitis.

19.3 Pathophysiology/ Predisposing Factors

Candida species are the most common cause of invasive fungal infections in humans. Candida exists predominantly as unicellular yeasts with

J. Gueudry
Department of Ophthalmology, Charles Nicolle University Hospital, Rouen, France

B. Bodaghi (✉)
Department of Ophthalmology, DHU Vision and Handicaps, University of Paris VI Pitié-Salpêtrière Hospital, 47 bd de l'Hôpital, Paris 75013, France
e-mail: bahram.bodaghi@psl.aphp.fr

S.-P. Chee, M. Khairallah (eds.), *Emerging Infectious Uveitis*, DOI 10.1007/978-3-319-23416-8_19

small, thin-walled ovoid cells that reproduce by budding. There are over 20 species that can cause infection in humans, and *Candida albicans* is by far the most common. *Candida albicans* is a commensal microorganism, isolated from approximately 70 % of the healthy population [16]. It can be found in the intestinal and urogenital tracts and the oral cavities. However, in some circumstances, the same strains of *Candida albicans* can become pathogenic. These infections can be superficial and affect the skin or mucous membrane (such as oropharyngeal and esophageal candidiasis) or can invade the bloodstream and involve any organ. Invasive candidiasis includes candidemia, disseminated candidiasis, endocarditis, meningitis, endophthalmitis, and other deep organ involvement. *Candida albicans* is the fourth leading cause of nosocomial bloodstream infections, with a high mortality rate (range from 37 to 59 %) [17].

Three major components of the pathogenesis of invasive candidiasis can be identified, including the increase of fungal colonization, typically resulting from the use of broad-spectrum antimicrobial agents, the breakdown of normal mucosal and skin barriers (e.g., indwelling vascular catheters, recent surgery or trauma, or severe mucositis associated with cytotoxic chemotherapy and radiation), and the immune dysfunction (e.g., neutropenia). Moreover, *Candida* species can adhere to intravascular catheters or other prosthetic devices.

Hence, three high-risk groups for ocular candidiasis can be distinguished. The first one includes recent major gastrointestinal surgery, abortion, cancer and chemotherapy, broad-spectrum antibiotics use, indwelling catheters, parenteral alimentation, debilitating diseases (e.g., diabetes mellitus), immunosuppressive drugs, prolonged neutropenia, organ transplantation, or a combination of these, such as prolonged length of stay in an intensive care unit [18–20]. The second one concerns newborn infants in the neonatal ICU, especially in case of low-weight-birth infants [21, 22]. The third one is the group of intravenous drug users [23–29]. In this context, ocular infection may be isolated without evidence of systemic candidiasis (Fig. 19.1).

Possible sources of infection have been explored. In the mid-1980s, in France, an outbreak of candidiasis followed the introduction on the drug market of a new brown heroin [30], which had poor water solubility. This drug had to be dissolved in lemon juice or another acidic solvent. The hypothesis that the lemon juice used to dissolve the heroin might have been contaminated with *Candida albicans* carried by drug users was suggested [31, 32]. Moreover, lemon juice has been shown to be a good growth medium for yeasts [33, 34]. However, it has also been suggested that yeasts may be present in saliva used for drug dissolution or transmitted by needle licking before injecting the heroin [24, 26]. Finally, endogenous *Candida* endophthalmitis may occur rarely in healthy, immunocompetent patients without any risk factors [35].

Contrary to superficial fungal infections, disseminated candidiasis, especially ocular infections such as *Candida* chorioretinitis or endophthalmitis, is uncommon among HIV-infected patients. An explanation would be that immunity against systemic candidiasis is not dependent on cell-mediated immunity, but depends mainly on neutrophil cellular activity, which is not severely disturbed in HIV infection [36, 37].

In the USA and Europe, an ophthalmic examination is recommended for all candidemic patients to rule out intraocular involvement [14]. In the current era of widespread prophylactic antifungal therapy, ocular fungal infection is rare, and some studies highlighted that the usefulness of routine ophthalmic consultations for all fungemic patients is relatively low [12, 13].

19.4 Clinical Features

19.4.1 Systemic Disease

Superficial mycoses include oropharyngeal, vaginal and cutaneous candidiasis, and paronychia and onychomycosis. Invasive candidiasis can involve virtually any organ and hence have a variety of clinical manifestations. *Candida* species may cause endocarditis, vertebral osteomyelitis, meningitis, cerebral abscess, endophthalmitis,

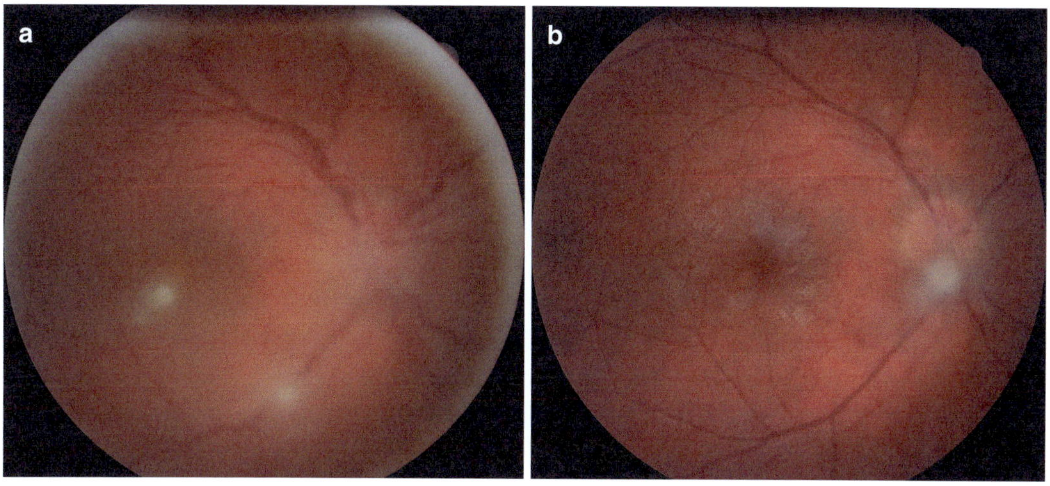

Fig. 19.1 Endogenous *Candida albicans* endophthalmitis in a 28-year-old male with a history of intravenous drug abuse. Note vitreous haze from vitritis, vitreous white fluffy lesions, and edematous optic disc (**a**). At 6 months, favorable clinical response after vitrectomy, one intravitreal amphotericin B injection, and systemic fluconazole treatment (**b**)

septic arthritis, involvement of the kidney, pneumonia, etc. This is why a positive blood culture for *Candida* species should always be considered and antifungal therapy is nowadays recommended for any episode of candidemia [14, 38].

A syndrome was reported in heroin addicts treated for systemic *Candida albicans* infections including cutaneous lesions (scalp nodules and pustulosis in hairy zones), ocular localizations (mainly chorioretinitis), and osteoarticular involvement (vertebrae, costal cartilage, knees, and sacroiliac) [30].

19.4.2 Ocular Disease

Patients may be asymptomatic and patients who are seriously ill may not be able to voice any visual changes. In other cases, symptoms are due to chorioretinal or vitreous involvement and may include floaters and blurred vision and scotoma, without pain in early stages. A red painful eye with photophobia arises from anterior uveitis and decreased vision resulting from macular chorioretinal involvement or dense vitritis. *Candida* chorioretinitis lesions are initially located at the level of the choroid and/or retina and spread into the vitreous cavity in the late phase. Early, the characteristic findings are creamy, white, well-circumscribed lesions, associated or not with retinal hemorrhages or perivascular sheathing, associated with overlying vitreous cellular inflammation. Lesions may be singular or multiple and posterior or peripheral. Occlusive retinal vasculitis is an uncommon complication of *Candida* infection [39]. Retinal hemorrhages may surround small necrotic lesions and appear similar to Roth spots. The vitreous exudates may assume a "string-of-pearls" or fluff ball appearance (Fig. 19.2). Chorioretinal lesions may become difficult to see at the late stage due to vitritis.

The anterior segment initially may be normal. Over time, patients may develop anterior uveitis with ciliary injection, non-granulomatous keratic precipitates, posterior synechiae, flare, cells, and, in severe cases, hypopyon (Fig. 19.3). Resolution of the acute chorioretinitis may result in permanent pigmentary scarring. Epiretinal membrane, vitreoretinal traction, macular hole, choroidal neovascularization, or retinal detachment may occur. Rare cases of spontaneous healing have been described [40–42].

Unlike endogenous fungal endophthalmitis, the vast majority of fungi identified in exogenous cases are molds. However, *Candida* species may be isolated in such situations, up to 29.8 % in a

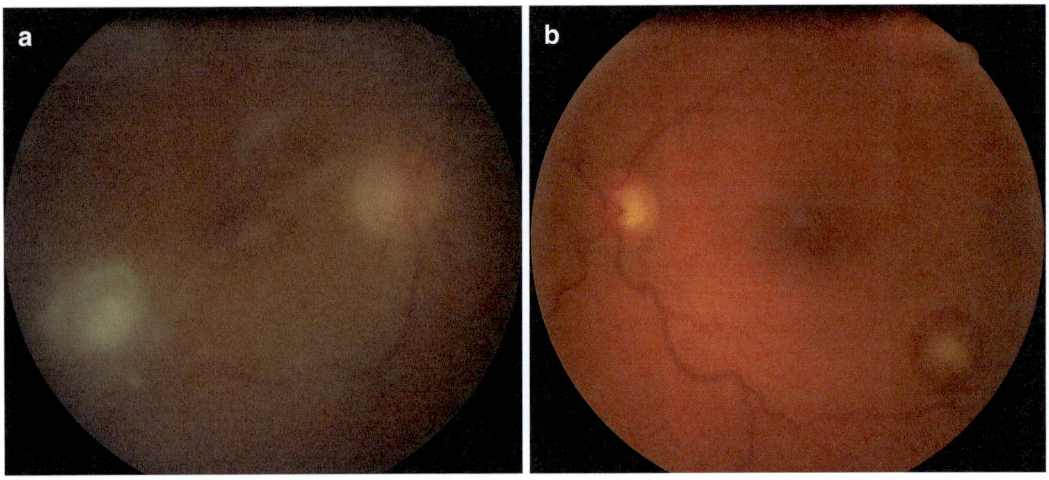

Fig. 19.2 *Candida albicans* endophthalmitis. Note typical fluff ball appearance of vitreous exudates (**a**) and "pseudo" Roth spots (**b**)

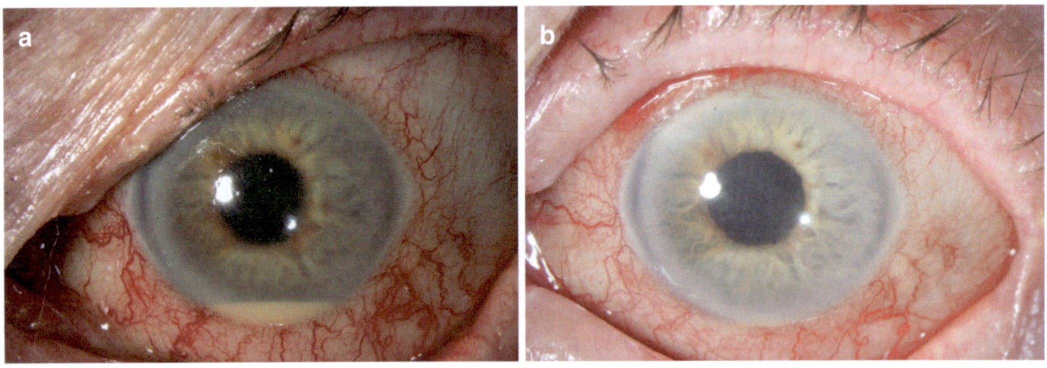

Fig. 19.3 *Candida albicans* endophthalmitis following a gastrointestinal surgery. Note the hypopyon (**a**). At 7 days, favorable clinical response after vitrectomy, one intravitreal amphotericin B injection, and systemic fluconazole treatment (**b**)

recent study [43]. In comparison with bacterial endophthalmitis, exogenous fungal endophthalmitis often presents with a latency period of weeks to months after intraocular inoculation with insidious course [44]. Typically, there are infiltrates in the anterior vitreous and fibrinous exudate in the anterior chamber. Confirmation of clinically fungal exogenous endophthalmitis is obtained by aspiration of aqueous humor and vitreous for microbiological analysis. Twenty-two isolates from patients with postsurgical endophthalmitis due to *Candida parapsilosis* as a result of exposure to a contaminated ocular irrigating solution were published by McCray et al. [45].

On fluorescein angiography, active lesions were early hypofluorescent and progressively became totally hyperfluorescent. Active choroidal inflammations appear as hypofluorescent spots on indocyanine green angiography without additional lesions than in fluorescein angiography [46].

OCT can clearly show the progression of chorioretinal lesions. Thus, OCT findings can show early lesions as a dome-shaped protrusion of the outer retina and pigment epithelium, then lesions involve the inner retinal layer as a hyper-reflective lesion, and finally, late-stage lesions appear like well-circumscribed, hyper-reflective,

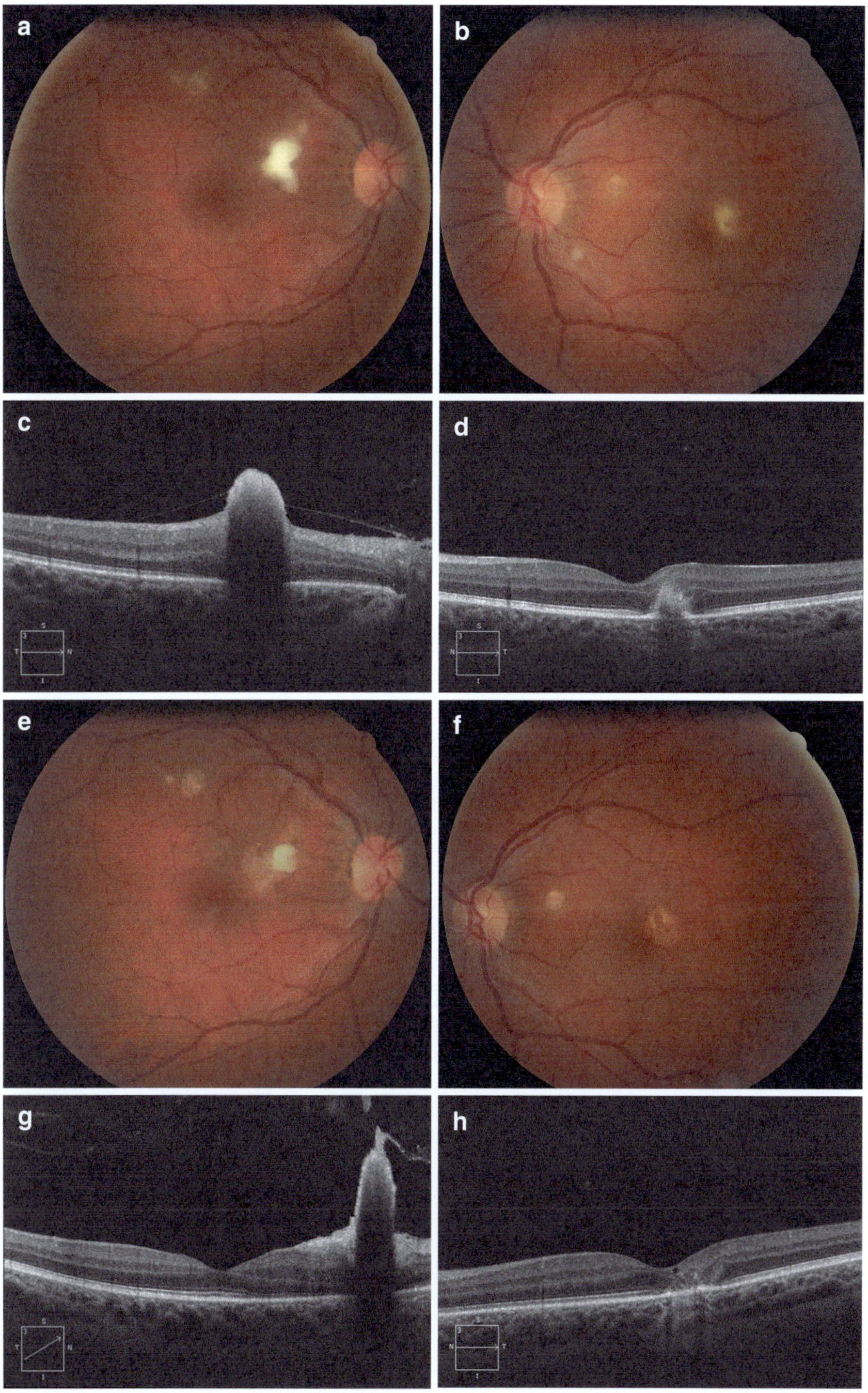

Fig. 19.4 Endogenous *Candida albicans* chorioretinitis in a patient with a history of indwelling central venous catheter in the context of pancreatic cancer (blood cultures were positive). Note creamy white lesions in the right (**a**) and the left eye (**b**). Ocular coherence tomography (OCT) findings show a well-circumscribed, hyperreflective, dome-shaped elevation overlying the retina with dense shadowing obscuring the underlying structures in the right eye (**c**) and a lesion of the outer retina and pigment epithelium in the left eye (**d**). At 2 months, favorable clinical response after systemic fluconazole treatment in the right eye (**e**) and in the left eye (**f**). OCT findings show persistent vitreoretinal traction in the right eye (**g**) and a paramacular chorioretinal thinning in the left eye (**h**)

dome-shaped elevation overlying the retina with dense shadowing obscuring the underlying structures [47]. OCT can also demonstrate large fluffy balls extending into the vitreous body and dense vitritis (Fig. 19.4). Hence, OCT is useful for monitoring progression of *Candida* endophthalmitis and its response to therapy, as well as in retinal complication detection.

19.5 Diagnosis

It is important to maintain a high index of suspicion of endogenous *Candida* ocular infection. Actually, the diagnosis of *Candida* endophthalmitis is usually based on the appearance of typical fundus lesions in a patient with disseminated *Candida* infection or significant risk factors. However, *Candida* blood culture may be negative even when disseminated disease is present, presumably because some patients only have transient or intermittent fungemia [48]. In this way, Martinez-Vazques et al. reported seven blood-positive cultures in 15 cases (47 %) of *C. albicans* endophthalmitis in intravenous drug abusers [27]. Moreover, isolation of *Candida* species from at least one extra-digestive site (urine, mouth, throat, upper and lower respiratory system, postoperative aspiration, or other suspected sites such as intravenous lines and indwelling catheters) supports the presumptive diagnosis [49]. *Candida* colonization is a reliable independent risk factor for candidemia [50, 51] and a colonization index (number of colonized sites/number of sampled sites) >0.5 is associated with an increased risk of candidemia with identification of the same *Candida* species in the colonized sites and bloodstream [52].

Vitreous biopsy can help to confirm the diagnosis of endophthalmitis. However, the yield of positive cultures from vitreous samples is variable, ranging from 26 to 68 % in literature [18, 27, 53, 54]. Vitreous specimens obtained by vitrectomy might be more sensitive than specimens obtained by needle biopsy, probably because the majority of *Candida* is present in vitreous near the retina and only sampled during vitrectomy from posterior vitreous near the retina and not by vitreous tap [55]. Henderson et al. confirmed that anterior chamber tap for culture was a poor diagnostic method in an experimental model [56]. Furthermore, polymerase chain reaction (PCR) has shown to be of high specificity for fungal detection in vitreous [57], even though PCR on humor aqueous seems to be not as sensitive as on vitreous [58]. Hence, PCR may allow a rapid diagnosis of fungal endophthalmitis. The use of serologic tests for circulating antibodies or antigens may be useful in providing a presumptive diagnosis of invasive fungal infection. However, the utility of these approaches remains to define in fungal endophthalmitis [59].

It is important to keep in mind that an infectious disease expert should be consulted because a complete medical workup for other sites of involvement is needed.

19.5.1 Differential Diagnosis

The differential diagnosis of *Candida* endophthalmitis includes endogenous bacterial endophthalmitis, endogenous endophthalmitis caused by other fungal organisms, toxoplasmic retinochoroiditis, primary intraocular lymphoma, and herpes virus family retinitis, in particular cytomegalovirus, multifocal choroiditis, and posterior uveitis.

19.6 Management

Four major categories of systemic antifungal agents used in candidiasis can be distinguished: the polyenes (amphotericin B deoxycholate and its lipid formulations), the triazoles (fluconazole, itraconazole, voriconazole, and posaconazole), the echinocandins (caspofungin, anidulafungin, and micafungin), and the flucytosine. It is important to keep in mind that in fungal endophthalmitis treatment, achieving adequate concentrations of antifungal agents in the choroid, retina, and vitreous is crucial to success.

Amphotericin B has long been considered the standard of therapy for intraocular fungal infections. Very few resistances were described and only *Candida lusitaniae* is frequently resistant to amphotericin B [60]. However, several studies noted the poor penetration of both amphotericin B deoxycholate (AmB-d) and its lipid formulations into the vitreous [61, 62]. Furthermore, amphotericin B use has been limited due to its systemic adverse effects, such as nephrotoxicity, fever, and hypotension. Amphotericin B has been injected directly into the vitreous as adjunctive treatment in severe fungal endophthalmitis [63, 64]. However, toxicity to the retina has been reported in rabbits with doses between 1 and 10 μg [65–67]. Experimental studies suggested reduced toxicity with intravitreal injections of liposomal amphotericin B [68, 69]. Amphotericin B intravitreal injection doses typically administered in humans are 5 or 10 μg/0.1 mL.

Flucytosine ocular penetration appears to be good, but this drug should not be used as monotherapy due to its propensity for the selection of resistant organisms. Hence, flucytosine is an adjunctive agent that can be used in combination with amphotericin B for the treatment of *Candida* endophthalmitis. Flucytosine is active against most *Candida* species, with the exception of *C. krusei* [14].

Fluconazole, an older generation of triazole, is most commonly used in ocular candidiasis due to its excellent efficacy, its low toxicity, and its good intraocular penetration [70–72]. Studies in humans have shown good response rates associated with amphotericin intravitreal injection [63] or not [73–76]. However, fluconazole had a limited spectrum of antifungal activity, and resistances were noted in immunosuppressed hosts who received long-term treatment. Fluconazole is active against all *Candida* species, except *C. krusei*, some strains of inherently resistant *C. glabrata*, and strains of *C. albicans*, which acquired resistance. Fluconazole treatment failures have been reported in endophthalmitis, even in cases of *Candida albicans* [77, 78]. Fluconazole is available in both intravenous and oral formulations.

Itraconazole has broader activity, but suffers from irregular absorption. It is not usually used in such cases. Furthermore, oral itraconazole has limited penetration into eyes with fungal endophthalmitis [79].

Voriconazole is a second-generation triazole available since 2002 with an extended spectrum of activity, including *C. krusei*, *C. glabrata*, and certain molds. Although voriconazole was highly active against *C. glabrata*, resistance to voriconazole has been reported. Moreover, voriconazole inhibited 90 % of clinical isolates of *Candida* species at a concentration six to eight times less than that determined for fluconazole [80]. Voriconazole is available in both intravenous and oral formulations. Voriconazole has excellent oral bioavailability achieving therapeutic aqueous and vitreous levels in the noninflamed human eye [81]. Despite these advantages, only a small number of patients who had *Candida* endophthalmitis treated with systemic voriconazole are described in the literature [82–84]. The most common adverse effects of voriconazole reported are disturbances of vision (photopsia, disturbed color vision, and blurring of vision), skin rashes, and elevations in hepatic enzyme level. The patients should be warned of the risk of photosensitization. The potential for drug interactions with voriconazole is high.

Voriconazole is also considered for intravitreal injection. Experimental studies showed no significant toxicity [85, 86], suggesting that an intravitreal voriconazole concentration up to 25 μg/mL is safe and that a dose of 100 μg could be used safely for intravitreal injection in humans [85]. Several reports have been published about the safety and efficacy of intravitreal voriconazole in fungal endophthalmitis [82, 87]. Voriconazole intravitreal injections may be safer than amphotericin B injections and may immediately achieve high vitreal concentrations [88].

Like voriconazole, posaconazole has excellent in vitro activity against most *Candida* species. However, very few data are available concerning its interest in fungal endophthalmitis management [89, 90].

Echinocandins ocular penetration is very poor in animal studies [91–93]. Furthermore, clinical failure of caspofungin in the management of *Candida albicans* endophthalmitis associated with poor vitreous penetration has been reported [94].

Currently, no clear guidelines exist about the role of early vitrectomy in ocular candidiasis management. Vitrectomy may be useful to decrease infection load, to increase intraocular diffusion of systemic antifungal treatment, to limit healing vitreous retraction, and to provide vitreous samples for the analysis of intraocular fluid. Some studies suggest that early vitrectomy may be useful in reducing the risk of retinal detachment [54, 95]. Furthermore, antifungal drug intravitreal injection may be performed at the conclusion of the surgery. However, evidences for vitrectomy remain modest. Moreover, early vitrectomy in an infected eye could lead to specific complications, such as retinal detachment or intraocular hemorrhage. In this context, early vitrectomy might be considered for patients with severe vitritis or in patients with no clinical improvement despite the antifungal treatment [27, 82].

Finally, systemic corticosteroids should be avoided in *Candida* endophthalmitis [54].

Although there are no prospective studies for the treatment of *Candida* endophthalmitis, recommendations exist. Current Infectious Diseases Society of America (IDSA) guidelines for the management of endogenous *Candida* endophthalmitis published in 2009 and current European Society of Clinical Microbiology and Infectious Diseases guidelines for ocular candidiasis published in 2012 still recommend intravenous AmB-d and oral flucytosine, possibly with vitrectomy and intravitreal AmB-d, as therapy for patients with sight-threatening infections or when the susceptibility of the isolate is unknown. They also recommend fluconazole alone for less severe cases [14, 96]. Nowadays, newer antifungals are changing this conventional approach to ocular candidiasis. Recently, recommendations have been suggested concerning *Candida* endophthalmitis treatment encouraging an increased role for fluconazole and voriconazole and a decreased role for AmB-d [88]. In these recommendations, either fluconazole (12 mg/kg loading dose, then 6–12 mg/kg daily) or voriconazole (6 mg/kg for 2 doses, then 4 mg/kg twice daily) may be used. Intravitreal injection of antifungal agents (voriconazole or AmB-d) should be considered if there is significant vitritis and, in cases of macular involvement, to achieve high vitreal concentrations as quickly as possible. It is recommended that treatment should be continued for at least 4–6 weeks, until complete resolution of visible lesions.

19.7 Prognosis

The visual outcome of *Candida* endophthalmitis is variable, depending on the stage of the disease. Previous studies have reported variable visual outcomes, with 15–60 % of eyes developing severe visual loss [55, 97]. Data from a more recent review by Sallam et al. indicated that a third of patients (33 %) develop severe visual loss (visual acuity of <20/200) and 50 % of patients develop visual loss (visual acuity worse than 20/40). In this study, poor initial visual acuity and centrally located lesions were associated with an increased risk of permanent visual loss. The authors suggested that early vitrectomy within 1 week of presentation significantly reduced the risk of retinal detachment, but had no effect on final visual outcomes [54]. Furthermore, patients with candidemia have a high overall mortality rate, which may approach 50 %, associated with the severity of fungal infection and with their underlying medical problems.

Conclusion

Fungal endophthalmitis is a sight-threatening disease most commonly caused by *Candida* species. *Candida* endophthalmitis most often results from hematogenous dissemination. Although the use of prophylactic systemic antifungal therapy decreases the prevalence of ocular involvement in fungemia, it is important to be on the lookout for endogenous *Candida* ocular infection, particularly in immunocompromised or diabetic patients, those with indwelling catheter, or among intravenous drug users. The diagnosis of *Candida* endophthalmitis is mainly clinical and is usually based on the appearance of typical fundus lesions. Further trials are needed to define the role of voriconazole, a drug with more side effects and drug interactions than fluconazole.

Core Messages

- *Candida* endophthalmitis is a vision-threatening condition.
- Endogenous *Candida* ocular infections may occur in immunocompromised or diabetic patients, those with indwelling catheter, or among intravenous drug users.
- Management and treatment should be instituted in collaboration with an infectious disease expert for systemic involvement management.
- Current treatments include systemic fluconazole or voriconazole due to their good intraocular penetration, associated or not with early vitrectomy or antifungal intravitreal injection.

References

1. Ness T, Pelz K, Hansen LL (2007) Endogenous endophthalmitis: microorganisms, disposition and prognosis. Acta Ophthalmol Scand 85(8):852–856
2. Schiedler, V., I.U. Scott, H.W. Flynn, Jr., et al. Culture-proven endogenous endophthalmitis: clinical features and visual acuity outcomes. Am J Ophthalmol 2004, 4, 137: 725–731
3. Connell PP, O'Neill EC, Fabinyi D et al (2011) Endogenous endophthalmitis: 10-year experience at a tertiary referral centre. Eye (Lond) 25(1):66–72
4. Lynn WA, Lightman S (2004) The eye in systemic infection. Lancet 364(9443):1439–1450
5. Brooks RG (1989) Prospective study of Candida endophthalmitis in hospitalized patients with candidemia. Arch Intern Med 149(10):2226–2228
6. Parke DW 2nd, Jones DB, Gentry LO (1982) Endogenous endophthalmitis among patients with candidemia. Ophthalmol 89(7):789–796
7. Griffin JR, Pettit TH, Fishman LS et al (1973) Blood-borne Candida endophthalmitis. A clinical and pathologic study of 21 cases. Arch Ophthalmol 89(6):450–456
8. Feman SS, Nichols JC, Chung SM et al (2002) Endophthalmitis in patients with disseminated fungal disease. Trans Am Ophthalmol Soc 100:67–70 discussion 70–1
9. Donahue SP, Greven CM, Zuravleff JJ et al (1994) Intraocular candidiasis in patients with candidemia. Clinical implications derived from a prospective multicenter study. Ophthalmol 101(7):1302–1309
10. Huynh N, Chang HY, Borboli-Gerogiannis S (2012) Ocular involvement in hospitalized patients with candidemia: analysis at a Boston tertiary care center. Ocul Immunol Inflamm 20(2):100–103
11. Oude Lashof AM, Rothova A, Sobel JD et al (2011) Ocular manifestations of candidemia. Clin Infect Dis 53(3):262–268
12. Ghodasra DH, Eftekhari K, Shah AR et al (2014) Outcomes, impact on management, and costs of fungal eye disease consults in a tertiary care setting. Ophthalmol 121(12):2334–2339
13. Dozier CC, Tarantola RM, Jiramongkolchai K et al (2011) Fungal eye disease at a tertiary care center: the utility of routine inpatient consultation. Ophthalmol 118(8):1671–1676
14. Pappas PG, Kauffman CA, Andes D et al (2009) Clinical practice guidelines for the management of candidiasis: 2009 update by the Infectious Diseases Society of America. Clin Infect Dis 48(5):503–535
15. Durand ML (2013) Endophthalmitis. Clin Microbiol Infect 19(3):227–234
16. Mavor AL, Thewes S, Hube B (2005) Systemic fungal infections caused by Candida species: epidemiology, infection process and virulence attributes. Curr Drug Targets 6(8):863–874
17. Wisplinghoff H, Bischoff T, Tallent SM et al (2004) Nosocomial bloodstream infections in US hospitals: analysis of 24,179 cases from a prospective nationwide surveillance study. Clin Infect Dis 39(3):309–317
18. Tanaka M, Kobayashi Y, Takebayashi H et al (2001) Analysis of predisposing clinical and laboratory findings for the development of endogenous fungal endophthalmitis. A retrospective 12-year study of 79 eyes of 46 patients. Retina 21(3):203–209
19. Shah CP, McKey J, Spirn MJ et al (2008) Ocular candidiasis: a review. Br J Ophthalmol 92(4):466–468
20. Pappas PG (2006) Invasive candidiasis. Infect Dis Clin North Am 20(3):485–506
21. Baley JE, Kliegman RM, Fanaroff AA (1984) Disseminated fungal infections in very low-birth-weight infants: clinical manifestations and epidemiology. Pediatrics 73(2):144–152
22. Johnson DE, Thompson TR, Green TP et al (1984) Systemic candidiasis in very low-birth-weight infants (less than 1500 grams). Pediatrics 73(2):138–143
23. Bisbe J, Miro JM, Latorre X et al (1992) Disseminated candidiasis in addicts who use brown heroin: report of 83 cases and review. Clin Infect Dis 15(6):910–923
24. Cassoux N, Bodaghi B, Lehoang P et al (2002) Presumed ocular candidiasis in drug misusers after intravenous use of oral high dose buprenorphine (Subutex). Br J Ophthalmol 86(8):940–941
25. Collignon PJ, Sorrell TC (1983) Disseminated candidiasis: evidence of a distinctive syndrome in heroin abusers. Br Med J (Clin Res Ed) 287(6396):861–862
26. Hirsbein D, Attal P, Gueudry J et al (2008) Endogenous Candida endophthalmitis in drug misusers injecting intravenous buprenorphine. J Fr Ophtalmol 31(2):180–183
27. Martinez-Vazquez C, Fernandez-Ulloa J, Bordon J et al (1998) *Candida albicans* endophthalmitis in

brown heroin addicts: response to early vitrectomy preceded and followed by antifungal therapy. Clin Infect Dis 27(5):1130–1133

28. Servant JB, Dutton GN, Ong-Tone L et al (1985) Candidal endophthalmitis in Glaswegian heroin addicts: report of an epidemic. Trans Ophthalmol Soc U K 104(Pt 3):297–308
29. Sorrell TC, Dunlop C, Collignon PJ et al (1984) Exogenous ocular candidiasis associated with intravenous heroin abuse. Br J Ophthalmol 68(11):841–845
30. Dupont B, Drouhet E (1985) Cutaneous, ocular, and osteoarticular candidiasis in heroin addicts: new clinical and therapeutic aspects in 38 patients. J Infect Dis 152(3):577–591
31. Leen CL, Brettle RP (1991) Fungal infections in drug users. J Antimicrob Chemother 28(Suppl A):83–96
32. Shankland GS, Richardson MD, Dutton GN (1986) Source of infection in candida endophthalmitis in drug addicts. Br Med J (Clin Res Ed) 292(6528):1106–1107
33. Newton-John HF, Wise K, Looke DF (1984) Role of the lemon in disseminated candidiasis of heroin abusers. Med J Aust 140(13):780–781
34. Podzamczer D, Ventin M, Sauca G et al (1986) Contaminated lemons as possible source of infection in heroin abusers with disseminated candidiasis. Eur J Clin Microbiol 5(4):477
35. Kostick DA, Foster RE, Lowder CY et al (1992) Endogenous endophthalmitis caused by *Candida albicans* in a healthy woman. Am J Ophthalmol 113(5):593–595
36. Jabs DA (1995) Ocular manifestations of HIV infection. Trans Am Ophthalmol Soc 93:623–683
37. Miailhes P, Labetoulle M, Naas T et al (2001) Unusual etiology of visual loss in an HIV-infected patient due to endogenous endophthalmitis. Clin Microbiol Infect 7(11):641–645
38. Pappas PG, Rex JH, Sobel JD et al (2004) Guidelines for treatment of candidiasis. Clin Infect Dis 38(2):161–189
39. Sanli E, Pandya VB, McDonald RJ et al (2013) Ocular candidiasis complicated by branch retinal vein occlusion. Br J Ophthalmol 97(3):375–376
40. Le Thien L, Fajnkuchen F, Chaine G (1998) Candida chorioretinitis in drug addicts. Apropos of 2 cases. J Fr Ophtalmol 21(5):387–392
41. Dellon AL, Stark WJ, Chretien PB (1975) Spontaneous resolution of endogenous Candida endophthalmitis complicating intravenous hyperalimentation. Am J Ophthalmol 79(4):648–654
42. McDonald HR, De Bustros S, Sipperley JO (1990) Vitrectomy for epiretinal membrane with Candida chorioretinitis. Ophthalmol 97(4):466–469
43. Silva RA, Sridhar J, Miller D et al (2015) Exogenous fungal endophthalmitis: an analysis of isolates and susceptibilities to antifungal agents over a 20-year period (1990–2010). Am J Ophthalmol 159(2):257–64 e1
44. Wykoff CC, Flynn HW Jr, Miller D et al (2008) Exogenous fungal endophthalmitis: microbiology and clinical outcomes. Ophthalmol 115(9):1501–7, 07 e1–2
45. McCray E, Rampell N, Solomon SL et al (1986) Outbreak of *Candida parapsilosis* endophthalmitis after cataract extraction and intraocular lens implantation. J Clin Microbiol 24(4):625–628
46. Baglivo E, Seghelmeble C, Bagnoud M et al (2003) Indocyanine green angiographic features in endogenous Candida chorioretinis. Klin Monbl Augenheilkd 220(3):179–181
47. Cho M, Khanifar AA, Chan RV (2011) Spectral-domain optical coherence tomography of endogenous fungal endophthalmitis. Retin Cases Brief Rep 5(2):136–140
48. Sallam A, Lynn W, McCluskey P et al (2006) Endogenous Candida endophthalmitis. Expert Rev Anti Infect Ther 4(4):675–685
49. Timsit JF, Azoulay E, Cornet M et al (2013) EMPIRICUS micafungin versus placebo during nosocomial sepsis in Candida multi-colonized ICU patients with multiple organ failures: study protocol for a randomized controlled trial. Trials 14:399
50. Lau AF, Kabir M, Chen SC et al (2015) Candida colonization as a risk marker for invasive candidiasis in mixed medical-surgical ICUs: development and evaluation of a simple, standard protocol. J Clin Microbiol 53(4):1324–1330
51. Leon C, Ruiz-Santana S, Saavedra P et al (2009) Usefulness of the "Candida score" for discriminating between Candida colonization and invasive candidiasis in non-neutropenic critically ill patients: a prospective multicenter study. Crit Care Med 37(5):1624–1633
52. Pittet D, Monod M, Suter PM et al (1994) Candida colonization and subsequent infections in critically ill surgical patients. Ann Surg 220(6):751–758
53. Connell, P.P., E.C. O'Neill, F.M. Amirul Islam, et al. Endogenous endophthalmitis associated with intravenous drug abuse: seven-year experience at a tertiary referral center. Retina 2010; 30(10): 1721–1725
54. Sallam A, Taylor SR, Khan A et al (2012) Factors determining visual outcome in endogenous Candida endophthalmitis. Retina 32(6):1129–1134
55. Zhang YQ, Wang WJ (2005) Treatment outcomes after pars plana vitrectomy for endogenous endophthalmitis. Retina 25(6):746–750
56. Henderson DK, Edwards JE Jr, Ishida K et al (1979) Experimental hematogenous Candida endophthalmitis: diagnostic approaches. Infect Immun 23(3):858–862
57. Okhravi N, Adamson P, Mant R et al (1998) Polymerase chain reaction and restriction fragment length polymorphism mediated detection and speciation of Candida spp causing intraocular infection. Invest Ophthalmol Vis Sci 39(6):859–866
58. Anand A, Madhavan H, Neelam V et al (2001) Use of polymerase chain reaction in the diagnosis of fungal endophthalmitis. Ophthalmol 108(2):326–330
59. Penn RL, Lambert RS, George RB (1983) Invasive fungal infections. The use of serologic tests in diagnosis and management. Arch Intern Med 143(6):1215–1220
60. Atkinson BJ, Lewis RE, Kontoyiannis DP (2008) *Candida lusitaniae* fungemia in cancer patients: risk factors for amphotericin B failure and outcome. Med Mycol 46(6):541–546

61. Fisher JF, Taylor AT, Clark J et al (1983) Penetration of amphotericin B into the human eye. J Infect Dis 147(1):164
62. O'Day DM, Head WS, Robinson RD et al (1985) Intraocular penetration of systemically administered antifungal agents. Curr Eye Res 4(2):131–134
63. Essman TF, Flynn HW Jr, Smiddy WE et al (1997) Treatment outcomes in a 10-year study of endogenous fungal endophthalmitis. Ophthalmic Surg Lasers 28(3):185–194
64. Weishaar PD, Flynn HW Jr, Murray TG et al (1998) Endogenous Aspergillus endophthalmitis. Clinical features and treatment outcomes. Ophthalmol 105(1):57–65
65. Axelrod AJ, Peyman GA, Apple DJ (1973) Toxicity of intravitreal injection of amphotericin B. Am J Ophthalmol 76(4):578–583
66. Baldinger J, Doft BH, Burns SA et al (1986) Retinal toxicity of amphotericin B in vitrectomised versus non-vitrectomised eyes. Br J Ophthalmol 70(9):657–661
67. Souri EN, Green WR (1974) Intravitreal amphotericin B toxicity. Am J Ophthalmol 78(1):77–81
68. Barza M, Baum J, Tremblay C et al (1985) Ocular toxicity of intravitreally injected liposomal amphotericin B in rhesus monkeys. Am J Ophthalmol 100(2):259–263
69. Cannon JP, Fiscella R, Pattharachayakul S et al (2003) Comparative toxicity and concentrations of intravitreal amphotericin B formulations in a rabbit model. Invest Ophthalmol Vis Sci 44(5):2112–2117
70. O'Day DM, Foulds G, Williams TE et al (1990) Ocular uptake of fluconazole following oral administration. Arch Ophthalmol 108(7):1006–1008
71. Tod M, Lortholary O, Padoin C et al (1997) Intravenous penetration of fluconazole during endophthalmitis. Clin Microbiol Infect 3(1):143–144
72. Urbak SF, Degn T (1994) Fluconazole in the management of fungal ocular infections. Ophthalmol 208(3):147–156
73. Christmas NJ, Smiddy WE (1996) Vitrectomy and systemic fluconazole for treatment of endogenous fungal endophthalmitis. Ophthalmic Surg Lasers 27(12):1012–1018
74. Luttrull JK, Wan WL, Kubak BM et al (1995) Treatment of ocular fungal infections with oral fluconazole. Am J Ophthalmol 119(4):477–481
75. del Palacio A, Cuetara MS, Ferro M et al (1993) Fluconazole in the management of endophthalmitis in disseminated candidosis of heroin addicts. Mycoses 36(5–6):193–199
76. Rex JH, Bennett JE, Sugar AM et al (1994) A randomized trial comparing fluconazole with amphotericin B for the treatment of candidemia in patients without neutropenia. Candidemia Study Group and the National Institute. N Engl J Med 331(20):1325–1330
77. Nomura J, Ruskin J (1993) Failure of therapy with fluconazole for candidal endophthalmitis. Clin Infect Dis 17(5):888–889
78. Chang YF, Yang CS, Lee FL et al (2012) Voriconazole for Candida endophthalmitis. Ophthalmol 119(11):2414–15 e4
79. Mochizuki K, Niwa Y, Ishida K et al (2013) Intraocular penetration of itraconazole in patient with fungal endophthalmitis. Int Ophthalmol 33(5):579–581
80. Mandras N, Tullio V, Allizond V et al (2009) In vitro activities of fluconazole and voriconazole against clinical isolates of Candida spp. determined by disk diffusion testing in Turin, Italy. Antimicrob Agents Chemother 53(4):1657–1659
81. Hariprasad SM, Mieler WF, Holz ER et al (2004) Determination of vitreous, aqueous, and plasma concentration of orally administered voriconazole in humans. Arch Ophthalmol 122(1):42–47
82. Breit SM, Hariprasad SM, Mieler WF et al (2005) Management of endogenous fungal endophthalmitis with voriconazole and caspofungin. Am J Ophthalmol 139(1):135–140
83. Varma D, Thaker HR, Moss PJ et al (2005) Use of voriconazole in candida retinitis. Eye (Lond) 19(4):485–487
84. Jang GJ, Kim KS, Shin WS et al (2005) Treatment of candida chorioretinitis with voriconazole. Korean J Ophthalmol 19(1):73–76
85. Gao H, Pennesi ME, Shah K et al (2004) Intravitreal voriconazole: an electroretinographic and histopathologic study. Arch Ophthalmol 122(11):1687–1692
86. Kernt M, Neubauer AS, De Kaspar HM et al (2009) Intravitreal voriconazole: in vitro safety-profile for fungal endophthalmitis. Retina 29(3):362–370
87. Kramer M, Kramer MR, Blau H et al (2006) Intravitreal voriconazole for the treatment of endogenous Aspergillus endophthalmitis. Ophthalmol 113(7):1184–1186
88. Riddell Jt, Comer GM, Kauffman CA (2011) Treatment of endogenous fungal endophthalmitis: focus on new antifungal agents. Clin Infect Dis 52(5):648–653
89. Arnoldner MA, Kheirkhah A, Jakobiec FA et al (2014) Successful treatment of Paecilomyces lilacinus keratitis with oral posaconazole. Cornea 33(7):747–749
90. Sponsel WE, Graybill JR, Nevarez HL et al (2002) Ocular and systemic posaconazole(SCH-56592) treatment of invasive Fusarium solani keratitis and endophthalmitis. Br J Ophthalmol 86(7):829–830
91. Groll AH, Gullick BM, Petraitiene R et al (2001) Compartmental pharmacokinetics of the antifungal echinocandin caspofungin (MK-0991) in rabbits. Antimicrob Agents Chemother 45(2):596–600
92. Groll AH, Mickiene D, Petraitis V et al (2001) Compartmental pharmacokinetics and tissue distribution of the antifungal echinocandin lipopeptide micafungin (FK463) in rabbits. Antimicrob Agents Chemother 45(12):3322–3327
93. Groll AH, Mickiene D, Petraitiene R et al (2001) Pharmacokinetic and pharmacodynamic modeling of anidulafungin (LY303366): reappraisal of its efficacy in neutropenic animal models of opportunistic

mycoses using optimal plasma sampling. Antimicrob Agents Chemother 45(10):2845–2855
94. Gauthier GM, Nork TM, Prince R et al (2005) Subtherapeutic ocular penetration of caspofungin and associated treatment failure in *Candida albicans* endophthalmitis. Clin Infect Dis 41(3):e27–e28
95. Smiddy WE (1998) Treatment outcomes of endogenous fungal endophthalmitis. Curr Opin Ophthalmol 9(3):66–70
96. Cornely OA, Bassetti M, Calandra T et al (2012) ESCMID* guideline for the diagnosis and management of Candida diseases 2012: non-neutropenic adult patients. Clin Microbiol Infect 18(Suppl 7):19–37
97. Binder MI, Chua J, Kaiser PK et al (2003) Endogenous endophthalmitis: an 18-year review of culture-positive cases at a tertiary care center. Medicine (Baltimore) 82(2):97–105

20 Emerging Infectious Uveitis: *Aspergillus* and Other Fungi

Avni V. Patel and Dean Eliott

20.1 Introduction

Intraocular fungal infection is uncommon but can have devastating visual consequences. Fungi may infect the eye either endogenously, through hematogenous spread from a systemic infection, or exogenously, due to trauma or surgery. The diagnosis and management of ocular fungal infection is challenging to even the most experienced clinician.

20.2 Epidemiology and Pathophysiology

Fungi are eukaryotic organisms that are pervasive in the environment. Human exposure to these organisms is common, but ocular infection is infrequent and depends on the presence of predisposing conditions, the virulence of the organism, and the immunocompetence of the host. Although fungi may be a rare cause of intraocular infection, the incidence of fungal endophthalmitis in the United States is increasing. This may be due to the growing number of immunocompromised patients receiving chemotherapy and immunomodulatory treatments as well as the use of newer broad-spectrum antimicrobials, which alter the normal human microbial flora and predispose to opportunistic infection [1, 2]. In a study of 102 cancer patients undergoing ophthalmologic examination for fungemia at a large oncology center in the United States, 23 % had evidence of fungal endophthalmitis [3].

Fungi are categorized into yeasts, molds, and those which have features of both. Yeasts are single-celled forms while molds form multicellular hyphae. Yeasts include *Candida* and *Cryptococcus* species, and molds include *Aspergillus* and *Fusarium*. Dimorphic fungi, such as *Histoplasma and Coccidioides*, grow as both a yeast and a mold depending on certain conditions (the yeast form of *Coccidioides* is called a spherule). The dimorphic fungi typically grow as yeast in the human and animal host. While *Candida* species are the most common cause of fungal endophthalmitis, *Aspergillus* is the most common mold isolate and the second most common cause of fungal infections overall [4]. *Candida* endophthalmitis is discussed in detail in another chapter of this book.

Fungal infections may occur in the eye either through endogenous or exogenous sources. Endogenous fungal endophthalmitis refers to an intraocular infection which develops via hematogenous dissemination from a systemic infection. Risk factors for endogenous infection include immunosuppression, intravenous drug use, prolonged hyperalimentation, chronic pulmonary disease, malignancy, organ transplantation, diabetes mellitus, alcoholism, and chronic indwelling catheter such as in the setting of

A.V. Patel, MD, MBA • D. Eliott, MD (✉)
Massachusetts Eye and Ear Infirmary, Harvard Medical School, Boston, MA, USA
e-mail: dean_eliott@meei.harvard.edu

S.-P. Chee, M. Khairallah (eds.), *Emerging Infectious Uveitis*, DOI 10.1007/978-3-319-23416-8_20

hemodialysis [5]. In an autopsy study of 85 liver transplant recipients, *Aspergillus* endophthalmitis was noted in 7% [6].

Exogenous endophthalmitis is associated with three main modalities of infection: penetrating trauma, intraocular dissemination from ocular surface disease, or intraocular surgery [7]. A variety of fungi have been associated with endophthalmitis after trauma or intraocular surgery. Aspergillus species have also been identified as the most common cause of postoperative endophthalmitis. In a case series of 113 eyes with largely posttraumatic and postsurgical endophthalmitis from India, *Aspergillus* was isolated in 54.4% of the cases [2].

20.3 *Aspergillus*

There are more than 200 species of *Aspergillus*, including *A. flavus*, *A. niger*, *A. nidulans*, and *A. terreus*; however the most common ocular pathogen is *A. fumigatus*. *Aspergillus* is a ubiquitous saprophytic mold found in soil, decaying vegetation, and water. The conidia or asexual spores of *Aspergillus* organisms are airborne, making inhalation an important route of entry into humans. The reported risk factors for disseminated aspergillosis include chronic pulmonary disease, chronic immunosuppression (particularly following liver transplantation), and treatment with systemic corticosteroids [6, 8]. Rare cases have been reported in immunocompetent patients [9].

20.4 Clinical Features of *Aspergillus* Infection

20.4.1 Systemic

The spectrum of systemic disease caused by *Aspergillus* is broad, and it ranges from acute invasive aspergillosis in severely immunocompromised patients to allergic bronchopulmonary aspergillosis in patients with asthma and cystic fibrosis. Invasive aspergillosis can rarely occur outside the sinopulmonary tract, but in addition to eye infections it has been reported in diseases of the skin, central nervous system, and gastrointestinal tract. *Aspergillus* is also a known to be a cause of fungal endocarditis, most commonly seen in patients with prosthetic heart valves [10].

20.4.2 Ophthalmic

Patients with *Aspergillus* endophthalmitis present with the rapid onset of severe pain and decreased visual acuity. The central macula and posterior pole are often involved. On ophthalmologic evaluation, one might see a characteristic confluent central yellowish macular infiltrate in the choroid and subretinal space (Fig. 20.1). In addition to the macular lesion, gravitational layering of an inflammatory exudate may be seen in the preretinal or subhyaloid space [8]. The degree of inflammation may vary from subretinal or subhyaloid infiltrate alone to full thickness retinal involvement with hemorrhages [11]. As the infection spreads, vitreous involvement is often seen, and in later stages of the disease variable involvement of the anterior segment has been described with cells, flare, and occasionally hypopyon.

In comparison with *Candida, Aspergillus* more commonly invades retinal and choroidal

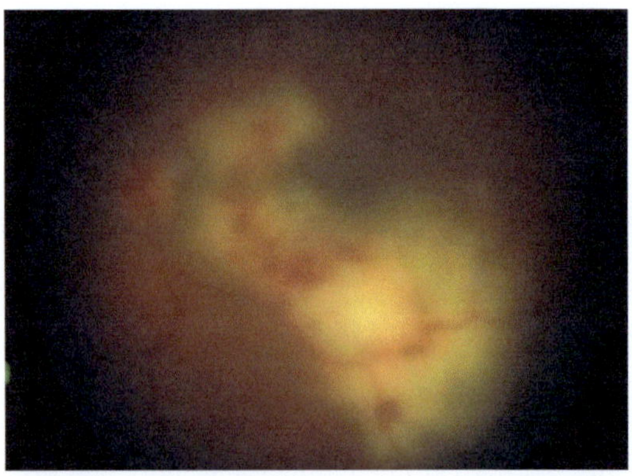

Fig. 20.1 A color fundus photo from young man with a history of intravenous drug abuse with endogenous *Aspergillus* endophthalmitis shows vitreous haze and a confluent macular lesion with retinal hemorrhages (This image was published in *Ophthalmology*, Yanoff and Duker, Fungal Endophthalmitis, 735–739, Copyright Elsevier (2013))

vasculature. As a result, retinal or choroidal vascular occlusion and exudative retinal detachment may be present with *Aspergillus* endophthalmitis and account for poorer visual outcomes compared with cases of *Candida* endophthalmitis [12].

20.5 Other Fungal Infections

20.5.1 *Fusarium*

Fusarium is a filamentous mold commonly found on plants and in soil. It is the most common fungal intraocular infection resulting from keratitis with contiguous spread from the ocular surface [7]. During an outbreak of *Fusarium* keratitis occurring due to one brand of contact lenses from 2004 to 2006, 6% of the keratitis patients progressed to endophthalmitis [13]. It has also been reported as a rare cause of fungal endophthalmitis following cataract surgery [14].

Endogenous spread of *Fusarium* is infrequent, and those cases that have been reported are limited to immunocompromised patients with disseminated fungal infection. In immunocompromised patients, *Fusarium* may cause sinusitis, pneumonia, and cellulitis at sites of skin breakdown or onychomycosis. Ocular disease typically manifests as a more localized inflammation or fungal mass confined to the anterior chamber or anterior vitreous, but disease can extend to the posterior vitreous in severe cases. While rare, these cases are often severe, presenting with a robust inflammatory reaction in the anterior chamber, vitritis, and varying degrees of retinal ischemia and necrosis [15] (Fig. 20.2).

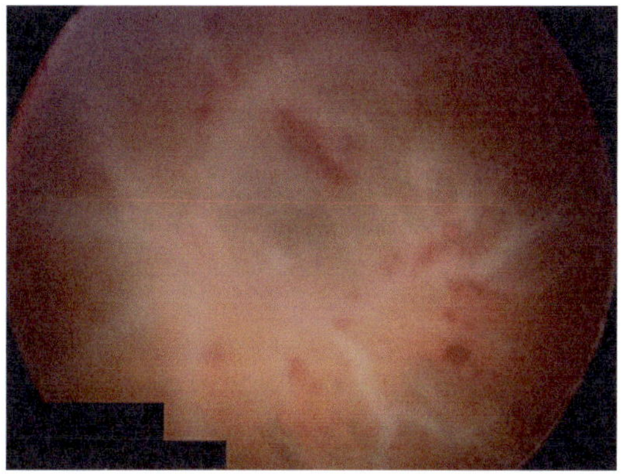

Fig. 20.2 A color fundus photo from a 70-year-old female with *Fusarium* endophthalmitis. Note vitreous haze from vitritis and severe vasculitis. (Courtesy of Lucia Sobrin, MD) (This image was published in *Ophthalmology*, Yanoff and Duker, Fungal Endophthalmitis, 735–739, Copyright Elsevier (2013))

20.5.2 *Histoplasma*

Histoplasma capsulatum is a thermally dimorphic fungus which grows as a mold in soil and as a yeast in human or animal hosts. When involved in eye infections, it typically affects a relatively young population, usually in the third or fourth decade of life. The fungus is endemic to the Central United States including the Ohio River Valley and Mississippi River Valley. Like many of the other fungal pathogens, its route of inoculation is most commonly through the respiratory tract. Humans usually acquire the infection via inhalation of spores (conidia) from soil that is contaminated with bat or bird droppings. While healthy patients may be asymptomatic, immunocompromised patients present with fever, pancytopenia, hepatosplenomegaly, and oropharyngeal or gastrointestinal lesions. Adrenal, brain, and skin lesions may additionally be seen in these patients [16]. Ocular clinical manifestations include punched-out choroidal scars, peripapillary pigmented degeneration, and macular choroidal neovascularization (CNV) or disciform scarring. The ocular disease is marked by little or no vitreous inflammation. As most cases of ocular histoplasmosis occur in healthy patients who are largely asymptomatic, regular follow-up for the possible occurrence of CNV is required [17, 18].

Histoplasma capsulatum is a very rare cause of endogenous endophthalmitis and when present occurs mostly in immunocompromised patients, such as those with AIDS, causing severe visual loss. Endogenous *Histoplasma* endophthalmitis is usually characterized by a granulomatous chorioretinitis and rarely by subretinal [22] and intraretinal exudates and retinal detachment [19].

20.5.3 *Coccidioides*

Coccidioides immitis is a dimorphic fungus found in dust in the endemic areas of the San Joaquin Valley of California, Arizona, and some parts of Central and South America. Agricultural and construction workers are among those at greatest risk for infection. Infection occurs through the inhalation of spores and in most patients leads to a self-limited disease. However, those patients who are re-exposed to the fungus may develop a chronic respiratory disease [20].

Coccidioides is a rare cause of endophthalmitis, and when it does cause intraocular infection, spread is hematogenous to the choroid. Cases of acute infection manifest with a multifocal choroiditis with scattered small lesions, vascular sheathing, exudative retinal detachment, and vitritis [21]. Other patients may remain asymptomatic and present only with chorioretinal scars [22].

20.5.4 *Cryptococcus*

Cryptococcus neoformans is an encapsulated yeast causing opportunistic infection in AIDS patients or other severely immunocompromised patients. Pigeons play an important role in its pathogenesis as the *Cryptococcus* spores survive up to 2 years in pigeon droppings. Human infection is acquired via the respiratory tract through the inhalation of spores. The fungus is then disseminated hematogenously and has a predilection for the central nervous system, most commonly resulting in fungal meningitis [23]. The organism reaches the eye either by direct extension from the optic nerve sheath or via hematogenous spread to the choroid. Ocular cryptococcosis is very rare, manifesting as a multifocal choroiditis with discrete, yellowish white lesions of differing size. Other manifestations include optic nerve edema, vascular sheathing, and exudative retinal detachment [24].

20.6 Diagnosis of *Aspergillus* and Other Fungal Infections

Early in the course of fungal infection, clinical manifestations may be subtle and variable, rendering a definitive diagnosis challenging. Therefore, the ability to make a prompt diagnosis of ocular fungal infection relies on a high index of suspicion and an appreciation of any predisposing conditions or risk factors that may make a patient more susceptible to fungal infection.

In the absence of an established source of infection or evidence of fungemia, it is important to obtain blood cultures as well as cultures from multiple sites and bodily fluids, including wounds and catheter tips. Cardiac imaging is recommended to rule out valvular vegetations which may be a source of septic emboli. A vitreous aspirate should be obtained and sent for special stains and culture. While this is the gold standard for the diagnosis of fungal endophthalmitis, the rates of positive cultures from vitreous sampling vary from 40 to 77 % [25]. In general, vitreous samples taken from vitrectomy are more likely to produce a positive culture result compared to an anterior chamber or vitreous tap [8].

Once a fluid sample has been obtained, most organisms can be identified by direct microscopy. *Aspergillus* will appear as septate hyphae branching at 45° angles (Fig. 20.3). Several special stains allow for improved visualization of fungal elements. Potassium hydroxide or KOH dissolves human cells and calcofluor white stains the cell wall of the fungi causing them to fluoresce. Both of these stains allow for easier detection of fungal elements. Calcofluor white is particularly useful in cases of fungal endophthalmitis resulting from keratitis [26]. Hematoxylin and eosin (H&E), periodic acid-Schiff (PAS), and Gomori methenamine silver (GMS) are among the stains used to detect fungi in cytologic

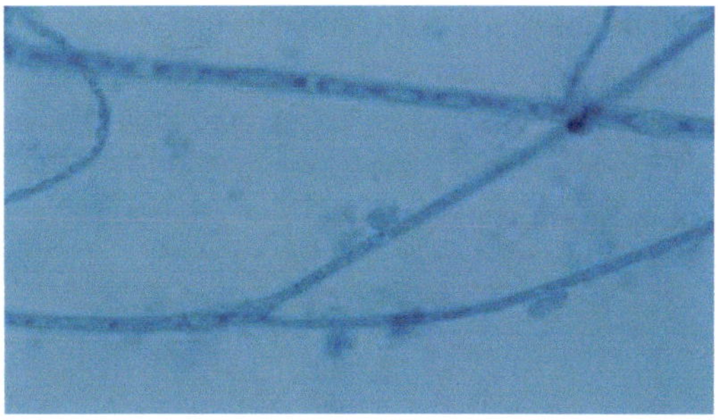

Fig. 20.3 Vitreous biopsy from a patient with *Aspergillus* endophthalmitis with multiple *Aspergillus* filaments in undiluted vitreous specimen staining with alcian blue (This image was published in *Ophthalmology*, Yanoff and Duker, Fungal Endophthalmitis, 735–739, Copyright Elsevier (2013))

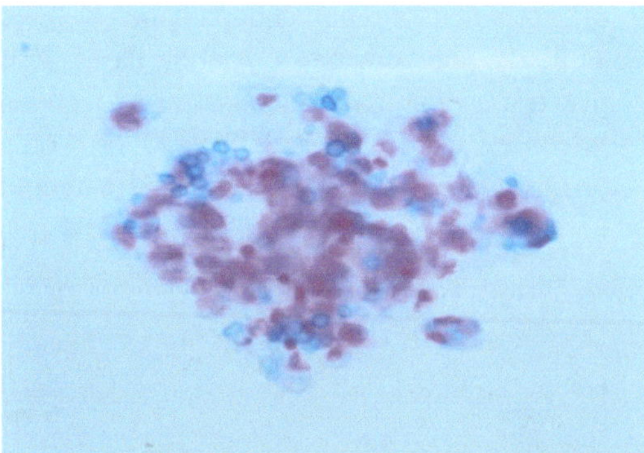

Fig. 20.4 Vitreous specimen from 69-year-old male with endogenous cryptococcal endophthalmitis. Note cryptococci staining with alcian blue (This image was published in *Ophthalmology*, Yanoff and Duker, Fungal Endophthalmitis, 735–739, Copyright Elsevier (2013))

preparations [27]. GMS is particularly helpful in cases of intraocular coccidioidomycosis, while India ink and mucicarmine are useful in cases where cryptococcal infection is suspected [21, 24] (Fig. 20.4).

In addition to these various stains, vitreous cultures should always be performed as they may aide in determining the susceptibility to various antifungal agents. More recent studies have shown polymerase chain reaction (PCR) detection of fungal species in vitreous samples to be highly specific and sensitive in the prompt diagnosis of fungal infection [28].

20.7 Differential Diagnosis (Figure)

Differential Diagnosis

- Bacterial endophthalmitis
- Toxoplasma chorioretinitis
- Intraocular lymphoma/leukemia
- Sarcoidosis
- Syphilis
- Tuberculosis
- Cytomegalovirus
- Viral retinitis

20.8 Management

The management of intraocular fungal infection involves both systemic and local treatment options. Previously, intravenous amphotericin B was widely used in the treatment of fungal infections; however due to limited intraocular penetration and multiple systemic toxicities including renal failure, this has since fallen out of favor. Systemic treatment with an alternative antifungal or in combination with intravitreal treatment is now the preferred management option. Azoles are an alternative antifungal class and newer-generation triazoles such as fluconazole and voriconazole provide greater than 90 % bioavailability, excellent intraocular penetration from the systemic circulation, and broad-spectrum antifungal activity [29, 30]. Further, fluconazole is very well tolerated, and the only major side effect is gastrointestinal upset. Voriconazole is a second-generation azole derived from fluconazole and, like fluconazole, may be given orally or intravenously. Systemic voriconazole, with and without intravitreal adjuvant treatment, has been shown to produce a more rapid response than other antifungals [29]. It is the treatment of choice for *Aspergillus* infections and is also active against *Fusarium.*

Fluconazole is given as a 12 mg/kg loading dose followed by a 6–12 mg/kg daily dose, and voriconazole is given as 6 mg/kg for 2 doses, then 4 mg/kg twice daily. Oral therapy may be used following an initial response to the IV formulation at a dose of 200 mg twice daily for both fluconazole and voriconazole. Systemic treatment is given for 4 to 6 weeks with the total course of treatment determined by clinical response [29].

For most cases of *Aspergillus* endophthalmitis and for sight-threatening fungal infection with macular involvement, intravitreal injection is recommended in addition to systemic treatment. Either amphotericin (5 μg/0.1 mL) or voriconazole (100 μg/0.1 mL) can be given as an intravitreal injection. While amphotericin has a longer half-life and there is more experience treating with this agent, voriconazole has been successfully employed in cases of resistant *Aspergillus* infection [31]. Response to therapy guides the need for repeat injections.

Pars plana vitrectomy is considered in cases of fungal infection with abscesses that are not amenable to penetration by systemic antifungal agents, with significant vitreous involvement, or with lack of improvement with intravitreal treatment [25, 32]. Vitrectomy may aide in decreasing the burden of infectious organisms. Vitrectomy should be combined with sampling the vitreous for culture and PCR as well as the administration of antifungal agents. It is important to note that the half-life of intravitreal antifungals may be decreased when given in a vitrectomized eye.

Close follow-up initially to evaluate the response to treatment and the need for further intervention is recommended. Collaboration with infectious disease colleagues is essential to providing safe and efficacious treatment as patients may require long term follow-up to monitor for drug interactions, toxicity, and systemic response to therapy.

Prognosis/Conclusion

The prognosis for patients with ocular fungal infection is guarded and depends on the extent of intraocular involvement, type of fungal infection, timing, and type of intervention. Prompt therapy is helpful in reducing ocular morbidity, and close monitoring to assess for the need for further treatment is crucial.

Factors associated with poor final visual acuity in these patients are macular involvement, poor visual acuity on initial examination, and retinal detachment. Retinal detachment has been reported to occur in up to 29% of patients with fungal endophthalmitis [25]. The visual outcomes in patients with *Aspergillus* infection, especially those with endogenous endophthalmitis, are often poor given the predilection for macular involvement. Visual acuity in patients with endogenous *Aspergillus* endophthalmitis is often worse than 20/200 in the majority of eyes and 20/50 or better in only 7% of eyes [8]. Cases of exogenous fungal endophthalmitis have similarly poor outcomes. Among cases with penetrating trauma as a cause for exogenous infection, nearly all have 20/400 or worse vision, while cases which begin as a fungal keratitis have a better prognosis [7].

Core Messages

- Ocular infection with *Aspergillus* or other fungi generally leads to poor visual outcomes.
- *Aspergillus* organisms infect the eye via hematogenous spread to the choroid, usually from a primary lung infection, in cases of endogenous endophthalmitis.
- For most cases of *Aspergillus* endophthalmitis and for sight-threatening fungal infection with macular involvement, intravitreal injection is recommended in addition to systemic treatment.
- The ability to make a prompt diagnosis of ocular fungal infection relies on a high index of suspicion and an appreciation of any predisposing conditions or risk factors that may make a patient more susceptible to fungal infection.

References

1. Essman TF, Flynn HW, Smiddy WE et al (1997) Treatment outcomes in a 10-year study of endogenous fungal endophthalmitis. Ophthalmic Surg Lasers 28(3):185–194
2. Chakrabarti A, Shivaprakash MR, Singh R et al (2008) Fungal endophthalmitis: fourteen years' experience from a center in India. Retina 28(10):1400–1407
3. Lamaris GA, Esmaeli B, Chamilos G et al (2008) Fungal endophthalmitis in a tertiary care cancer center: a review of 23 cases. Eur J Clin Microbiol Infect Dis 27(5):343–347
4. Ness T, Pelz K, Hansen LL (2007) Endogenous endophthalmitis: microorganisms, disposition and prognosis. Acta Ophthalmol Scand 85(8):852–856
5. Sridhar J, Flynn HW, Kuriyan AE, Miller D, Albini T (2013) Endogenous fungal endophthalmitis: risk factors, clinical features, and treatment outcomes in mold and yeast infections. J Ophthalmic Inflamm Infect 3(1):60
6. Hunt LKE, Glasgow BJ (1996) Aspergillus endophthalmitis. Ophthalmology 103(5):757–767
7. Wykoff CC, Flynn HW, Miller D, Scott IU, Alfonso EC (2008) Exogenous fungal endophthalmitis: microbiology and clinical outcomes. Ophthalmology 115(9):1501–1507, 1507.e1–e2
8. Weishaar PD, Flynn IHW, Murray ITG et al (1998) Endogenous Aspergillus endophthalmitis clinical features and treatment outcomes. Ophthalmology 105:57–65
9. Logan S, Rajan M, Graham E, Johnson E, Klein J (2010) A case of Aspergillus endophthalmitis in an immuncompetent woman: intra-ocular penetration of oral voriconazole: a case report. Cases J 3:31
10. Aspergillosis — NEJM. http://www.nejm.org/doi/full/10.1056/NEJMra0808853. Accessed 2 March 2015
11. Rao NA, Hidayat AA (2001) Endogenous mycotic endophthalmitis: variations in clinical and histopathologic changes in candidiasis compared with aspergillosis. Am J Ophthalmol 132(2):244–251
12. Jampol LM, Dyckman S, Maniates V, Tso M, Daily M, O'Grady R (1988) Retinal and choroidal infarction from Aspergillus: clinical diagnosis and clinicopathologic correlations. Trans Am Ophthalmol Soc 86:422–440
13. Epstein AB (2007) In the aftermath of the Fusarium keratitis outbreak: What have we learned? Clin Ophthalmol 1(4):355–366
14. Cakir M, Imamoğlu S, Cekiç O et al (2009) An outbreak of early-onset endophthalmitis caused by Fusarium species following cataract surgery. Curr Eye Res 34(11):988–995
15. Rezai KA, Eliott D, Plous O, Vazquez JA, Abrams GW (2005) Disseminated Fusarium infection presenting as bilateral endogenous endophthalmitis in a patient with acute myeloid leukemia. Arch Ophthalmol 123(5):702–703
16. Goodwin RA, Shapiro JL, Thurman GH, Thurman SS, Des Prez RM (1980) Disseminated histoplasmosis: clinical and pathologic correlations. Medicine (Baltimore) 59(1):1–33
17. Oliver A, Ciulla TA, Comer GM (2005) New and classic insights into presumed ocular histoplasmosis syndrome and its treatment. Curr Opin Ophthalmol 16(3):160–165
18. Thuruthumaly C, Yee DC, Rao PK (2014) Presumed ocular histoplasmosis. Curr Opin Ophthalmol 25(6):508–512
19. Gonzales CA, Scott IU, Chaudhry NA et al (2000) Endogenous endophthalmitis caused by Histoplasma capsulatum var. capsulatum: a case report and literature review. Ophthalmol 107(4):725–729
20. Stone JL, Kalina RE (1993) Ocular coccidioidomycosis. Am J Ophthalmol 116(2):249–250
21. Vasconcelos-Santos DV, Lim JI, Rao NA (2010) Chronic coccidioidomycosis endophthalmitis without concomitant systemic involvement: a clinicopathological case report. Ophthalmol 117(9):1839–1842
22. Rodenbiker HT, Ganley JP, Galgiani JN, Axline SG (1981) Prevalence of chorioretinal scars associated with coccidioidomycosis. Arch Ophthalmol 99(1):71–75
23. Rex JH, Larsen RA, Dismukes WE, Cloud GA, Bennett JE (1993) Catastrophic visual loss due to Cryptococcus neoformans meningitis. Medicine (Baltimore). 72(4):207–224
24. Henderly DE, Liggett PE, Rao NA (1987) Cryptococcal chorioretinitis and endophthalmitis. Retina 7(2):75–79
25. Lingappan A, Wykoff CC, Albini TA et al (2012) Endogenous fungal endophthalmitis: causative organisms, management strategies, and visual acuity outcomes. Am J Ophthalmol 153(1):162–166.e1
26. Kalkanci A, Ozdek S (2011) Ocular fungal infections. Curr Eye Res 36(3):179–189
27. Guarner J, Brandt ME (2011) Histopathologic diagnosis of fungal infections in the 21st century. Clin Microbiol Rev 24(2):247–280
28. Hidalgo JA, Alangaden GJ, Eliott D et al (2000) Fungal endophthalmitis diagnosis by detection of Candida albicans DNA in intraocular fluid by use of a species-specific polymerase chain reaction assay. J Infect Dis 181(3):1198–1201
29. Riddell J, Comer GM, Kauffman CA (2011) Treatment of endogenous fungal endophthalmitis: focus on new antifungal agents. Clin Infect Dis 52(5):648–653
30. Savani DV, Perfect JR, Cobo LM, Durack DT (1987) Penetration of new azole compounds into the eye and efficacy in experimental Candida endophthalmitis. Antimicrob Agents Chemother 31(1):6–10
31. Kramer M, Kramer MR, Blau H, Bishara J, Axer-Siegel R, Weinberger D (2006) Intravitreal voriconazole for the treatment of endogenous Aspergillus endophthalmitis. Ophthalmology 113(7):1184–1186
32. Christmas NJ, Smiddy WE (1996) Vitrectomy and systemic fluconazole for treatment of endogenous fungal endophthalmitis. Ophthalmic Surg Lasers 27(12):1012–1018

21 The Zika Virus: Review of Ocular Findings

Maurício Maia, Juliana Prazeres, Bruno de Paula Freitas, João Rafael de Oliveira Dias, Camila V. Ventura, and Rubens Belfort Jr.

The Zika virus (ZIKV), an emerging mosquito-borne pathogen, was described first in 1947 after being isolated from Rhesus monkeys in a Ugandan forest. In 1952, the pathogen then was isolated for the first time in humans in Uganda and Tanzania [1, 2].

ZIKV belongs to the genus *Flavivirus*, from the *Flaviviridae* family, and is related closely to other flaviviruses including dengue, yellow fever, and West Nile viruses.

The most common route of ZIKV transmission is by mosquitoes from the *Culicidae* family and the *Aedes* genus, especially by the *Aedes aegypti*, which is usually found in urban areas. Direct interhuman transmission, most likely by sexual intercourse, breastfeeding, and perinatal transmission, also has been described [3–5]. The ZIKV also has been detected in human saliva, blood, semen, and urine [6, 7].

In 2007, the first ZIKV outbreak outside of Africa and Asia was reported on Yap Island, Micronesia, and caused relatively mild disease in that population [8]. In 2013, a large outbreak was reported on the archipelago of French Polynesia [9], and by May 2015, the first local transmission of the ZIKV with autochthonous cases was reported in Brazil. It is estimated that about 440,000–1,300,000 cases of ZIKV disease occurred in Brazil in 2015 [10]. Last update: By December 1 2016, 48 countries and territories in the Americas have confirmed local mosquito-borne transmission of ZIKV disease since 2015. By February 2016, 22 countries and territories subsequently identified autochthonous transmission within the region, reflecting the virus's capacity to cause large-scale outbreaks where the biologic vector is present [11].

On February 1, 2016, the World Health Organization announced that the ZIKV outbreak constitutes a "Public Health Emergency of International Concern" [12]. World Health Organization. Regional Zika epidemiological update (Americas) July 29, 2016. http://www.paho.org/hq/index.php?option=com_content&view=article&id=11599:regional-zika-epidemiological-update-americas&Itemid=41691&lang=en. Accessed December 14, 2016. The outbreak was described as "an extraordinary event which is determined to constitute a public health risk to other States through the international spread of

M. Maia, MD, PhD (✉) • J. Prazeres, MD • J.R. de Oliveira Dias, MD • R. Belfort Jr., MD, PhD
Department of Ophthalmology and Visual Sciences, Paulista School of Medicine, Federal University of São Paulo, Vision Institute IPEPO, São Paulo, Brazil
e-mail: maiamauricio@terra.com.br; retina@femanet.com.br

B. de Paula Freitas, MD
Roberto Santos Hospital, Salvador, Brazil

C.V. Ventura, MD
Department of Ophthalmology and Visual Sciences, Paulista School of Medicine, Federal University of São Paulo, Vision Institute IPEPO, São Paulo, Brazil

Altino Ventura Foundation, Recife, Brazil

Pernambuco's Eye Hospital (HOPE), Recife, Brazil

S.-P. Chee, M. Khairallah (eds.), *Emerging Infectious Uveitis*, DOI 10.1007/978-3-319-23416-8_21

disease and to potentially require a coordinated international response."

For a half century, the ZIKV infection was associated with mild and self-limited symptoms (headache, rash, joint pain, and conjunctivitis). However, recently an association between the ZIKV infection during pregnancy and microcephaly in newborns was first suspected 6 months after the onset of the ZIKV outbreak in Brazil, because there was an unusual increase in newborns with microcephaly reported in Brazil [13, 14]. In 2015, 1248 new suspected cases were registered, corresponding to a prevalence of 99.7 per 100,000 live births, which represents a 20-fold increase from 2014 to 2015 [15]. Furthermore, the Brazilian Ministry of Health updated these data in January 2016 and reported a total of 3174 newborns with microcephaly, the majority of whom were in northeastern Brazil [16].

This hypothesis was strengthened by the fact that the ZIKV was detected in the amniotic fluid of two pregnant women of babies with microcephaly and the tissue of a newborn with microcephaly who died after birth [17]. Another study in Brazil tested blood and urine specimens for the ZIKV by reverse transcriptase-polymerase chain reaction (RT-PCR) assays in pregnant women in whom a rash developed within 5 days. Fetal ultrasonography was performed in 42 women who were ZIKV-positive and in all women who were ZIKV-negative. Fetal abnormalities were detected by Doppler ultrasonography in 12 of the 42 ZIKV-positive women and none of the 16 ZIKV-negative women [18]. Mlakar et al. [19] detected the ZIKV in fetal brain tissue on RT-PCT after autopsy performed on a fetus with microcephaly; the mother reported having a febrile illness associated with rash in the first trimester of pregnancy while she was in Brazil.

Congenital Zika syndrome (CZS) manifestations that extend beyond the central nervous system have been observed, including ophthalmologic findings distinct from other congenital conditions [20]. The first report of possible congenital ocular lesions related to the ZIKV was published in December 2015 in Recife, Brazil [21]. This case series found ocular lesions in three infants born with microcephaly. The same group described retinal lesions in 10 newborn infants with a diagnosis of microcephaly and ophthalmology abnormalities in February 2016 [22]. Another study conducted in Salvador, Brazil, suggested a prevalence of 34.5 % of vision-threatening lesions in a case series of patients presenting with microcephaly, possibly associated with the ZIKV congenital infection [23].

21.1 Diagnosis and Ocular Features

A diagnosis of Zika during pregnancy should be considered after the appearance of symptoms of fever, arthralgia, rash, and conjunctivitis in people living in endemic areas or in those who traveled within the previous 2 weeks to an area with ongoing transmission. RT-PCT and serology tests should be performed in pregnant women living in high-risk areas, since it is estimated that 80 % of patients with the ZIKV infection are asymptomatic or oligosymptomatic. In addition, the ZIKV infection occurs in areas in which *A. aegypti* is endemic and where the mosquito is the biologic vector of three distinct viral diseases: the ZIKV, dengue fever, and Chikungunya virus [24, 25]. The signs and symptoms in patients infected with these three distinct viruses are similar.

Currently, the evidence of the presence of the ZIKV infection relies on molecular detection of RT-PCR (positive only for a brief period of viremia) and also IgM and IgG serology specific to Zika antibodies. However, interpretation of serology results is complex due to cross-reactivity among the flaviviruses. It is essential to have more sensitive and specific serologic tests, without cross-reactivity with other infections, particularly dengue fever, yellow fever, and other flaviviruses [26].

The first report of ocular lesions associated with presumed ZIKV congenital infections was in Recife, Brazil, and described ophthalmologic findings in three children with microcephaly born after the ZIKV outbreak in Brazil. One mother reported a rash and arthralgia during the first trimester of pregnancy. The mothers had no ocular lesions, but the three infants had unilateral ocular findings involving the macula. Macular pigment mottling was described in all three children.

Well-defined macular chorioretinal atrophy was detected in one infant [21].

In February 2016, the same group published the ocular abnormalities of 10 infants who had been diagnosed clinically with ZIKV-related microcephaly. Seven (70.0 %) mothers reported symptoms during pregnancy (arthralgia, malaise, and rash); of these, six (85.7 %) mothers reported having symptoms during the first trimester. The mothers did not report ocular symptoms such as conjunctivitis during pregnancy, and their ocular examination did not show ophthalmologic abnormalities. Ocular findings included macular pigment mottling and/or chorioretinal atrophy in 15 (75.0 %) eyes. Optic nerve abnormalities such as optic disc hypoplasia, pallor, and/or increased cup-to-disc ratio were reported in nine (45.0 %) eyes. All infants had normal anterior segment structures; horizontal nystagmus was observed in one infant. No patient had inflammatory signs such as uveitis or vasculitis [22].

In addition to the studies in Recife, the study conducted in Salvador, Brazil, evaluated the ocular findings in infants with microcephaly associated with presumed intrauterine ZIKV infection. Twenty-three (79.3 %) of twenty-nine mothers reported suspected ZIKV infection signs and symptoms (rash, fever, arthralgia, headache, itch, and malaise) during pregnancy, 18 (62.0 %) in the first trimester, four in the second trimester, and one in the third trimester. All mothers denied signs or symptoms of conjunctivitis and all had normal findings on ocular examination. Ophthalmologic abnormalities were present in 17 (29.3 %) eyes of 10 children (34.5 %), and bilateral findings were seen in 7 of 10 patients presenting with ocular lesions. The most common lesions were focal retinal pigment mottling and chorioretinal atrophy in 11 (64.7 %) of 17 eyes with abnormalities, followed by optic nerve abnormalities (optic disc hypoplasia and severe optic disc cupping) in eight (47.1 %) eyes. One infant had anterior segment findings, i.e., bilateral iris coloboma and lens subluxation, in one eye. No infants had vasculitis or active uveitis [23].

In all of these, serologic examinations ruled out other congenital infections such as toxoplasmosis, rubella, cytomegalovirus, herpes simplex virus, syphilis, and human immunodeficiency virus.

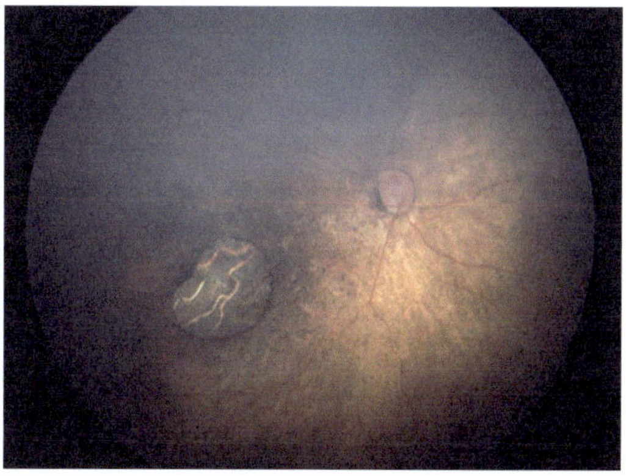

Fig. 21.1 Wide-angle fundus image (Retcam, Clarity Medical Systems, Pleasanton, CA, USA) of the right eye of an infant with a well-defined macular chorioretinal atrophic lesion associated with macular pigment mottling

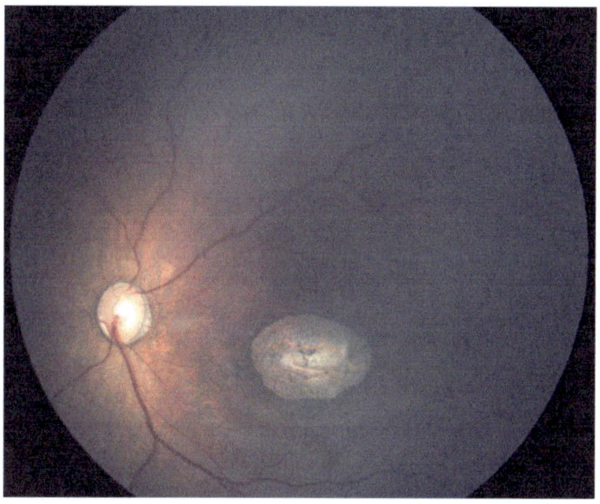

Fig. 21.2 Wide-angle fundus image (Retcam, Clarity Medical Systems, Pleasanton, CA, USA) of the left right eye of an infant with a chorioretinal scar and perilesional pigmentary mottling in the macular region

In summary, the main ophthalmologic findings in infants with suspected ZIKV-related microcephaly were focal pigment mottling (Figs. 21.1 and 21.2), chorioretinal atrophy (Figs. 21.1 and 21.2), and optic nerve abnormalities (optic disc hypoplasia and severe optic disc cupping) [21–23].

According to the studies conducted so far, chorioretinal atrophy and focal pigment mottling occurred predominantly in the posterior pole, especially the macular area [21–23]. It was also observed that some chorioretinal lesions had an excavated appearance (colobomatous-like) [23]. No signs of active uveitis or vasculitis were observed. Most mothers who reported symptoms had them predominantly in the first trimester of pregnancy, and no expectant mother had conjunctivitis [21–23].

The current data suggested that even asymptomatic or oligosymptomatic pregnant patients presumably infected with ZIKV might have children with CZS manifestations such as ophthalmologic lesions. Another important consideration is whether children without microcephaly born from mothers infected during pregnancy develop ocular lesions as a spectrum of CZS and if these patients need to be screened in areas with ongoing ZIKV transmission.

21.2 Recommendations

Screening approaches are essential for pregnant women who reside in regions where the ZIKV is present and include PCR, serology tests, and ultrasound and amniocentesis in some patients.

Pregnant women who live in areas of ongoing ZIKV transmission and women who traveled to these areas who present with a dengue-like illness (rash, fever, myalgias, and arthralgias) should undergo an RT-PCR test on serum collected within 7 days of symptom onset. Viremia decreases over time and a negative RT-PCR result from serum collected 5–7 days after symptom onset does not exclude the ZIKV infection. Pregnant women who live in risk areas for the ZIKV infection and do not report symptoms can undergo a ZIKV IgM test during prenatal care. If negative, repeat testing can be considered during the second trimester. The CDC recommends that men who live in or travel to an area with active Zika virus transmission and who have a pregnant partner should use condoms every time they have sex or not have sex for the duration of the pregnancy [27].

IgM antibodies to the ZIKV, dengue viruses, and other flaviviruses have strong cross-reactivity. More accurate IgM and IgG assays are essential to stratify the risk in women of childbearing age and facilitate targeted prenatal screening. This is even more important where abortion for this situation is legal.

Infants that abnormalities are consistent with Congenital Zika Syndrome or laboratory evidence of Zika virus infection of mothers presumably infected with the ZIKV during pregnancy should undergo at least one ocular examination that includes an a complete ophthalmological evaluation, including the anterior and posterior segment assessment and indirect ophthalmoscopy under pharmacologic mydriasis. Anterior segment changes should be described, and optic nerve, retinal, and choroidal abnormalities should be registered with a wide-field digital imaging system. Children who have macular lesions and a high probability of low vision should be referred to a specialist. The current data suggested that even asymptomatic or oligosymptomatic pregnant patients presumably infected with the ZIKV might have microcephalic newborns with retinal and optic disc lesions. It is unknown whether the ZIKV congenital infection might cause future ocular abnormalities.

Due to the difficulties in controlling the mosquito vector, the development of a vaccine against ZIKV seems to be essential for long-term control of new cases. In addition, for those existing cases of CZS, more information is needed in order to fully understand their needs and manage their disabilities.

Core Messages

Zika virus congenital infection may cause microcephaly and ocular abnormalities in 29-45% of newborns. Majority of lesions are bilateral and may affect the macula. Early diagnosis and visual as well as cognitive rehabilitation are necessary.

The best prevention is the control of the biologic vector Aedes aegypti and to avoid pregnant in endemic areas. The use of insect repellents is high recommended in such situations and adults that had the diagnosis of Zika infection should avoid sexual reaction or use condom for 3-6 months. Care must be take in blood tranfusion from endemic areas.

References

1. Dick GW, Kitchen SF, Haddow AJ (1952) Zika virus. I: isolations and serological specificity. Trans R Soc Trop Med Hyg 46:509–520
2. Dick GW (1952) Zika virus, II: pathogenicity and physical properties. Trans R Soc Trop Med Hyg 46:521–534
3. Foy BD, Kobylinski KC, Chilson Foy JL et al (2011) Probable non-vector-borne transmission of Zika virus, Colorado, USA. Emerg Infect Dis 17:880–882
4. Besnard M, Lastère S, Teissier A, Cao-Lormeau V, Musso D (2014) Evidence of perinatal transmission of Zika virus, French Polynesia, December 2013 and February 2014. Euro Surveill 19:20751
5. Lanciotti RS, Kosoy OL, Laven JJ et al (2008) Genetic and serologic properties of Zika virus associated with an epidemic, Yap State, Micronesia, 2007. Emerg Infect Dis 14:1232–1239
6. Musso D, Roche C, Nhan TX, Robin E, Teissier A, Cao-Lormeau VM (2015) Detection of Zika virus in saliva. J Clin Virol 68:53–55
7. Gourinat AC, O'Connor O, Calvez E, Goarant C, Dupont-Rouzeyrol M (2015) Detection of Zika virus in urine. Emerg Infect Dis 21:84–86
8. EB H (2009) Zika virus outside Africa. Emerg Infect Dis 15:1347–1350
9. Cao-Lormeau V-M (2014) Zika Virus, French Polynesia, South Pacific, 2013. Emerg Infect Dis 20:1960
10. Zanluca C, de Melo VC, Mosimann AL, Dos Santos GI, Dos Santos CN, Luz K (2015) First report of autochthonous transmission of Zika virus in Brazil. Mem Inst Oswaldo Cruz 110:569–572
11. Yakob L, Walter T (2016) Zika virus outbreak in the Americas: the need for novel mosquito control methods. Lancet Glob Health 4(3):e148–e149
12. World Health Organization (WHO) WHO director-general summarizes the outcome of the emergency committee regarding clusters of microcephaly and Guillain-Barré syndrome. http://www.who.int/mediacentre/news/statements/2016/emergency-committee-zika-microcephaly/en/. Accessed 1 Feb 2016
13. Fauci AS, Morens DM (2016) Zika virus in the Americas – yet another arbovirus threat. N Engl J Med 374:601–604
14. Schuler-Faccini L, Ribeiro EM, Feitosa IM et al (2016) Possible association between Zika virus infection and microcephaly – Brazil, 2015. MMWR Morb Mortal Wkly Rep 65:59–62
15. Centro de Operações de Emergências em Saúde Pública sobre Microcefalias Monitoramento dos casos de microcefalias no Brasil. http://portalsaude.saude.gov.br/images/pdf/2015/novembro/30/coes-microcefalias---informe-epidemiol--gico---se-47.pdf. Accessed 26 Dec 2015
16. Ministério da Saúde Microcefalia: 3174 casos são investigados em 20 estados e no Distrito Federal. http://portalsaude.saude.gov.br/index.php/o-ministerio/principal/secretarias/job/webradio/21527-microcefalia-3174-casos-sao-investigados-em-20-estados-e-no-distrito-federal. Accessed 9 Jan 2016
17. Centro de Operações de Emergências em Saúde Pública sobre Microcefalias (COES) Monitoramento dos casos de microcefalia no Brasil até a Semana Epidemiológica 47. Informe Epidemiológico – Semana Epidemiológica 47. 2015. http://portalsaude.saude.gov.br/images/pdf/2015/novembro/30/coes-microcefalias---informe-epidemiol—gico—se-47.pdf. Accessed 9 Jan 2016
18. Brasil P, Pereira JP Jr, Raja Gabaglia C, et al (2016) Zika virus infection in pregnant women in Rio de Janeiro – preliminary report. N Engl J Med 375(24):2321–2334
19. Mlakar J, Korva M, Tul N et al (2016) Zika virus associated with microcephaly. N Engl J Med 374(10): 951–958
20. Costa F, Sarno M, Khouri R et al (2016) Emergence of congenital Zika syndrome: viewpoint from the front lines. Ann Intern Med 164(10):689–691
21. Ventura CV, Maia M, Bravo-Filho V, Gois AL, Belfort R Jr (2016) Zika virus in Brazil and macular atrophy in a child with microcephaly. Lancet 387:228
22. Ventura CV, Maia M, Ventura BV et al (2016) Ophthalmologic assessment of ten infants with microcephaly and presumable intra-uterus zika virus infection. Arq Bras Oftalmol 79:1–3
23. de Paula Freitas B, de Oliveira Dias JR, Prazeres J, et al (2016) Ocular findings in infants with microcephaly associated with presumed Zika virus congenital infection in Salvador, Brazil. JAMA Ophthalmol
24. CDC (2015) Chikungunya virus: clinical evaluation & disease. US Department of Health and Human Services, CDC, Atlanta. www.cdc.gov/chikungunya/hc/clinicalevaluation.html. Accessed 9 Jan 2016
25. World Health Organization (2009) Dengue: guidelines for diagnosis, treatment, prevention and control. World Health Organization, Geneva/Switzerland. http://apps.who.int/iris/bitstream/10665/44188/1/9789241547871_eng.pdf. Accessed 9 Jan 2016
26. Barreto ML, Barral-Netto M, Stabeli R et al (2016) Zika virus and microcephaly in Brazil: a scientific agenda. Lancet 387(10022):919–921
27. Oduyebo T, Petersen EE, Rasmussen SA et al (2016) Update: Interim guidelines for health care providers caring for pregnant women and women of reproductive age with possible Zika virus exposure – United States, 2016. MMWR Morb Mortal Wkly Rep 65:122–127

MIX
Papier aus verantwortungsvollen Quellen
Paper from responsible sources
FSC® C105338

If you have any concerns about our products,
you can contact us on
ProductSafety@springernature.com

In case Publisher is established outside the EU,
the EU authorized representative is:
Springer Nature Customer Service Center GmbH
Europaplatz 3, 69115 Heidelberg, Germany

Printed by Libri Plureos GmbH
in Hamburg, Germany